# THE CONSUMER'S GUIDE TO
# DRUG INTERACTIONS

# THE CONSUMER'S GUIDE TO
# DRUG
# INTERACTIONS

## Jeffrey R. Schein, M.S.,
### and
## Philip Hansten, Pharm.D.

**Collier Books**
Macmillan Publishing Company
New York

Maxwell Macmillan Canada
Toronto

Maxwell Macmillan International
New York    Oxford    Singapore    Sydney

Collier Books
Macmillan Publishing Company
866 Third Avenue
New York, NY 10022

Maxwell Macmillan Canada, Inc.
1200 Eglinton Avenue East
Suite 200
Don Mills, Ontario M3C 3N1

Macmillan Publishing Company is part of the Maxwell Communication Group of Companies.

Library of Congress Cataloging-in-Publication Data
Schein, Jeffrey.
The consumer's guide to drug interactions —
Jeffrey R. Schein and Philip D. Hansten.
p.    cm.
Includes index.
ISBN 0-02-028865-4
1. Drug interactions—Handbooks, manuals, etc.
I. Hansten, Philip D. II. Title
RM302.S35   1993                       92–41050
615´.7045—dc20                              CIP

Macmillan books are available at special discounts for bulk purchases for sales promotions, premiums, fund-raising, or educational use. For details, contact:

Special Sales Director
Macmillan Publishing Company
866 Third Avenue
New York, NY 10022

Designed by Michael Mendelsohn

First Collier Books Edition 1993

10  9  8  7  6  5  4  3  2  1

Printed in the United States of America

The goal of *The Consumer's Guide to Drug Interactions* is to present information on drug interactions to the general reader in an accurate and readable manner. This publication is not intended to provide personal medical advice or to substitute for consultation with a physician. Rather, the authors encourage readers to discuss their health-related concerns with their personal physician and pharmacist.

# CONTENTS

# ACKNOWLEDGMENTS

Approximately five years ago, Phil Hansten (P.H.) called me (J.S.) to check whether I would be interested in co-authoring a book on drug interactions for the consumer. I would like to thank Phil for that opportunity. While the task involved in writing such a book has been great, the efforts of both authors have been characterized by mutual pleasure and respect, both for each other and for the subject.

We wish to acknowledge all of the contributing reviewers who generously devoted their time and energy to help ensure that the book is accurate and practical. Their efforts are greatly appreciated. I (J.S.) would like to acknowledge two reviewers in particular, who warrant special recognition: Dr. Jonathan Klahr and Dr. Mitchell Cappell. Dr. Klahr, a skilled rheumatologist and good friend, provided detailed, practical information to the chapter on pain-relieving medications. Dr. Cappell meticulously critiqued the chapter concerning medications for the stomach and intestine. Their valuable input—as well as the comments provided from all of the contributing reviewers—enhanced the usefulness of this book.

Lastly, and most importantly, we wish to thank our families for their understanding and sacrifice. Without the patience, practical help, and loving support of Lee Ann Schein, this book would never have become a reality. Likewise, without the invaluable support, patience, and encouragement of Ruth Hansten, the data for this book would not have been meticulously reviewed. In a book this size and kind, it is difficult to thank all of those who helped us. We beg pardon of any omissions.

JEFFREY R. SCHEIN                                    PHILIP D. HANSTEN, PHARM.D.
Highland Park, NJ                                    Bainbridge Island, WA

# CONTRIBUTING REVIEWERS

## Chapter 1

**Robert M. Julien, M.D., Ph.D.**
Staff Anesthesiologist
St. Vincent Hospital and Medical
Center
Portland, OR

**Jonathan Klahr, M.D.**
Attending Rheumatologist
Long Island Jewish Medical Center
New Hyde Park, NY

Private Practice, Rheumatology
Cedarhurst, NY

**Kathleen M. Foley, M.D.**
Chief, Pain Service
Department of Neurology
Memorial Sloan-Kettering Cancer
Center
New York, NY

Professor of Neurology, Neuroscience,
and Clinical Pharmacology
Cornell University Medical College
New York, NY

## Chapter 2

**Elliott Frank, M.D.**
Chief, Infectious Diseases Section
Department of Medicine
Jersey Shore Medical Center
Neptune, NJ

Clinical Associate Professor of
Medicine
UMDNJ-Robert Wood Johnson
Medical School
New Brunswick, NJ

## Chapter 3

**Margaret L. Soderberg-Warner, M.D.**
Assistant Clinical Professor of
Pediatrics
Department of Pediatric
Immunology/Allergy
UCLA Medical Center
Los Angeles, CA

**Donald N. Leibner, M.D.**
Private Practice, Allergy and
Asthma
East Brunswick, NJ

Attending Allergist
Department of Pediatrics and
Medicine
Robert Wood Johnson University
Hospital
and
St. Peter's Medical Center
New Brunswick, NJ

## Chapter 4

**Donald N. Leibner, M.D.**
Private Practice, Allergy and
Asthma
East Brunswick, NJ

Attending Allergist
Departments of Pediatrics and
Medicine
Robert Wood Johnson University
Hospital
and
St. Peter's Medical Center
New Brunswick, NJ

xi

**Sandra M. Gawchik, D.O.**
Co-Director, Asthma and Allergy
Associates
Crozer-Chester Medical Center
Chester, PA

Chairman, Division of Allergy and
Clinical Immunology
Department of Pediatrics
Philadelphia College of Osteopathic
Medicine
Philadelphia, PA

*Chapter 5*

**Mitchell S. Cappell, M.D., Ph.D.**
Director, Gastrointestinal Motility and
Laser Endoscopy Unit
Department of
Medicine/Gastroenterology
UMDNJ-Robert Wood Johnson
Medical School
New Brunswick, NJ

*Chapter 6*

**James T. Willerson, M.D.**
Professor and Chairman
Department of Internal Medicine
University of Texas Medical School at
Houston

Director, Cardiology Research
Texas Heart Institute
Houston, TX

**Brian F. Hoffman, M.D.**
Professor of Pharmacology
Chairman, Department of
Pharmacology
Associate Dean
College of Physicians and Surgeons of
Columbia University
New York, NY

*Chapter 7*

**Claude J. M. Lenfant, M.D.**
Director, National Heart, Lung, and
Blood Institute
National Institutes of Health
Bethesda, MD

**Ray W. Gifford, Jr., M.D.**
Senior Vice-Chairman,
Division of Medicine
Senior Physician,
Hypertension and Nephrology
The Cleveland Clinic Foundation
Cleveland, OH

*Chapter 8*

**Marian D. Damewood, M.D.**
Associate Professor
Department of Gynecology and
Obstetrics
Division of Reproductive
Endocrinology
The Johns Hopkins University School
of Medicine
Baltimore, MD

Director, In Vitro Fertilization Program
The Johns Hopkins University School
of Medicine
Baltimore, MD

**Edward S. Horton, M.D.**
Chairman, Department of Medicine
University of Vermont
Burlington, VT

Former President (1990–1991),
American Diabetes Association

*Chapter 9*

**James W. Jefferson, M.D.**
Professor of Psychiatry
Director, Center for Affective
Disorders
Co-Director, Lithium and Obsessive
Compulsive Information Centers
University of Wisconsin Medical
School
Madison, WI

*Chapter 10*

*Sleep-Inducing Drugs*

**Floyd Bloom, M.D.**
Chairman, Department of
Neuropharmacology
The Scripps Research Institute
Department of Neuropharmacology
LaJolla, CA

*Anti-Anxiety Drugs*

**Thomas W. Uhde, M.D.**
Chief, Section on Anxiety and
Affective Disorders
Biological Psychiatry Branch
National Institute of Mental Health
National Institutes of Health
Bethesda, MD

Clinical Professor
Department of Psychiatry
Uniformed Services University of the
Health Sciences
School of Medicine
Bethesda, MD

# INTRODUCTION

There are times when you, or a family member, may need to take more than one medication at a time. Whenever this happens, there is the risk that one drug will affect how the other drug acts. Usually this results in only minor changes that you don't even notice, but occasionally the outcome is more serious. Nobody knows exactly how often drug interactions cause problems in the population at large, but we do know that certain combinations of drugs increase your risk of adverse effects.

## What Is a Drug Interaction?

A drug interaction is a change in the effect of one drug when you take a second drug concomitantly. This change may be desirable, adverse, or inconsequential. An example of a desirable drug interaction is cancer treatment: patients with cancer often receive combinations of drugs that act in concert to fight the malignancy.

In this book, we are almost entirely concerned with adverse drug interactions; that is, those in which the effect of the interaction leads to an adverse event, such as an unwanted side effect (for example, nausea) or a decrease in the effectiveness of the drug. Most adverse drug interactions result in an increase or decrease in the effect of one of the drugs. But sometimes a combination of drugs results in a whole new reaction that is not seen with either of the drugs alone.

### Increased effect of a medication

One of the most common drug interactions involves one drug causing an "increased effect" of another medication. This doesnot mean that the drug works better; rather, it indicates an abnormal, exaggerated effect. This exaggerated effect may be associated with various undesirable symptoms, such as sweating, nausea, rapid heartbeat, etc.; the type of symptoms that develop, as well as their severity, depends on the specific drugs being taken as well as individual variability of your own body. If severe undesirable symptoms develop, the increased effect is termed a "toxic" effect. For example, when cimetidine (Tagamet®)—a drug used to treat stomach and intestinal ulcers—is taken with theophylline—a medication used to relieve asthma—the result may be an increased amount of theophylline in the blood, possibly resulting in theophylline toxicity with symptoms such as nausea, vomiting, diarrhea, headache, irritability, restlessness, nervousness, rapid heartbeat, insomnia, tremor, and seizure.

### Decreased effect of a medication

Another very common drug interaction involves just the converse of what we described above. One drug may *decrease* the effectiveness of another drug. The end result depends on the degree of the decreased effect. If the decrease is small, the drug may still retain most of its pharmacologic activity. If the decrease is large, however, the effectiveness of the drug may be greatly diminished, or it may not work at all. For example, if ciprofloxacin (Cipro®), an antibiotic used to treat various bacterial infections, is combined with antacids that contain aluminum or magnesium (such as Maalox® or Mylanta®), the bacteria-fighting ability of ciprofloxacin is substantially decreased.

## How Do Drugs Interact?

To better understand how drugs interact with each other, let's follow a drug on its journey through your body. Since most drugs are taken orally, the starting point can be a tablet or capsule in your mouth being washed down into your stomach with a glass of water. (By the way, it's a good idea to wash down a medication with a full glass of water to make sure it doesn't spend too much time in your esophagus. This can be irritating to the lining of your esophagus.) Once the drug appears in your stomach, it starts to dissolve in the fluids there. Most drugs are not absorbed in the stomach to any great extent, but rather are emptied into the small intestine, where the enormous surface area is better able to absorb various items, such as medications or nutrients from food.

Once absorbed, the drug is distributed throughout your body in the bloodstream, often hitching a ride on blood proteins (such as albumin). Some of the drug goes to the tissues and organs, where it will produce its beneficial effect, usually by attaching to specific chemical landing pads called "receptors." By this time the body has also begun the process of eliminating the drug. Some drugs are soluble enough in water so that they are excreted by your kidneys and appear in the urine without any alteration by your body. Most drugs, however, must be altered by your body before your kidneys can get rid of them.

The premier organ for preparing drugs for elimination by your kidneys is your liver. Your liver is a versatile organ that has many functions, but one important one is ridding your body of foreign substances (which is a good way to look at drugs!). Your liver contains substances called "enzymes," hard-working chemicals that are very good at altering drug molecules so that they can be eliminated. The liver usually accomplishes this by taking the drug molecule into the liver cell, and then either removing certain parts of the drug molecule or adding chemical groups onto the drug molecule. The altered drug, now more water soluble and called a "metabolite," is then expelled from the liver cell back into the bloodstream. The liver has now accomplished its mission to rid the body of this alien substance; the metabolite has lost most of its ability to produce effects (good or bad) in the body, and it can now be eliminated in the urine.

Now that you know what the normal processes are, we can talk about how drug interactions interfere with these processes. Before we begin this discussion, we should define two terms: "object drug" and "precipitant drug." These terms arise in any discussion of drug interaction mechanisms. If you look at almost any drug interaction, one medication can be considered the object drug and one medication can be considered the precipitant drug. Their definitions are as follows:

**Object Drug:** The drug whose effect is altered by the interaction.
**Precipitant Drug:** The drug that *causes,* or precipitates, the altered effect in the object drug.

Think of the precipitant drug being the bat, and the object drug being the ball.

## Drug interactions in the stomach and intestine

Some precipitant drugs bind with object drugs in the stomach or intestine and inhibit their ability to be absorbed into your bloodstream. For example, if you are taking the antibiotic ciprofloxacin, most antacids will bind with it and will dramatically reduce the amount of antibiotic getting into your bloodstream. The bacteria romping and reproducing in your system have a reprieve while the antibiotic is sailing down your intestine only to be excreted in your stool. Antacids bind tightly with some drugs such as ciprofloxacin and tetracyclines, thus dramatically reducing their absorption. With many other drugs, however, antacids bind only weakly and the effect on the object drug is fairly small. Medicines other than antacids that can sometimes bind drugs in the stomach and intestine include cholestyramine (Questran®), colestipol (Colestid®), and antidiarrheal agents such as kaolin-pectin (Donnagel-PG®) and attapulgite (Donnagel®).

## Drug interactions in the liver

The liver is the site of many important drug interactions. Some precipitant drugs, called "enzyme inhibitors," slow down the drug-metabolizing machinery in the liver, so that certain enzymes in the liver cannot metabolize drug molecules properly. This results in accumulation of the object drug in the blood, and may increase the risk of side effects and toxicity. Examples of enzyme inhibitors are cimetidine (Tagamet®), ciprofloxacin (Cipro®), diltiazem (Cardizem®), erythromycin (E-Mycin®, Erythrocin®), ketoconazole (Nizoral®), and verapamil (Calan®, Isoptin®).

Other drugs, called "enzyme inducers," have the opposite effect on drug metabolism in the liver; they speed up drug metabolism by adding more machinery (enzymes) to the system. This results in more rapid elimination of the object drug, and tends to reduce its effect. Examples of enzyme inducers are anticonvulsants such as carbamazepine (Tegretol®), phenobarbital, phenytoin (Dilantin®), primidone (Mysoline®), and the antibiotic rifampin (Rifadin®, Rimactane®).

### Drug interactions in the kidney

The kidney is not a common site of drug interactions compared with the liver, but kidney drug interactions can be important. The kidney is important in the elimination of some drugs, such as lithium carbonate (Lithane®, Lithobid®) and methotrexate (Mexate®). When another drug interferes with this process, lithium or methotrexate accumulates in the body and serious toxicity can result.

## Subtle Drug Interactions

It's important to understand that serious consequences may ensue not only when two drugs interact, but also when one of the two interacting drugs is either reduced in dosage or discontinued altogether. For example, when propoxyphene (Darvon®), a pain-relieving medication, is given with carbamazepine (Tegretol®), a drug used to control seizures, the result is an increased amount of carbamazepine in the body, which may lead to carbamazepine toxicity with symptoms such as drowsiness, dizziness, nausea, vomiting, incoordination, headache, involuntary rapid movement of the eyeball, and blurred vision.

Generally, when an interaction such as this occurs, your doctor will adjust the dose of the medication to alleviate adverse side effects (in this case, the doctor may choose to reduce the dose of the carbamazepine so that drug toxicity will not occur) while ensuring the drug is working properly. Getting just the right amount in your body so that the drug can do its job properly without serious side effects is called "titrating" the dose (only your doctor should do this). However, in our case of a person taking carbamazepine and propoxyphene simultaneously, this "correct amount"—also called the therapeutic dose—was attained while the person was taking one drug (propoxyphene) that affected the concentration of the other drug (carbamazepine). What do you suppose would happen if propoxyphene is discontinued, or its dosage changed? The therapeutic dose of the anti-seizure drug would no longer be a true therapeutic dose, but rather will become *sub*therapeutic, or less than the dose needed to control seizure. (Remember, the amount of the antiseizure drug in the body was initially elevated due to the presence of the pain-relieving drug).

## Are Drug Interactions Preventable?

In virtually every case, adverse drug interactions can be prevented. If you are receiving (or about to receive) interacting drugs, there are several ways to try to avoid problems. Sometimes the best way is simply for your doctor to avoid giving the interacting drugs. For most disorders there are several different medicines that can be used for treatment, and it may be possible to select an alternative to one of the interacting drugs. If the patient truly needs both interacting drugs, other preventive measures may be needed. Sometimes the dose of the object drug is adjusted to correct for the alteration caused by the drug interaction. Sometimes the doctor will monitor your response to the object drug more carefully in order to catch the interaction before it does any damage. Sometimes the interaction can be prevented by spacing the doses of the interacting drugs appropriately, or by giving one of the drugs by a different route of administration. Using these and other methods, you can usually prevent the adverse effects of drug interactions. But as you will soon see, prevention must be a cooperative effort between you, your doctor, and your pharmacist.

## How Can You Avoid Drug Interaction Problems?

Over the past twenty years, doctors and pharmacists have increased their efforts to detect and prevent adverse drug interactions. The first line of defense, however, is the patient. There are several things that you can do to minimize the likelihood that you will be one of the unlucky ones.

1. *Do not take drugs unless they are necessary.* Sometimes the obvious needs repeating: the more drugs you take, the greater the chance that you will eventually take a combination that doesn't mix well. Unfortunately, some people have had severe reactions involving drugs that weren't truly necessary to start with. For example, a 1989 report in the *Journal of Clinical Psychiatry* described four woman with depression taking phenelzine (Nardil®) who had severe hypertensive reactions after using nonprescription cold products containing decongestants. One woman taking phenelzine died after taking a cold medication containing a decongestant called phenylpropanolamine. Phenelzine belongs to a class of antidepressants called monoamine oxidase inhibitors, second-line drugs in the treatment of depression that are not frequently used. It is obvious, however, that people taking monoamine oxidase inhibitors should avoid taking decongestant medicines for their colds. A box of tissues would have been a lot safer!

2. *Keep your doctors informed of all drugs you are taking.* If you have to go to specialists (for example, cardiologists, gastroenterologists, rheumatologists, etc.), you need to have a primary-care physician (usually a family physician or internal medicine physician) who is looking at the "big picture." It is important to keep this primary-care physician informed of all of the medications prescribed by the other doctors, dentists, and anyone else involved in your treatment. This is especially important if you go to a specialist without a referral from your primary physician, because such specialists may not always inform your primary physician of the medications they have prescribed. It is safest to assume that your specialists are not informing your primary physician of the drugs they have prescribed for you. That way the worst that can happen is that your family doctor is informed about your medicines twice, which is considerably better than not at all. You should make sure that the specialists you are seeing know all of the drugs you are taking. This will reduce the chance that one of them will give you a prescription for a drug that interacts adversely with one of the drugs you are already taking.

Unfortunately, drug interactions sometimes occur even when you are going to only one doctor, and even when you keep all of your doctors well informed of all your medicines. There are literally hundreds of drug interactions and new ones are discovered every month. Thus, it is impossible for even the best doctors to keep up with every single drug interaction that has ever been reported. Another important line of defense against drug interactions is your pharmacist.

3. *Use your pharmacist to help defend against drug interactions.* Pharmacists are trained in drug interactions and can work with your doctor to reduce the risk of adverse interactions. But, like your doctor, your pharmacist needs cooperation from you! If possible, go to the same pharmacy to have all of your prescriptions filled. That way, your pharmacist will have a complete record of all of your medications. A growing number of pharmacies have computerized drug interaction screening programs that produce alerts to the pharmacist if a new prescription you are having filled interacts with any of your other medications. Going to only one pharmacy is a particularly good idea when more than one doctor is prescribing medications for you. That way if your physicians are not communicating well with each other and prescribe interacting drugs, you still have another line of defense in your pharmacist.

4. *Ask questions!* It isn't realistic to expect that your doctor and pharmacist will always remember to tell you every precaution about drug interactions for every new drug you receive. When your doctor prescribes a new medication for you, ask him or her whether there are any nonprescription drugs that you should avoid while taking this drug. If you drink alcohol it is a good idea to ask whether you have to reduce your alcohol intake or abstain from alcohol altogether. Your pharmacist is also a good source for this kind of information, so don't be afraid to ask.

5. *Follow directions carefully when taking your medications.* Everyone knows that following directions increases the chances that the medication will do what it

is supposed to and *decreases* the chances that it will cause adverse side effects. But following directions can also reduce your risk of an adverse drug interaction. For example, if you have been advised to take your ciprofloxacin (Cipro®) two hours before taking your antacid, that is to make sure that the ciprofloxacin gets absorbed into your blood before the antacid has a chance to bind with the ciprofloxacin and prevent its absorption.

It is also important not to *stop* taking a medication before you are supposed to without checking with the doctor who prescribed it. Sometimes a person is stabilized on two interacting drugs, and everything is fine because the doses have been adjusted to compensate for the interaction. In this situation stopping the precipitant drug may throw the object drug out of whack and you may have an adverse effect. This is probably what happened to one boy who was receiving theophylline for his asthma along with carbamazepine (Tegretol®) for seizures. Carbamazepine enhances the ability of the liver to inactivate theophylline, so a larger dose of theophylline was required. When the carbamazepine was stopped, the theophylline blood concentrations skyrocketed, resulting in a severe reaction and permanent brain damage in this unfortunate child. Many other examples of severe drug interactions due to *stopping* an interacting drug have been described in medical and pharmacy journals. The lesson is clear; stopping a drug on your own can be chancy, so check with your doctor or pharmacist.

6. *Don't take other people's medicine.* If you needed one more reason to resist taking your husband's or neighbor's prescription medicine, here it is. When you take up someone's offer to sample a medicine that worked well for that person, you circumvent the normal machinery for detecting drug interactions. Neither your doctor nor your pharmacist can protect you from an interaction involving a drug that he or she doesn't know you are taking.

7. *Become an informed consumer of health care.* The fact that you are reading this book is a good sign! The practice of medicine and the use of drugs to treat disease have become so complicated that it is simply not possible for any one doctor or pharmacist to know every bit of information about every single drug. Gone are the days when all the doctor had was morphine, aspirin, and penicillin. Many wonderful new drugs are available that have made a tremendous positive impact on people's lives. But these medications have their darker side as well. Try to keep yourself informed about all of the medicines you are taking. If you read something troubling about one of your drugs, ask your doctor or pharmacist about it. Don't act on your own without checking it out! There are countless articles and books for the consumer these days about medicines; many are good, some are not so good. So be sure to get a "second opinion" from your health care professional before you do anything.

# Important Note to Readers

The goal of *The Consumer's Guide to Drug Interactions* is to present information on drug interactions to the general reader in an accurate and readable manner. This publication is *not* intended to provide personal medical advice or to substitute for consultation with a physician. Rather, the authors encourage readers to discuss their health-related concerns with their personal physician and pharmacist.

New drug interactions and/or additional information about drug interactions are discovered virtually every day. If a drug interaction is not mentioned in this book, the reader should *not* assume that an interaction will not occur. Furthermore, the way the human body responds to a specific medication may vary from one person to another; such variation may also occur with drug interactions.

Knowledge concerning drug interactions is far from complete. Much more work needs to be conducted regarding the factors that contribute to drug interactions, the frequency of drug interactions, the likelihood of an interaction occurring, and which persons are especially susceptible to drug interactions and under which conditions.

# HOW TO USE THIS BOOK

The Index is key to the effective use of this book. The Index lists both generic and trade names of drugs. The generic name identifies the official medical name for the basic active ingredient. The trade name is selected by the drug manufacturer, which often chooses a name that is more easily pronounced and remembered than the generic name. Often, several trade name drugs may be available (each one produced by a different manufacturer) that contain the same generic substance. For example, aspirin is a generic name; Anacin®, Bayer®, Bufferin®, Empirin®, and Excedrin® are all trade name products that contain aspirin.

Although the authors have made a sincere attempt to include the major trade names of drug products, this is not an assurance that *all* drug trade names will be found here. Many new trade names are introduced into the market each year. Furthermore, listing all trade names for medications becomes unmanageable. The antibiotic erythromycin, for example, has more than twenty trade names; pseudoephedrine, a nasal decongestant, is found in more than forty combination-type medications.

We suggest the following method when looking up the names of drugs in the Index.

Step 1. If you know the trade name of your medication, look it up in the Index. If you find the name of your drug, fine. You may now turn to the page indicated in the Index to obtain detailed information. However, if you do not find the name of your drug, go to Step 2.

Step 2. Look up the generic name of the drug(s) you wish to find. If you don't know the generic name, look on the medication container or call your pharmacist or doctor. For over-the-counter medications, simply read the label, which identifies each generic ingredient.

Step 3. Make sure you check every drug that may interact with the one you're interested in. All drugs, as well as medications with which they interact, are presented in alphabetical order.

# What Does Clinically Significant Mean?

You'll notice that each entry in the book is accompanied by *one* of three graphics.

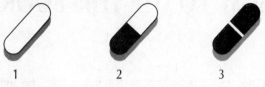

1        2        3

These graphics represent an estimate of the *clinical significance* of the drug interaction. This simply means that the interaction has an effect on the body, such as the development of symptoms (associated with excessive drug effect or decreased effect). On the other hand, a drug interaction may be observed and measured in the *laboratory* (for example, an increased amount of drug found in the blood), but the laboratory finding may not necessarily indicate that the interaction is associated with an observable change in the body. When the drug interaction leads to a change in the body, rather than just a laboratory result, we refer to the interaction as being *clinically significant.* The authors have attempted to limit most interactions to clinically significant ones, but we have also included some that we think will turn out to be clinically significant with further study.

A legend appears on many pages that list drug interactions and looks like this:

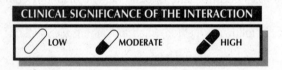

CLINICAL SIGNIFICANCE OF THE INTERACTION

LOW      MODERATE      HIGH

= The white capsule represents an interaction of **low** clinical significance. Interactions with this graphic may occur, but are of low clinical significance either because documentation is poor (e.g., few studies or poorly designed studies), the potential harm to the consumer is low, the interaction occurs infrequently, or a combination of these factors.

= The half-shaded capsule represents an interaction of **moderate** clinical significance. These interactions have more documentation than the low clinical significance interactions, yet more documentation is still needed. Potential harm to patients may be moderate.

= The black capsule represents an interaction of **high** or major clinical significance. These interactions are generally well documented, and in the population as a whole, they pose more potential harm to the consumer than the other interactions. These interactions tend to be more severe and more predictable relative to other interactions.

It is very important to remember that scientists cannot accurately predict the exact nature of a drug interaction in any given individual. Because of differences among individuals (such as general health, genetics, doses of medication used, environmental exposures, and many other individual variations), an interaction of "high" clinical significance may produce no ill effects *in a particular individual,* whereas an interaction of "low" clinical significance may lead to a severe adverse effect *in a particular individual.* The words "in a particular individual" are stressed because our discussion of clinical significance refers to the general population; individual differences may occur.

## CHAPTER 1

# PAIN-RELIEVING DRUGS

Throbbing, burning, aching, crushing—all of these words can describe an all-too common phenomenon: pain. Pain is actually a perception, not a sensation. In other words, no two people feel pain in precisely the same way; the same stimulus that elicits a mild reaction in one person may cause agony in another. Although pain is not well understood, both physical and psychological components play a role. That explains why an anxious or depressed person often has an increased sensation of pain.

Most "routine" pain is short-lasting—sore muscles from working too strenuously in the yard or a headache from not enough sleep. In these cases, the pain is self-limiting: with rest, it will go away by itself. On the other hand, pain may be long-term, and the underlying cause may need to be identified and treated. For example, rheumatoid arthritis is a disease in which certain joints—and tissues surrounding the joints—become inflamed, leading to pain and stiffness when these joints are moved. By reducing the inflammation, anti-inflammatory drugs relieve the *symptoms* (e.g., pain and stiffness), but these drugs do not cause a remission of the arthritis itself; other medications are needed to do that. Another example of long-term pain may be a cancerous tumor that is pushing against a nerve. Although drugs usually can relieve a moderate amount of pain in such a case, to fully eliminate the pain, the tumor must be either removed or shrunk to a smaller size.

Structures that sense pain are called *sensory receptors.* Found in the skin and in deeper tissues, these receptors are very fine, highly branched structures that are attached to a nerve cell (neuron). These receptors are sensitive to temperature and pressure. The specific receptor that causes pain is called the *nociceptor,* which is sensitive to severe stimulation, such as traumatic injury (for instance, a fall down a flight of stairs). Pain arises when these receptors are stimulated and pass on a "signal" of pain to surrounding nerves, which transmit the signal ultimately to the brain, where the signal is interpreted as pain.

When an injury occurs—say, a cut—certain chemicals, such as prostaglandin, bradykinin, and histamine, are produced. These chemicals play a role in causing nerves that surround the injured site to become stimulated and to begin transmitting the pain signal. Whether the stimulus is a cut or a cancerous tumor, prostaglandins transmit a message of pain to the spinal cord, which carries the signal to the brain. Pain is felt only if the brain receives and processes the signal that is sent. Researchers have focused on alleviating pain via two primary routes: either by inhibiting the chemicals that help to transmit pain signals to the brain or by blocking the ability of the spinal cord or brain to receive these signals.

## Medications Used to Relieve Pain

Medications used to relieve pain are called *analgesics*. One group of analgesics is made up of a family of drugs known as the nonsteroidal *anti-inflammatory* drugs (steroidal anti-inflammatory drugs, such as cortisone and prednisone, are also useful ·in relieving inflammation; these drugs are discussed in Chapter 8, "Hormonal Drugs," and in Chapter 4, "Drugs for Asthma and Other Breathing Disorders"). Nonsteroidal anti-inflammatory drugs block the production of prostaglandins and other inflammation-causing chemicals.

Many anti-inflammatory drugs have both analgesic and anti-inflammatory capabilities. These are often distinct characteristics. In low doses, some of these drugs may help to relieve pain but not inflammation, which often requires more prolonged use of the medication at higher doses. Generally, your doctor may recommend a particular anti-inflammatory medication at a particular dose in order to relieve pain, reduce inflammation, bring down a fever, or achieve a combination of these goals.

Anti-inflammatory drugs include diclofenac (Voltaren®), diflunisal (Dolobid®), etodolac (Lodine®), fenoprofen (Nalfon®), flurbiprofen (Ansaid®), ibuprofen (Advil®, Motrin®, Nuprin®, Rufen®), indomethacin (Indocin®), ketoprofen (Orudis®), ketorolac (Toradol®), meclofenamate (Meclomen®), nabumetone (Relafen®), naproxen (Naprosyn®), naproxen sodium (Anaprox®), oxaprozin (Daypro®), piroxicam (Feldene®), sulindac (Clinoril®), tolmetin (Tolectin®), and others.

Aspirin is also a nonsteroidal anti-inflammatory drug. Aspirin is found in an enormous number of products, especially cough/cold preparations. To name a few, in addition to aspirin-only brand-name products (such as Anacin®, Bayer®, Bufferin®, Ecotrin®, and others), aspirin is found in compounds such as Ascriptin®, Alka-Seltzer® Antacid and Pain Reliever, Excedrin® Extra Strength, Midol® (original formula), 4-Way® Cold Tablets, Empirin® with Codeine, Fiorinal®, Percodan®, Vanquish®, Cama® Arthritis Pain Reliever, Sine-Off® (aspirin formula), and many others.

Acetaminophen relieves pain and brings down a fever, but does nothing for inflammation. As a result, acetaminophen will not relieve the stiffness, redness, or swelling that is caused by inflammation. In addition to brand-name products containing acetaminophen only (such as Anacin-3®, Panadol®, Tempra®, and Tylenol®), this analgesic is found in compounds such as Sinutab®, Vicks Formula 44M® Multi-Symptom Cough Mixture, Vicks Nyquil®, Comtrex®, Coricidin® and Coricidin® "D"® Tablets, Drixoral® Plus, Contac® Severe Cold Formula Caplets, Contac® Nighttime Cold Medicine, Vanquish®, Extra-Strength Datril®, Excedrin P.M.®, and many others.

*Narcotic* analgesics (also called *opiates* or *opioids* because they are derived from the opium poppy plant) are another group of pain-relieving drugs. These medications interfere with the brain's ability to receive messages of pain from the spinal cord. For pain to "register" in the brain, the pain signal must pass from one brain cell to another. Each cell that receives such a signal contains many opiate receptors, the actual sites where the signal is received. Narcotic drugs occupy these sites so that the pain signal cannot be received. Think of a lock and key. The key is the pain signal, and the lock is the opiate receptor. Narcotic drugs plug up the "lock" so that the key, or pain signal, cannot be inserted.

Narcotics are often more powerful pain-relieving agents than acetaminophen or anti-inflammatory drugs. Although the narcotics are excellent pain-relieving drugs, they have several significant side effects. One is depression of certain sites in the central nervous system, possibly leading to drowsiness, decreased alertness (including an impaired ability to concentrate and think clearly), and slowed reaction time. As a result, operating dangerous machinery (including driving a car) may be hazardous while taking narcotic analgesics. One of the most important—and potentially lethal—side effects of narcotic use is depression of respiration, which may cause death when an overdose of these drugs is taken. Other side effects include nausea and constipation.

Morphine and codeine are narcotics. Codeine relieves mild to moderate pain and is found in a variety of combination products, such as cough suppressants. Codeine is often paired with a nonnarcotic pain reliever, such as aspirin or acetaminophen. Morphine is a much more potent narcotic that is used for more severe types of pain.

Although morphine and codeine are naturally derived opiates because they are produced directly from the seeds of the opium plant, scientists have also discovered how to synthetically manufacture narcotics. The synthetic opiates include butorphanol (Stadol®), hydromorphone (Dilaudid®), levorphanol (Levo-Dromoran®), meperidine (Demerol®, Mepergan®), methadone (Dolophine®), and pentazocine (Talwin®).

Other narcotic analgesics are not derived directly from the opium plant, nor are they entirely prepared in the laboratory. These drugs—oxymorphone (Numorphan®), oxycodone (Percodan®, Percocet®), hydrocodone bitartrate (Vicodin®), nalbuphine (Nubain®), and others—are "semisynthetic" medications. Researchers use natural sources (such as plants) as a starting point, then manipulate the chemical structure in the laboratory to come up with a new compound.

## Which Type of Analgesic Should Be Used?

The type of pain-relieving medication a doctor decides to prescribe depends on several factors, some of which include the severity of the pain, its cause, current or past medical conditions of the patient, and the type of pain that is being experienced. Depending upon which part of the body has been injured, the perception of pain can vary substantially. The skin, for instance, is extremely sensitive to sharp, burning, or freezing stimuli. None of these sensations, however, elicits the same dramatic effect when applied to an internal organ such as the stomach or intestines. Pain occurs in these organs when other stimuli are present, such as stretching and bloating, as when one eats excessively.

Generally, each kind of pain has an appropriate drug for its treatment. However, not all persons respond to the same drug in the same way, so your doctor may need to prescribe or recommend one pain-relieving medication, but later switch you to another drug before successfully alleviating your pain. For example, the pain associated with an inflammatory arthritis (such as rheumatoid arthritis) often responds better to an anti-inflammatory pain reliever than to a narcotic; however, some persons may not respond to the anti-inflammatory drug, but obtain significant relief from a narcotic.

| PAIN-RELIEVING DRUG | INTERACTING DRUG | RESULT |
|---|---|---|

Acetaminophen

Alcohol

Drinking excessive amounts of alcohol for a prolonged period of time has been associated with liver damage. Some evidence suggests that the combination of drinking alcohol (over a prolonged period of time) with high doses—or overdoses—of acetaminophen may lead to an increased susceptibility to liver damage.

**Recommendation:** If you drink a lot of alcohol (i.e., several drinks a day), it would be good idea to avoid taking acetaminophen regularly unless advised to do so by your doctor.

---

Acetaminophen

Anticoagulants (oral), such as dicumarol and warfarin (**Coumadin®, Panwarfin®**)

[for the prevention of blood clots]

Acetaminophen usually does not cause problems in persons taking oral anticoagulants, but a few cases of increased anticoagulant effect have been reported.

**Recommendation:** Although acetaminophen is often recommended as a pain reliever in people taking oral anticoagulants and usually causes no problems, it would be prudent to take acetaminophen only when you really need it and make sure you do not exceed the recommended doses. Aspirin is much more likely to interact with oral anticoagulants than acetaminophen; thus, aspirin is not a good alternative.

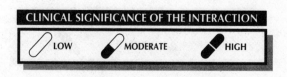

CLINICAL SIGNIFICANCE OF THE INTERACTION

LOW    MODERATE    HIGH

| PAIN-RELIEVING DRUG | INTERACTING DRUG | RESULT |
|---|---|---|
| Acetaminophen  | Barbiturates:<br><br>• amobarbital (**Amytal**®)<br>• butabarbital (**Butisol**®)<br>• butalbital<br>• pentobarbital (**Nembutal**®)<br>• phenobarbital (**Luminal**®, **Solfoton**®)<br>• primidone (**Mysoline**®)<br>• secobarbital (**Seconal**®),and others<br><br>[used to treat insomnia and anxiety; certain barbiturates are used to prevent seizures] | Persons who regularly take barbiturates may have a reduced effect of the acetaminophen. In addition, when too much acetaminophen is taken, this interaction may increase the likelihood of toxicity and the risk of liver damage. Symptoms of toxicity include nausea, vomiting, diarrhea, sweating, loss of appetite, and abdominal pain.<br><br>**Recommendation:** If you are taking barbiturates, be sure not to take more than the recommended amount of acetaminophen per day. It would also be wise to avoid taking acetaminophen for prolonged periods unless your doctor has advised you to do so. |
| Acetaminophen  | Charcoal<br>[for relief of gas] | Large amounts of activated charcoal may reduce serum acetaminophen concentrations in the body by reducing the amount of acetaminophen that is absorbed into the blood.<br><br>**Recommendation:** If you are taking an activated charcoal preparation, take it at least two hours before or after taking acetaminophen. |
| Acetaminophen  | Cholestyramine (**Questran**®)<br><br>[for treatment of high cholesterol levels] | Cholestyramine markedly reduces plasma concentrations of acetaminophen, thereby reducing the effect of the acetaminophen.<br><br>**Recommendation:** Take acetaminophen at least one hour before or several hours after taking cholestyramine. |

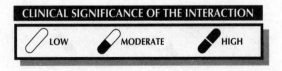

CLINICAL SIGNIFICANCE OF THE INTERACTION

LOW      MODERATE      HIGH

| PAIN-RELIEVING DRUG | INTERACTING DRUG | RESULT |
|---|---|---|
| Aspirin  | **Acetazolamide (Diamox®)** [for treatment of excess body fluid, glaucoma, and certain convulsive disorders] | Aspirin may increase the concentration of acetazolamide in the blood, possibly leading to central nervous system toxicity. Symptoms of central nervous system toxicity include lethargy, confusion, sleepiness, anorexia (an abnormal and persistent loss of appetite), and ringing or a clicking sound in the ears. **Recommendation:** If you are taking acetazolamide, try to limit your intake of aspirin. If you do take aspirin, be alert for the symptoms described above. |
| Aspirin  | Alcohol | Alcohol may enhance two of the adverse side effects that are related to aspirin use: (1) damage to the lining of the stomach, particularly minor bleeding of the stomach lining; and (2) increased time for blood to clot. **Recommendation:** Whenever possible, avoid aspirin use within eight to ten hours of moderate to heavy alcohol consumption. |
| Aspirin  | Antacids that contain aluminum or magnesium, such as **Gaviscon®, Gelusil®, Maalox®, Mylanta®, Phillips' Milk of Magnesia®**, and others [for relief of acid indigestion, heartburn, and abdominal pain caused by too much acid in the stomach] | With large doses of aspirin, this interaction could result in a reduced concentration of aspirin in the body, which could lead to a decreased effect of the aspirin. Aspirin is in a chemical class known as salicylates. When these salicylates are taken in large doses with antacids, this interaction could result in a reduced effect of the salicylate. Some salicylate medications include choline salicylate (Arthropan®), magnesium salicylate (Magsal®), sodium salicylate (Pabalate®), and salsalate (Disalcid®). |

| PAIN-RELIEVING DRUG | INTERACTING DRUG | RESULT |
| --- | --- | --- |

Aspirin

Anticoagulants (oral), such as dicumarol and warfarin (**Coumadin®, Panwarfin®**)

[for the prevention of blood clots]

Use of aspirin in persons taking an oral anticoagulant increases the risk of bleeding. Such bleeding is evidenced by blood in the urine, coughing up of blood, black stool (or red blood in stool), vomiting of blood or substance resembling coffee grounds, bruising, or other bleeding.

In doses of even 75 milligrams a day, aspirin has been shown to impair the body's ability to stop bleeding. Combined with an anticoagulant—which inactivates certain substances in the blood, leading to the prevention of blood clotting—use of aspirin exacerbates the impairment of the body's ability to clot blood. As a result, abnormal bleeding may occur, particularly in the stomach because aspirin can irritate the stomach's lining.

**Recommendation:** Avoid using aspirin-containing products when taking an oral anticoagulant, unless specifically instructed to do so by the physician who prescribed the anticoagulant. If a mild pain reliever is needed, acetaminophen may be preferable to aspirin. (Of course, discuss your personal medical condition with your doctor.)

**Note:** Occasionally doctors prescribe aspirin and warfarin together *intentionally,* but only when they feel that the increased risk of bleeding is outweighed by the stronger anticoagulant effect.

Aspirin

Antidiabetic drugs:

- acetohexamide (**Dymelor®**)
- chlorpropamide (**Diabinese®**)
- glipizide (**Glucotrol®**)
- glyburide (**DiaBeta®, Micronase®**)
- insulin (**Humulin®, Lente®, Novolin®**, and others)

Aspirin may increase the blood sugar–lowering (hypoglycemic) effect of antidiabetic drugs. Symptoms of an excessively low amount of sugar in the blood include increased heart rate, cold sweats, trembling, nausea, hunger, mental confusion, and, in severe cases, coma.

**Recommendation:** Occasional use of aspirin probably has little effect on antidiabetic drugs with the possible

| PAIN-RELIEVING DRUG | INTERACTING DRUG | RESULT |
|---|---|---|

*(cont.)*

**Aspirin**

Antidiabetic drugs:

- tolazamide (**Tolinase®**)
- tolbutamide (**Orinase®**), and others

[for treatment of diabetes mellitus, a condition that results in excessively high amounts of sugar in the blood and urine]

exception of chlorpropamide. Consult with your doctor before taking larger amounts of aspirin.

---

**Aspirin**

Captopril (**Capoten®**)

[for treatment of high blood pressure and congestive heart failure]

Repeated doses of aspirin decrease the antihypertensive effect of captopril in some persons.

Not much is known about the effect of aspirin on ACE inhibitors (the chemical class to which captopril belongs) other than captopril, but they may also interact. Other ACE inhibitors include benazepril (Lotensin®), enalapril (Vasotec®), fosinopril (Monopril®), lisinopril (Prinivil®, Zestril®), and ramipril (Altace®), and others.

**Recommendation:** Occasional doses of aspirin probably do not affect captopril. If aspirin is used often, however, blood pressure should be monitored frequently to ensure the aspirin is not interfering with the antihypertensive effect.

---

**Aspirin**

Corticosteroids:

- betamethasone (**Celestone®**)
- cortisone (**Cortone®**)
- dexamethasone (**Decadron®**)

Corticosteroids (especially when taken orally or by injection) may reduce the concentration of aspirin in the blood, leading to a decrease in the effectiveness of the aspirin.

This interaction may be important in persons taking large amounts of aspirin, such as arthritis sufferers. *(cont.)*

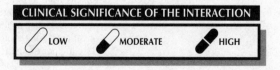

**CLINICAL SIGNIFICANCE OF THE INTERACTION**

LOW   MODERATE   HIGH

9

| PAIN-RELIEVING DRUG | INTERACTING DRUG | RESULT |
|---|---|---|

(cont.)
Aspirin

Corticosteroids
• hydrocortisone
(**Cortef®, Hydro-
cortone®, Solu-
Cortef®**)
• prednisolone
(**Cortalone®, Delta-
Cortef®**)
• prednisone
(**Deltasone®, Liquid
Pred®, Prednicen-M®**),
and others
[for relieving inflamma-
tion and suppressing
allergic reactions]

Aspirin toxicity could result if persons taking moderate to high doses of
aspirin suddenly discontinued corticosteroid therapy. Signs of aspirin
toxicity include hearing loss, ringing
in the ears, rapid breathing, rapid
heart rate, nausea, vomiting, agitation, slurred speech, hallucinations,
disorientation, and seizures.

**Recommendation:** If you are taking
moderate to high doses of aspirin
(3,000 milligrams per day or more in
an adult) for a prolonged period of
time (more than a week), check with
your doctor if oral or injected corticosteroids are started, stopped, or
changed in dosage. Your aspirin
blood level is likely to be affected.

Aspirin

Heparin (**Calciparine®,
Liquaemin®**)

[for the prevention and
control of blood clots]

Use of aspirin by persons taking heparin increases the risk of bleeding.
Such bleeding is evidenced by blood
in the urine, coughing up of blood,
black stool (or red blood in stool),
vomiting of blood or substance resembling coffee grounds, bruising, or
other bleeding.

**Recommendation:** Avoid this combination unless instructed otherwise by
your doctor. Acetaminophen is often
an adequate substitute for aspirin to
relieve pain or reduce fever.

Aspirin

Methotrexate (**Mexate®**)

[for treatment of certain
cancers, such as breast,
lung, and certain forms
of leukemia; also used
for treatment of psoriasis
and rheumatoid arthritis]

Increased effect of the methotrexate,
possibly leading to methotrexate toxicity. Symptoms of toxicity include
fever, sores in the mouth and on the
skin, bleeding, vomiting, diarrhea,
and severe reduction in the number
of white blood cells produced by the
bone marrow.

It's important to note that the risk of
toxicity from this interaction is much
greater when methotrexate is given in
high doses, such as for the treatment
of cancer. Using aspirin with low-
dose methotrexate therapy—which is

| PAIN-RELIEVING DRUG | INTERACTING DRUG | RESULT |
|---|---|---|

*(cont.)*
Aspirin

Methotrexate

used to treat arthritis and psoriasis—poses a smaller risk of inducing methotrexate toxicity. However, caution is still warranted. .

**Recommendation:** Avoid taking aspirin and aspirin-containing products while taking methotrexate unless the doctor who prescribed the methotrexate specifically advises you to do so. (Make sure *all* of your doctors are aware of *all* of the drugs you are taking.)

---

Aspirin

Nitroglycerin **(Deponit®, Minitran®, Nitro-Bid®, Nitrodisc®, Nitro-Dur®, Nitrogard®, Nitrong®, Nitrostat®)**

[used to relieve the pain of an angina attack]

The effect of the nitroglycerin is enhanced. Nitroglycerin dilates blood vessels by causing the muscles that surround them to relax. This interaction may result in excessive dilatation of blood vessels, which may lead to headaches and low blood pressure. The low blood pressure may cause dizziness and/or fainting.

This result is based on the interaction of aspirin with nitroglycerin taken under the tongue. The effect of aspirin on an oral form of nitroglycerin is not known.

---

Aspirin

Phenytoin **(Dilantin®)**

[for the prevention of seizures]

Large doses of aspirin (i.e., more than 2,000 milligrams a day) could lead to phenytoin intoxication in some people, symptoms of which include double vision, incoordination, uncontrolled eye movements, and mental impairment.

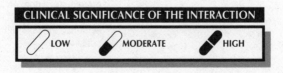

CLINICAL SIGNIFICANCE OF THE INTERACTION

LOW    MODERATE    HIGH

11

| PAIN-RELIEVING DRUG | INTERACTING DRUG | RESULT |
| --- | --- | --- |

Aspirin

Probenecid **(Benemid®)**

[for reduction of uric acid levels in the body to prevent gout and gouty arthritis; also used to increase the effectiveness of certain antibiotics]

Large amounts of aspirin can reduce the effectiveness of probenecid in ridding the body of excess uric acid.

Taking a small dose of aspirin, however—such as an occasional one or two aspirins—probably does not influence the effectiveness of probenecid.

---

Aspirin

Sulfinpyrazone **(Anturane®)**

[for the treatment—particularly prevention—of gout]

Large amounts of aspirin can reduce the effectiveness of sulfinpyrazone in ridding the body of excess uric acid.

Taking a small dose of aspirin, however—such as an occasional one or two aspirins—does not influence the effectiveness of sulfinpyrazone.

---

Aspirin

Valproic acid **(Depakene®)**

[for the treatment of seizures]

When more than a few doses of aspirin are taken, an increase in the concentration of valproic acid—possibly leading to toxicity—has been noted. Symptoms of valproic toxicity include drowsiness, nausea, vomiting, tremor, confusion, excessive weight gain, and hair loss.

---

Diclofenac **(Voltaren®)**

Anticoagulants (oral), such as dicumarol and warfarin **(Coumadin®, Panwarfin®)**

[for the prevention of blood clots]

Three potential problems may arise: (1) all nonsteroidal anti-inflammatory drugs (NSAIDs), a group of drugs including diclofenac, can increase the risk of bleeding in your stomach lining (usually minor, but occasionally will cause severe bleeding); (2) all NSAIDs can interfere with the action of platelets (small substances in the blood that help stop bleeding); (3) although clinical tests suggest that diclofenac is unlikely to increase the blood-thinning effect of oral anticoagulants, the possibility should be considered.

| PAIN-RELIEVING DRUG | INTERACTING DRUG | RESULT |
|---|---|---|

*(cont.)*

**Diclofenac** | **Anticoagulants** |

If bleeding occurs, it may show up as black stool (or red blood in stool), vomiting of blood or a substance resembling coffee grounds, blood in the urine, coughing up of blood, bruising, or other bleeding.

**Recommendation:** Except under exceptional circumstances, it is best to avoid taking any NSAID while taking an oral anticoagulant because of the increased risk of bleeding.

**Diclofenac (Voltaren®)**

Lithium (**Cibalith-S®, Eskalith®, Lithane®, Lithobid®**, and others)

[for manic-depressive disorder]

May lead to higher levels of lithium in the blood, which could lead to lithium toxicity. Symptoms of lithium toxicity include: muscle twitching, dizziness, blurred vision, vomiting or severe nausea, persistent diarrhea, confusion, weakness, coarse trembling of hands or legs, and slurred speech.

**Recommendation:** If you are taking lithium, do not start or stop taking diclofenac (a nonsteroidal anti-inflammatory drug) without consulting with your doctor. Sulindac (Clinoril®), a drug in the same class as diclofenac, appears to produce a slight *decrease* in the amount of lithium in the body, and does not seem to cause difficulties in people taking lithium. However, your doctor may wish to monitor your lithium levels when *any* nonsteroidal anti-inflammatory drug is started or stopped.

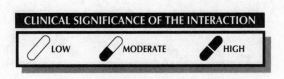

CLINICAL SIGNIFICANCE OF THE INTERACTION

LOW    MODERATE    HIGH

| PAIN-RELIEVING DRUG | INTERACTING DRUG | RESULT |
|---|---|---|

Diflunisal
**(Dolobid®)**

Antacids that contain aluminum, such as **Gaviscon®, Gelusil®, Kolantyl®, Maalox®, Mylanta®**, and others.

[for relief of acid indigestion, heartburn, and abdominal pain caused by too much acid in the stomach]

Decreased effect of the diflunisal when these two medications are taken on an empty stomach.

**Recommendation:** If you must take these two medications, take them with meals. When taken with food, this interaction typically does not occur.

---

Diflunisal
**(Dolobid®)**

Anticoagulants (oral), such as dicumarol and warfarin **(Coumadin®, Panwarfin®)**

[for the prevention of blood clots]

Three potential problems may arise: (1) all nonsteroidal anti-inflammatory drugs (NSAIDs), a group of drugs including diflunisal, can increase the risk of bleeding in your stomach lining (usually minor, but occasionally will cause severe bleeding); (2) all NSAIDs can interfere with the action of platelets (small substances in the blood that help stop bleeding); (3) some NSAIDs (especially phenylbutazone) can increase the blood-thinning effect of oral anticoagulants.

If bleeding occurs, it may show up as black stool (or red blood in stool), vomiting of blood or substance resembling coffee grounds, blood in the urine, coughing up of blood, bruising, or other bleeding.

**Recommendation:** Except under exceptional circumstances, it is best to avoid taking any NSAID while taking an oral anticoagulant because of the increased risk of bleeding.

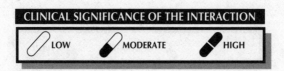

CLINICAL SIGNIFICANCE OF THE INTERACTION

LOW    MODERATE    HIGH

| PAIN-RELIEVING DRUG | INTERACTING DRUG | RESULT |
|---|---|---|

Etodolac **(Lodine®)**

Anticoagulants (oral), such as dicumarol and warfarin **(Coumadin®, Panwarfin®)**

[for the prevention of blood clots]

Three potential problems may arise: (1) all nonsteroidal anti-inflammatory drugs (NSAIDs), a group of drugs including etodolac, can increase the risk of bleeding in your stomach lining (usually minor, but occasionally will cause severe bleeding); (2) all NSAIDs can interfere with the action of platelets (small substances in the blood that help stop bleeding); (3) some NSAIDs (especially phenylbutazone) can increase the blood-thinning effect of oral anticoagulants.

If bleeding occurs, it may show up as black stool (or red blood in stool), vomiting of blood or substance resembling coffee grounds, blood in the urine, coughing up of blood, bruising, or other bleeding.

**Recommendation:** Except under exceptional circumstances, it is best to avoid taking any NSAID while taking an oral anticoagulant because of the increased risk of bleeding.

Fenoprofen **(Nalfon®)**

Anticoagulants (oral), such as dicumarol and warfarin **(Coumadin®, Panwarfin®)**

[for the prevention of blood clots]

Three potential problems may arise: (1) all nonsteroidal anti-inflammatory drugs (NSAIDs), a group of drugs including fenoprofen, can increase the risk of bleeding in your stomach lining (usually minor, but occasionally will cause severe bleeding); (2) all NSAIDs can interfere with the action of platelets (small substances in the blood that help stop bleeding); (3) some NSAIDs (especially phenylbutazone) can increase the blood-thinning effect of oral anticoagulants.

If bleeding occurs, it may show up as black stool (or red blood in stool), vomiting of blood or substance resembling coffee grounds, blood in the urine, coughing up of blood, bruising, or other bleeding.

**Recommendation:** Except under exceptional circumstances, it is best to avoid taking any NSAID while taking an oral anticoagulant because of the increased risk of bleeding.

15

Flurbiprofen **(Ansaid®)**

Anticoagulants (oral), such as dicumarol and warfarin **(Coumadin®, Panwarfin®)**

[for the prevention of blood clots]

Three potential problems may arise: (1) all nonsteroidal anti-inflammatory drugs (NSAIDs), a group of drugs including flurbiprofen can increase the risk of bleeding in your stomach lining (usually minor, but occasionally will cause severe bleeding); (2) all NSAIDs can interfere with the action of platelets (small substances in the blood that help stop bleeding); (3) some NSAIDs (especially phenylbutazone) can increase the blood-thinning effect of oral anticoagulants.

If bleeding occurs, it may show up as black stool (or red blood in stool), vomiting of blood or substance resembling coffee grounds, blood in the urine, coughing up of blood, bruising, or other bleeding.

**Recommendation:** Except under exceptional circumstances, it is best to avoid taking any NSAID while taking an oral anticoagulant because of the increased risk of bleeding.

Ibuprofen **(Advil®, Medipren®, Midol®, Motrin®, Nuprin®,** and **Rufen®)**

Anticoagulants (oral), such as dicumarol and warfarin **(Coumadin®, Panwarfin®)**

[for the prevention of blood clots]

Three potential problems may arise: (1) all nonsteroidal anti-inflammatory drugs (NSAIDs), a group of drugs including ibuprofen, can increase the risk of bleeding in your stomach lining (usually minor, but occasionally will cause severe bleeding); (2) all NSAIDs can interfere with the action of platelets (small substances in the blood that help stop bleeding); (3) some NSAIDs (especially phenylbutazone) can increase the blood-thinning effect of oral anticoagulants.

If bleeding occurs, it may show up as black stool (or red blood in stool), vomiting of blood or substance resembling coffee grounds, blood in the urine, coughing up of blood, bruising, or other bleeding.

| PAIN-RELIEVING DRUG | INTERACTING DRUG | RESULT |
|---|---|---|

(cont.)
Ibuprofen

Anticoagulants

**Recommendation:** Except under exceptional circumstances, it is best to avoid taking any NSAID while taking an oral anticoagulant because of the increased risk of bleeding.

Ibuprofen (**Advil**®, **Medipren**®, **Midol**®, **Motrin**®, **Nuprin**®, and **Rufen**®)

Lithium (**Cibalith-S**®, **Eskalith**®, **Lithane**®, **Lithobid**®, and others)

[for manic-depressive disorder]

May produce higher levels of lithium in the blood, which could lead to lithium toxicity. Symptoms of lithium toxicity include muscle twitching, dizziness, blurred vision, vomiting or severe nausea, persistent diarrhea, confusion, weakness, coarse trembling of hands or legs, and slurred speech.

**Recommendation:** If you are taking lithium, do not start or stop taking ibuprofen (a nonsteroidal anti-inflammatory drug) without consulting with your doctor. Sulindac (Clinoril®), a drug in the same class as ibuprofen, appears to produce a slight decrease in the amount of lithium in the body, and does not seem to cause difficulties in people taking lithium. However, your doctor may wish to monitor your lithium levels when *any* nonsteroidal anti-inflammatory drug is started or stopped.

Indomethacin (**Indocin**®)

Acebutolol, (**Sectral**®)

[for treatment of high blood pressure and angina]

Indomethacin (an anti-inflammatory drug, or NSAID) may reduce the antihypertensive or antianginal effect of acebutolol. This effect may occur with other NSAIDs, such as piroxicam (Feldene®), naproxen (Naprosyn®), and naproxen sodium (Anaprox®). Sulindac (Clinoril®) appears less likely to interfere with the antihypertensive effect of acebutolol.

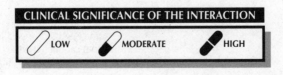

CLINICAL SIGNIFICANCE OF THE INTERACTION

LOW    MODERATE    HIGH

| PAIN-RELIEVING DRUG | INTERACTING DRUG | RESULT |
|---|---|---|

(cont.)
Indomethacin

Acebutolol

**Recommendation:** If you are taking any drug for hypertension, your doctor may wish to check your blood pressure if indomethacin (or any other nonsteroidal anti-inflammatory drug) is started or stopped. Changes in blood pressure may be gradual, over a week or two.

Indomethacin (**Indocin®**)

ACE inhibitors:

- benazepril (**Lotensin®**)
- captopril (**Capoten®**)
- enalapril (**Vasotec®**)
- fosinopril (**Monopril®**)
- lisinopril (**Prinivil®**, **Zestril®**)
- ramipril (**Altace®**)

[for high blood pressure and congestive heart failure]

Indomethacin (a nonsteroidal anti-inflammatory drug) may inhibit the antihypertensive effect of captopril and probably other ACE inhibitors. Other nonsteroidal anti-inflammatory drugs (NSAIDs)—with the possible exception of sulindac (Clinoril®)—probably have a similar effect. Other NSAIDs include diclofenac (Voltaren®), diflunisal (Dolobid®), etodolac (Lodine®), fenoprofen (Nalfon®), flurbiprofen (Ansaid®), ibuprofen (Advil®, Motrin®, Nuprin®, Rufen®), ketoprofen (Orudis®), ketorolac (Toradol®), meclofenamate (Meclomen®), nabumetone (Relafen®), naproxen (Naprosyn®), naproxen sodium (Anaprox®), piroxicam (Feldene®), and tolmetin (Tolectin®).

**Recommendation:** Your doctor may want to check your blood pressure if you start, stop, or change the dose of an NSAID.

Indomethacin (**Indocin®**)

Anticoagulants (oral), such as dicumarol and warfarin (**Coumadin®**, **Panwarfin®**)

[for the prevention of blood clots]

Three potential problems may arise: (1) all nonsteroidal anti-inflammatory drugs (NSAIDs), a group of drugs including indomethacin, can increase the risk of bleeding in your stomach lining (usually minor, but occasionally will cause severe bleeding); (2) all NSAIDs can interfere with the action of platelets (small substances in the blood that help stop bleeding); (3) some NSAIDs (especially phenylbutazone) can increase the blood-thinning effect of oral anticoagulants.

18

*(cont.)*
Indomethacin | Anticoagulants | (If bleeding occurs, it may show up as black stool (or red blood in stool), vomiting of blood or substance resembling coffee grounds, blood in the urine, coughing up of blood, bruising, or other bleeding.

**Recommendation:** Except under exceptional circumstances, it is best to avoid taking any NSAID while taking an oral anticoagulant because of the increased risk of bleeding.

Indomethacin **(Indocin®)**

Atenolol **(Tenormin®)**

[for treatment of high blood pressure and angina]

Indomethacin may reduce the antihypertensive or antianginal effect of atenolol. This effect may occur with other nonsteroidal anti-inflammatory agents (NSAIDs), besides indomethacin, such as diclofenac (Voltaren®), diflunisal (Dolobid®), etodolac (Lodine®), fenoprofen (Nalfon®), flurbiprofen (Ansaid®), ibuprofen (Advil®, Motrin®, Nuprin®, Rufen®), ketoprofen (Orudis®), ketorolac (Toradol®), meclofenamate (Meclomen®), nabumetone (Relafen®), naproxen (Naprosyn®), naproxen sodium (Anaprox®), piroxicam (Feldene®), sulindac (Clinoril®), and tolmetin (Tolectin®). Sulindac (Clinoril®) appears less likely to interfere with the antihypertensive effect of atenolol.

**Recommendation:** Your doctor may want to check your blood pressure if you start, stop, or change the dose of an NSAID. Changes in blood pressure may be gradual, over a week or two.

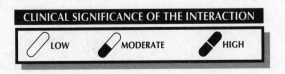

CLINICAL SIGNIFICANCE OF THE INTERACTION

LOW     MODERATE     HIGH

| PAIN-RELIEVING DRUG | INTERACTING DRUG | RESULT |
| --- | --- | --- |

Indomethacin **(Indocin®)**

Bumetanide **(Bumex®)**

[for treatment of high blood pressure and reduction of fluid retention, which can result from heart failure]

Indomethacin impairs the ability of bumetanide to lower blood pressure or to rid the body of excess fluid. Other nonsteroidal anti-inflammatory drugs (NSAIDs)—with the possible exception of sulindac (Clinoril®)—that may interact similarly include aspirin, diclofenac (Voltaren®), diflunisal (Dolobid®), etodolac (Lodine®), fenoprofen (Nalfon®), flurbiprofen (Ansaid®), ibuprofen (Advil®, Motrin®, Nuprin®, Rufen®), ketoprofen (Orudis®), ketorolac (Toradol®), meclofenamate (Meclomen®), nabumetone (Relafen®), naproxen (Naprosyn®), naproxen sodium (Anaprox®), piroxicam (Feldene®), and tolmetin (Tolectin®).

**Recommendation:** Your doctor may want to check your blood pressure if you start, stop, or change your dose of an NSAID.

Indomethacin **(Indocin®)**

Furosemide **(Lasix®)**

[for treatment of high blood pressure and reduction of fluid retention, which can result from heart failure]

Indomethacin may reduce the antihypertensive effect of furosemide. Some evidence indicates that most other nonsteroidal anti-inflammatory drugs may also decrease the effectiveness of furosemide. These drugs include diclofenac (Voltaren®), diflunisal (Dolobid®), etodolac (Lodine®), fenoprofen (Nalfon®), flurbiprofen (Ansaid®), ibuprofen (Advil®, Motrin®, Nuprin®, Rufen®), ketoprofen (Orudis®), ketorolac (Toradol®), meclofenamate (Meclomen®), nabumetone (Relafen®), naproxen (Naprosyn®), naproxen sodium (Anaprox®), piroxicam (Feldene®), sulindac (Clinoril®), and tolmetin (Tolectin®).

Large amounts of aspirin may also decrease the effectiveness of furosemide.

Some evidence indicates that sulindac (Clinoril®) is less likely to interfere with the effect of furosemide.

| PAIN-RELIEVING DRUG | INTERACTING DRUG | RESULT |
|---|---|---|

*(cont.)*
**Indomethacin** | Furosemide | **Recommendation:** Your doctor may want to check your blood pressure if you start, stop, or change your dose of NSAID.

Indomethacin **(Indocin®)**

Hydralazine **(Apresoline®)**

[for treatment of high blood pressure]

Indomethacin may lead to a reduced antihypertensive effect of hydralazine. Other nonsteroidal anti-inflammatory drugs (NSAIDs), besides indomethacin, that may lead to a similar interaction include diclofenac (Voltaren®), diflunisal (Dolobid®), etodolac (Lodine®), fenoprofen (Nalfon®), flurbiprofen (Ansaid®), ibuprofen (Advil®, Motrin®, Nuprin®, Rufen®), ketoprofen (Orudis®), ketorolac (Toradol®), meclofenamate (Meclomen®), nabumetone (Relafen®), naproxen (Naprosyn®), naproxen sodium (Anaprox®), piroxicam (Feldene®), sulindac (Clinoril®), and tolmetin (Tolectin®).

If this interaction occurs, your doctor may adjust your hydralazine dosage, switch you to (or add) another antihypertensive medication, or try using a different anti-inflammatory drug.

**Recommendation:** Your doctor may want to check your blood pressure if you start, stop, or change the dosage of an NSAID.

Indomethacin **(Indocin®)**

Lithium **(Cibalith-S®, Eskalith®, Lithane®, Lithobid®,** and others)

[for manic-depressive disorder]

May produce higher levels of lithium in the blood, which could lead to lithium toxicity. Symptoms of this toxicity include muscle twitching, dizziness, blurred vision, vomiting or severe nausea, persistent diarrhea,

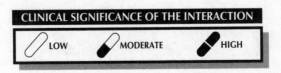

21

| PAIN-RELIEVING DRUG | INTERACTING DRUG | RESULT |
|---|---|---|

*(cont.)*
Indomethacin     Lithium

confusion, weakness, coarse trembling of hands or legs, and slurred speech.

**Recommendation:** If you are taking lithium, do not start or stop taking indomethacin without consulting with your doctor. Sulindac (Clinoril®), a drug in the same class as indomethacin, appears to produce a slight decrease in the amount of lithium in the body, and does not seem to cause difficulties in people taking lithium. However, your doctor may wish to monitor your lithium levels when *any* nonsteroidal anti-inflammatory drug (NSAID) is started or stopped.

---

Indomethacin **(Indocin®)**

Methotrexate **(Mexate®)**

[for treatment of certain cancers, such as breast, lung, and certain forms of leukemia; also used for treatment of psoriasis and rheumatoid arthritis]

Increased effect of the methotrexate, possibly leading to methotrexate toxicity. Symptoms of toxicity include fever, sores in the mouth and on the skin, bleeding, vomiting, diarrhea, and severe reduction in the number of white blood cells produced by the bone marrow.

It's important to note that the risk of toxicity from this interaction is much greater when methotrexate is given in high doses, such as for the treatment of cancer. Low-dose methotrexate therapy—which is used to treat arthritis and psoriasis—poses a smaller risk of inducing methotrexate toxicity. However, caution is still warranted.

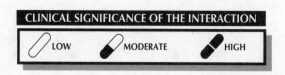

CLINICAL SIGNIFICANCE OF THE INTERACTION

LOW     MODERATE     HIGH

| PAIN-RELIEVING DRUG | INTERACTING DRUG | RESULT |
|---|---|---|

*(cont.)*
Indomethacin

Methotrexate

**Recommendation:** Avoid taking indomethacin—as well as other nonsteroidal anti-inflammatory drugs—when taking methotrexate unless the doctor who prescribed the methotrexate specifically advises you to do so. (Make sure *all* of your doctors are aware of *all* of the drugs you are taking.)

Indomethacin **(Indocin®)**

Pindolol **(Visken®)**

[for treatment of high blood pressure]

Reduction in the antihypertensive or antianginal effect. This effect may occur with other nonsteroidal anti-inflammatory agents (NSAIDs) besides indomethacin, such as piroxicam (Feldene®), naproxen (Naprosyn®), and naproxen sodium (Anaprox®). Sulindac (Clinoril®) appears less likely to interfere with the antihypertensive effect of pindolol.

**Recommendation:** Your doctor may want to check your blood pressure if you start, stop, or change the dosage of an NSAID.

Indomethacin **(Indocin®)**

Propranolol **(Inderal®)**

[for treatment of high blood pressure, angina pectoris, and irregular heartbeats; also used to prevent migraine headaches]

Reduction in the antihypertensive or antianginal effect of propranolol. This effect may occur with other nonsteroidal anti-inflammatory agents (NSAIDs) besides indomethacin, such as piroxicam (Feldene®) and naproxen (Anaprox®, Naprosyn®). Sulindac (Clinoril®) appears less likely to interfere with the antihypertensive effect of propranolol.

**Recommendation:** Your doctor may want to check your blood pressure if you start, stop, or change the dosage of an NSAID.

Indomethacin (**Indocin**®)

Thiazide and thiazide-like diuretics:

- chlorothiazide (**Diuril**®)
- hydrochlorothiazide (**Esidrix**®, **HydroDIURIL**®, **Oretic**®, and others)
- metolazone (**Diulo**®, **Zaroxolyn**®)
- chlorthalidone (**Hygroton**®)

[for treatment of high blood pressure and to reduce fluid retention in persons with congestive heart failure, kidney disorders, and premenstrual tension]

Mild reduction in the antihypertensive effect of the thiazide. This interaction may occur with other nonsteroidal anti-inflammatory drugs besides indomethacin, such as diclofenac (Voltaren®), diflunisal (Dolobid®), etodolac (Lodine®), fenoprofen (Nalfon®), flurbiprofen (Ansaid®), ibuprofen (Advil®, Motrin®, Nuprin®, Rufen®), ketoprofen (Orudis®), ketorolac (Toradol®), meclofenamate (Meclomen®), nabumetone (Relafen®), naproxen (Naprosyn®), naproxen sodium (Anaprox®), piroxicam (Feldene®), sulindac (Clinoril®), and tolmetin (Tolectin®).

**Recommendation:** Although this interaction usually does not cause problems, it would be prudent to have your blood pressure checked if you take indomethacin or other nonsteroidal anti-inflammatory drugs regularly.

Indomethacin (**Indocin**®)

Triamterene (**Dyrenium**®, **Dyazide**®, **Maxzide**®)

[for treatment of high blood pressure and reduction of fluid retention]

Can lead to kidney damage, even kidney failure. Avoid this combination.

May occur with diclofenac (Voltaren®) or ibuprofen (Advil®, Nuprin®, Motrin®)—drugs in the same class as indomethacin—but the evidence is less substantial than that of the indomethacin-triamterene interaction. Until more studies are completed, caution is warranted when any nonsteroidal anti-inflammatory drug is used with triamterene.

Other drugs—such as furosemide (Lasix®) and spironolactone (Aldactone®)—that like triamterene, are diuretics, have not been associated with kidney damage when given with indomethacin.

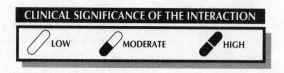

CLINICAL SIGNIFICANCE OF THE INTERACTION

LOW   MODERATE   HIGH

Ketoprofen
**(Orudis®)**

Anticoagulants (oral), such as dicumarol and warfarin **(Coumadin®, Panwarfin®)**

[for the prevention of blood clots]

Three potential problems may arise:(1) all nonsteroidal anti-inflammatory drugs (NSAIDs), a group of drugs including ketoprofen, can increase the risk of bleeding in your stomach lining (usually minor, but occasionally will cause severe bleeding);(2) all NSAIDs can interfere with the action of platelets (small substances in the blood that help stop bleeding);(3) some NSAIDs (especially phenylbutazone) can increase the blood-thinning effect of oral anticoagulants. If bleeding occurs, it may show up as black stool (or red blood in stool), vomiting of blood or substance resembling coffee grounds, blood in the urine, coughing up of blood, bruising, or other bleeding.

**Recommendation:** Except under exceptional circumstances, it is best to avoid taking any NSAID while taking an oral anticoagulant because of the increased risk of bleeding.

Ketoprofen
**(Orudis®)**

Methotrexate **(Mexate®)**

[for treatment of certain cancers, such as breast, lung, and certain forms of leukemia; also used for treatment of psoriasis and rheumatoid arthritis]

Ketoprofen may increase the toxicity of the methotrexate, symptoms of which include fever, sores in the mouth and on the skin, bleeding, vomiting, diarrhea, and severe reduction in the number of white blood cells produced by the bone marrow. It is recommended to avoid using ketoprofen—as well as other nonsteroidal anti-inflammatory drugs—when taking methotrexate. It's important to note that the risk of toxicity from this interaction is much greater when methotrexate is given in high doses, such as for the treatment of cancer. Low-dose methotrexate therapy—which is used to treat arthritis and psoriasis—poses a smaller risk of inducing methotrexate toxicity. However, caution is still warranted.

**Recommendation:** Avoid taking ketoprofen—as well as other nonsteroidal anti-inflammatory drugs—when taking methotrexate unless the doctor who prescribed the methotrexate specifically

| PAIN-RELIEVING DRUG | INTERACTING DRUG | RESULT |
|---|---|---|
| *(cont.)*<br>Ketoprofen | Methotrexate | advises you to do so. (Make sure *all* of your doctors are aware of *all* of the drugs you are taking.) |
| Ketoprofen **(Orudis®)**<br> | Probenecid **(Benemid®)**<br>[for reduction of uric acid levels in the body to prevent gout and gouty arthritis; also used to increase the effectiveness of certain antibiotics] | May increase the plasma concentration of ketoprofen in the blood, thereby increasing the incidence of ketoprofen side effects, such as dizziness, drowsiness, ringing in the ears, diarrhea, and kidney damage. |
| Meclofenamate **(Meclomen®)**<br> | Anticoagulants (oral), such as dicumarol and warfarin **(Coumadin®, Panwarfin®)**<br>[for the prevention of blood clots] | Three potential problems may arise: (1) all nonsteroidal anti-inflammatory drugs (NSAIDs), a group of drugs including meclofenamate, can increase the risk of bleeding in your stomach lining (usually minor, but occasionally will cause severe bleeding); (2) all NSAIDs can interfere with the action of platelets (small substances in the blood that help stop bleeding); (3) some NSAIDs (especially phenylbutazone) can increase the blood-thinning effect of oral anticoagulants. If bleeding occurs, it may show up as black stool (or red blood in stool), vomiting of blood or substance resembling coffee grounds, blood in the urine, coughing up of blood, bruising, or other bleeding.<br><br>**Recommendation:** Except under exceptional circumstances, it is best to avoid taking any NSAID while taking an oral anticoagulant because of the increased risk of bleeding. |
| Mefenamic acid **(Ponstel®)**<br> | Anticoagulants (oral), such as dicumarol and warfarin **(Coumadin®, Panwarfin®)**<br>[for the prevention of blood clots] | Three potential problems may arise: (1) all nonsteroidal anti-inflammatory drugs (NSAIDs), a group of drugs including mefenamic acid, can increase the risk of bleeding in your stomach lining (usually minor, but occasionally will cause severe bleeding); (2) all NSAIDs can interfere with the action of |

*(cont.)*
Mefenamic acid     Anticoagulants

platelets (small substances in the blood that help stop bleeding); (3) some NSAIDs (especially phenylbutazone) can increase the blood-thinning effect of oral anticoagulants. If bleeding occurs, it may show up as black stool (or red blood in stool), vomiting of blood or substance resembling coffee grounds, blood in the urine, coughing up of blood, bruising, or other bleeding.

**Recommendation:** Except under exceptional circumstances, it is best to avoid taking any NSAID while taking an oral anticoagulant because of the increased risk of bleeding

---

Meperidine **(Demerol®, Mepergan®)**

Barbiturates:

- amobarbital **(Amytal®)**
- butabarbital **(Butisol®)**
- butalbital
- pentobarbital **(Nembutal®)**
- phenobarbital **(Luminal®, Solfoton®)**
- primidone **(Mysoline®)**
- secobarbital **(Seconal®), and others**

[used to treat insomnia and anxiety; certain barbiturates are used to prevent seizures]

Barbiturates may increase the sedative effect of merperidine, leading to prolonged sedation, dizziness, drowsiness, or visual disturbances. Although much of the documentation on this interaction has been done on one barbiturate in particular, phenobarbital, other barbiturates are likely to act in the same way.

---

Meperidine **(Demerol®, Mepergan®)**

Chlorpromazine **(Thorazine®)**

[for treatment of various psychotic disorders, such as schizophrenia and mania]

May result in an excessive decrease in blood pressure levels (hypotension) and impaired breathing. The central nervous system may also be depressed excessively when these two medications are taken, with symptoms such as lethargy and prolonged sedation.

---

**CLINICAL SIGNIFICANCE OF THE INTERACTION**

LOW     MODERATE     HIGH

| PAIN-RELIEVING DRUG | INTERACTING DRUG | RESULT |
|---|---|---|

Meperidine (**Demerol**®, **Mepergan**®)

Cimetidine (**Tagamet**®)

[for relief of stomach and intestinal ulcers]

Cimetidine may increase the effect of meperidine, possibly leading to increased sedation and impaired breathing.

Ranitidine (Zantac®) and probably famotidine (Pepcid®) and nizatidine (Axid®) appear less likely to interact with narcotic analgesics.

---

Meperidine (**Demerol**®, **Mepergan**®)

Monoamine oxidase inhibitors:

- isocarboxazid (**Marplan**®)
- phenelzine (**Nardil**®)
- tranylcypromine (**Parnate**®)

[for the treatment of depression]

Can be very dangerous interaction. Some individuals receiving meperidine and a monoamine oxidase inhibitor may develop severe side effects, such as severe alterations in blood pressure (both excessively high blood pressure in some persons, and excessively low blood pressure in others), impaired breathing, rigidity, convulsions, coma, and death. Less severe side effects include excitation and sweating.

**Recommendation:** Avoid this combination. Also, do not use meperidine for three weeks following the cessation of an antidepressant from the monoamine oxidase inhibitor class.

---

Methadone (**Dolophine**®)

Barbiturates:

- amobarbital (**Amytal**®)
- butabarbital (**Butisol**®)
- butalbital
- pentobarbital (**Nembutal**®)
- phenobarbital (**Luminal**®, **Solfoton**®)
- primidone (**Mysoline**®)
- secobarbital (**Seconal**®), and others

[used to treat insomnia and anxiety; certain barbiturates are used to prevent seizures]

Barbiturates may cause the concentration of methadone in the blood to drop, possibly leading to a decreased effect of the methadone and sometimes to symptoms of methadone withdrawal.

| PAIN-RELIEVING DRUG | INTERACTING DRUG | RESULT |
|---|---|---|
| Methadone **(Dolophine®)** | Carbamazepine **(Tegretol®)** [for epilepsy, trigeminal neuralgia (spasms of pain in the face), and other disorders] | Carbamazepine may cause the concentration of methadone in the blood to drop, leading to a decreased effect of the methadone and sometimes to symptoms of methadone withdrawal. |
| Methadone **(Dolophine®)** | Phenytoin **(Dilantin®)** [for the prevention of seizures] | Phenytoin may cause the concentration of methadone in the blood to drop, leading to a decreased effect of the methadone and sometimes to symptoms of methadone withdrawal. |
| Methadone **(Dolophine®)** | Rifampin **(Rifadin®, Rimactane®)** [used in combination with at least one other drug, rifampin is used to treat tuberculosis; also used in the treatment of individuals who are carriers of meningitis] | Rifampin may cause the concentration of methadone in the blood to drop, leading to a decreased effect of the methadone and sometimes to symptoms of methadone withdrawal. |
| Naproxen **(Anaprox®, Naprosyn®)** | Anticoagulants (oral), such as dicumarol and warfarin **(Coumadin®, Panwarfin®)** [for the prevention of blood clots] | Three potential problems may arise: (1) all nonsteroidal anti-inflammatory drugs (NSAIDs), a group of drugs including naproxen, can increase the risk of bleeding in your stomach lining (usually minor, but occasionally will cause severe bleeding); (2) all NSAIDs can interfere with the action of platelets (small substances in the blood that help stop bleeding); (3) some NSAIDs (especially phenylbutazone) can increase the blood-thinning effect of oral anticoagulants. |

**CLINICAL SIGNIFICANCE OF THE INTERACTION**

LOW   MODERATE   HIGH

| PAIN-RELIEVING DRUG | INTERACTING DRUG | RESULT |
|---|---|---|

(cont.)
Naproxen | Anticoagulants | If bleeding occurs, it may show up as black stool (or red blood in stool), vomiting of blood or substance resembling coffee grounds, blood in the urine, coughing up of blood, bruising, or other bleeding.

**Recommendation:** Except under exceptional circumstances, it is best to avoid taking any NSAID while taking an oral anticoagulant because of the increased risk of bleeding.

Naproxen **(Anaprox®, Naprosyn®)** | Lithium **(Cibalith-S®, Eskalith®, Lithane®, Lithobid®, and others)**

[for manic-depressive disorder] | May produce higher levels of lithium in the blood, which could lead to lithium toxicity. Symptoms of this toxicity include muscle twitching, dizziness, blurred vision, vomiting or severe nausea, persistent diarrhea, confusion, weakness, coarse trembling of hands or legs, and slurred speech.

**Recommendation:** If you are taking lithium, do not start or stop taking naproxen without consulting with your doctor. Sulindac (Clinoril®) appears to produce a slight decrease in the amount of lithium in the body, and does not seem to cause difficulties in people taking lithium. However, your doctor may wish to monitor your lithium levels when *any* nonsteroidal anti-inflammatory drug is started or stopped.

Naproxen **(Anaprox®, Naprosyn®)** | Methotrexate **(Mexate®)**

[for treatment of certain cancers, such as breast, lung, and certain forms of leukemia; also used for treatment of psoriasis and rheumatoid arthritis] | May increase the effect of the methotrexate, possibly leading to methotrexate toxicity. Symptoms of toxicity include fever, sores in the mouth and on the skin, bleeding, vomiting, diarrhea, and severe reduction in the number of white blood

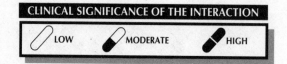

| CLINICAL SIGNIFICANCE OF THE INTERACTION | | |
|---|---|---|
| LOW | MODERATE | HIGH |

(*cont.*)
Naproxen

Methotrexate

cells produced by the bone marrow.

It's important to note that the risk of toxicity from this interaction is much greater when methotrexate is given in high doses, such as for the treatment of cancer. Low-dose methotrexate therapy—which is used to treat arthritis and psoriasis—poses a smaller risk of inducing methotrexate toxicity. However, caution is still warranted.

**Recommendation:** Avoid taking naproxen—as well as other non-steroidal anti-inflammatory drugs—with methotrexate unless the doctor who prescribed the methotrexate specifically advises you to do so. (Make sure *all* of your doctors are aware of *all* of the drugs you are taking.)

Narcotic analgesics:

- codeine
- hydrocodone (**Azdone®**)
- meperidine (**Demerol®, Mepergan®**)
- hydromorphone (**Dilaudid®**)
- oxycodone (**Percodan®, Percocet®**)
- oxymorphone (**Numorphan®**)
- pentazocine (**Talwin®**)
- propoxyphene (**Darvocet-N®, Darvon®, Wygesic®**)

Alcohol

Drinking even a small amount of alcohol while taking a narcotic analgesic may result in excessive sedation and a significant reduction in alertness. A large amount of alcohol taken with narcotic analgesics could result in coma or death.

**Recommendation:** Do not combine alcohol with narcotic analgesics. Such a combination could be extremely dangerous when sharp reactions are needed, such as when driving a car or operating machinery. This interaction is particularly dangerous when either the alcohol or the narcotic is used in excess or when an overdose of the narcotic agent is taken.

31

Nonsteroidal anti-inflammatory drugs:

- aspirin
- diclofenac (**Voltaren**®)
- diflunisal (**Dolobid**®)
- etodolac (**Lodine**®)
- fenoprofen (**Nalfon**®)
- flurbiprofen (**Ansaid**®)
- ibuprofen (**Advil**®, **Motrin**®, **Nuprin**®,**Rufen**®)
- indomethacin (**Indocin**®)
- ketoprofen (**Orudis**®)
- ketorolac (**Toradol**®)
- meclofenamate (**Meclomen**®)
- nabumetone (**Relafen**®)
- naproxen (**Naprosyn**®)
- naproxen sodium (**Anaprox**®)
- phenylbutazone (**Butazolidin**®)
- piroxicam (**Feldene**®)
- sulindac (**Clinoril**®)
- tolmetin (**Tolectin**®)

Prazosin (**Minipress**®)

[for treatment of high blood pressure]

Nonsteroidal anti-inflammatory drugs (NSAIDs) may reduce the effectiveness of several antihypertensive drugs (such as prazosin, captopril, and thiazide diuretics), resulting in an increase in blood pressure. Although certain studies indicate that specifically ibuprofen and indomethacin can reduce the effectiveness of prazosin, other NSAIDs may interact similarly.

If this interaction occurs, your doctor may adjust your prazosin dosage, switch you to (or add) another antihypertensive medication, or try using a different anti-inflammatory drug.

Some evidence indicates that one NSAID—sulindac (Clinoril®)—is less likely to interfere with the effect of antihypertensive medications.

**Recommendation:** Your doctor may want to check your blood pressure if you start, stop, or change the dosage of an NSAID.

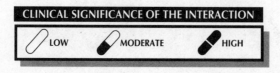

| CLINICAL SIGNIFICANCE OF THE INTERACTION |
| LOW | MODERATE | HIGH |

Pentazocine
**(Talwin®)**

Cigarette smoking

Smoking may cause a decreased pain-relieving effect of pentazocine. As a result, a larger dose of pentazocine may be required in smokers to achieve the same analgesic effect achieved in nonsmokers. (Of course, only your doctor should alter the dose of your medication.)

Phenylbutazone
**(Azolid®, Butazolidin®)**

Anticoagulants (oral), such as dicumarol and warfarin **(Coumadin®, Panwarfin®)**

[for the prevention of blood clots]

Three potential problems may arise: (1) all nonsteroidal anti-inflammatory drugs (NSAIDs), a group of drugs including phenylbutazone, can increase the risk of bleeding in your stomach lining (usually minor, but occasionally will cause severe bleeding); (2) all NSAIDs can interfere with the action of platelets (small substances in the blood that help stop bleeding); (3) phenylbutazone markedly increases the blood-thinning effect of oral anticoagulants.

If bleeding occurs, it may show up as black stool (or red blood in stool), vomiting of blood or substance resembling coffee grounds, blood in the urine, coughing up of blood, bruising, or other bleeding.

Phenylbutazone (Butazolidin®) can cause such severe bone-marrow depression (i.e., decrease in the number of white blood cells the bone marrow produces) that many doctors prescribe this drug very hesitantly, if at all.

**Recommendation:** Except under exceptional circumstances, it is best to avoid taking any NSAID while taking an oral anticoagulant because of the increased risk of bleeding. Phenylbutazone (Butazolidin®) in particular should not be used in persons taking oral anticoagulants except under extremely rare circumstances.

33

| PAIN-RELIEVING DRUG | INTERACTING DRUG | RESULT |
| --- | --- | --- |
| Phenylbutazone (**Azolid**®, **Butazolidin**®)  | Antidiabetic agents:<br>• chlorpropamide (**Diabinese**®)<br>• glipizide (**Glucotrol**®)<br>• glyburide (**DiaBeta**®, **Micronase**®)<br>• tolazamide (**Tolinase**®)<br>• tolbutamide (**Orinase**®)<br>and others<br><br>[for treatment of diabetes mellitus, a condition that results in excessively high amounts of sugar in the blood and urine] | Phenylbutazone increases the plasma concentration of several antidiabetic drugs, which leads to an enhanced reduction of sugar levels in the blood (a condition known as hypoglycemia). Symptoms of an excessive drop in blood sugar levels include increased heart rate, cold sweats, trembling, nausea, hunger, mental confusion, and, in severe cases, coma.<br><br>**Recommendation:** People taking oral antidiabetic agents should generally avoid phenylbutazone. If the combination is used, great care is needed to make sure the blood sugar does not get too low. |
| Phenylbutazone (**Azolid**®, **Butazolidin**®)  | Aspirin<br><br>(**Alka-Seltzer**® **Antacid and Pain Reliever, Anacin**®, **Ascriptin**®, **Bayer**®, **Bufferin**®, **Ecotrin**®, and many others) | Increased amount of uric acid in the blood.<br><br>Although this interaction is not significant enough to avoid concurrent use in most individuals, persons with a history of gout—a condition involving excessively high amounts of uric acid in the blood—may be advised by their physicians to avoid using these two drugs simultaneously. |
| Phenylbutazone (**Azolid**®, **Butazolidin**®)  | Lithium (**Cibalith-S**®, **Eskalith**®, **Lithane**®, **Lithobid**®, and others)<br><br>[for manic-depressive disorder] | May produce higher levels of lithium in the blood, which could lead to lithium toxicity. Symptoms of this toxicity include muscle twitching, dizziness, blurred vision, vomiting or severe nausea, persistent diarrhea, confusion, weakness, coarse trembling of hands or legs, and slurred speech.<br><br>**Recommendation:** If you are taking lithium, do not start or stop taking phenylbutazone without consulting with your doctor. Sulindac (Clinoril®), a drug in the same class as phenylbutazone, appears to produce a slight decrease in the amount of lithium |

| PAIN-RELIEVING DRUG | INTERACTING DRUG | RESULT |
|---|---|---|

*(cont.)*
Phenylbutazone — Lithium — in the body, and does not seem to cause difficulties in people taking lithium. However, your doctor may wish to monitor your lithium levels when *any* nonsteroidal anti-inflammatory drug is started or stopped

---

Phenylbutazone **(Azolid®, Butazolidin®)**

Methotrexate **(Mexate®)**

[for treatment of certain cancers, such as breast, lung, and certain forms of leukemia; also used for treatment of psoriasis and rheumatoid arthritis]

Can lead to an increased effect of methotrexate to the point of methotrexate toxicity. Symptoms of toxicity include fever, sores in the mouth and on the skin, bleeding, vomiting, diarrhea, and severe reduction in the number of white blood cells produced by the bone marrow.

It's important to note that the risk of toxicity from this interaction is much greater when methotrexate is given in high doses, such as for the treatment of cancer. Low-dose methotrexate therapy—which is used to treat arthritis and psoriasis—poses a smaller risk of inducing methotrexate toxicity. However, caution is still warranted.

**Recommendation:** If possible, avoid this combination.

---

Phenylbutazone **(Azolid®, Butazolidin®)**

Phenytoin **(Dilantin®)**

[for the prevention of seizures]

Phenylbutazone may increase the plasma levels of phenytoin, which may lead to uncontrolled eye movements, double vision, incoordination, and mental impairment.

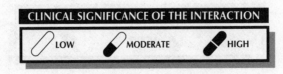

CLINICAL SIGNIFICANCE OF THE INTERACTION

LOW    MODERATE    HIGH

Piroxicam
**(Feldene®)**

Anticoagulants (oral), such as dicumarol and warfarin **(Coumadin®, Panwarfin®)**

[for the prevention of blood clots]

Three potential problems may arise: (1) all nonsteroidal anti-inflammatory drugs (NSAIDs), a group of drugs including piroxicam, can increase the risk of bleeding in your stomach lining (usually minor, but occasionally will cause severe bleeding); (2) all NSAIDs can interfere with the action of platelets (small substances in the blood that help stop bleeding); (3) some NSAIDs (especially phenylbutazone) can increase the blood-thinning effect of oral anticoagulants. If bleeding occurs, it may show up as black stool (or red blood in stool), vomiting of blood or substance resembling coffee grounds, blood in the urine, coughing up of blood, bruising, or other bleeding.

**Recommendation:** Except under exceptional circumstances, it is best to avoid taking any NSAID while taking an oral anticoagulant because of the increased risk of bleeding.

Piroxicam
**(Feldene®)**

Cholestyramine
**(Questran®)**

[for lowering cholesterol levels]

Cholestyramine may reduce the effectiveness of piroxicam, but more studies are needed to document this effect.

**Recommendation:** Separate the doses of cholestyramine and piroxicam as much as possible.

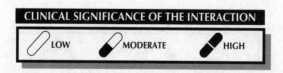

CLINICAL SIGNIFICANCE OF THE INTERACTION

LOW   MODERATE   HIGH

Piroxicam
(**Feldene**®)

Lithium (**Cibalith-S**®,
**Eskalith**®, **Lithane**®,
**Lithobid**®, and others)

[for manic-depressive
disorder]

May produce higher levels of lithium
in the blood, which could lead to
lithium toxicity. Symptoms of this
toxicity include muscle twitching,
dizziness, blurred vision, vomiting or
severe nausea, persistent diarrhea,
confusion, weakness, coarse trembling of hands or legs, and slurred
speech.

**Recommendation:** If you are taking
lithium, do not start or stop taking
piroxicam without consulting with
your doctor. Sulindac (Clinoril®), a
drug in the same class as piroxicam,
appears to produce a slight decrease
in the amount of lithium in the body,
and does not seem to cause difficulties in people taking lithium.
However, your doctor may wish to
monitor your lithium levels when
*any* nonsteroidal anti-inflammatory
drug is started or stopped.

Propoxyphene
(**Darvocet-N**®,
**Darvon**®, **Darvon**®
with A.S.A.®,
**Dolene**®, and
**Wygesic**®)

Carbamazepine
(**Tegretol**®)

[for epilepsy, trigeminal
neuralgia (spasms of pain
in the face), and other
disorders]

Propoxyphene has consistently been
shown to increase the amount of carbamazepine in the blood; this effect
may lead to carbamazepine toxicity
with symptoms such as drowsiness,
dizziness, nausea, vomiting, incoordination, headache, involuntary rapid
movement of the eyeball, and blurred
vision.

It's also important to be alert for a reduced effect of the carbamazepine
(as shown by reduced control of
seizures) if propoxyphene is suddenly
discontinued or reduced in dosage.

**Recommendation:** It would be best to
avoid taking propoxyphene if you are
on carbamazepine therapy.

37

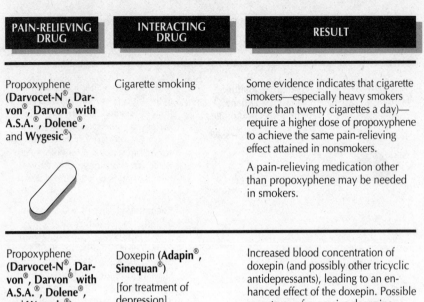

Propoxyphene **(Darvocet-N®, Darvon®, Darvon® with A.S.A.®, Dolene®, and Wygesic®)**

Cigarette smoking

Some evidence indicates that cigarette smokers—especially heavy smokers (more than twenty cigarettes a day)—require a higher dose of propoxyphene to achieve the same pain-relieving effect attained in nonsmokers.

A pain-relieving medication other than propoxyphene may be needed in smokers.

---

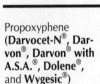

Propoxyphene **(Darvocet-N®, Darvon®, Darvon® with A.S.A.®, Dolene®, and Wygesic®)**

Doxepin **(Adapin®, Sinequan®)**

[for treatment of depression]

Increased blood concentration of doxepin (and possibly other tricyclic antidepressants), leading to an enhanced effect of the doxepin. Possible symptoms of excessive doxepine effect include lethargy, dry mouth, blurred vision, and constipation.

---

Propoxyphene (**Darvocet-N®, Darvon®, Darvon® with A.S.A.®, Dolene®, and Wygesic®)**

Metoprolol **(Lopressor®)**

[for treatment of high blood pressure and angina]

Can increase the concentration of metoprolol, leading to slowing of the heart rate and an increased likelihood of the occurrence of side effects, such as cold hands, cold feet, and lethargy.

---

Propoxyphene (**Darvocet-N®, Darvon®, Darvon® with A.S.A.®, Dolene®, and Wygesic®)**

Propranolol **(Inderal®)**

[for treatment of high blood pressure, angina pectoris, and irregular heartbeats; also used to prevent migraine headaches]

Can increase the concentration of propranolol, possibly leading to an excessive reduction in blood pressure, slowed heart rate, difficulty breathing, and cold hands and feet.

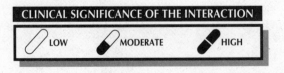

CLINICAL SIGNIFICANCE OF THE INTERACTION

LOW    MODERATE    HIGH

| PAIN-RELIEVING DRUG | INTERACTING DRUG | RESULT |
|---|---|---|

Sulindac **(Clinoril®)**

Anticoagulants (oral), such as dicumarol and warfarin **(Coumadin®, Panwarfin®)**

[for the prevention of blood clots]

Three potential problems may arise: (1) all nonsteroidal anti-inflammatory drugs (NSAIDs), a group of drugs including sulindac, can increase the risk of bleeding in your stomach lining (usually minor, but occasionally will cause severe bleeding); (2) all NSAIDs can interfere with the action of platelets (small substances in the blood that help stop bleeding); (3) some NSAIDs (especially phenylbutazone) can increase the blood-thinning effect of oral anticoagulants.

If bleeding occurs, it may show up as black stool (or red blood in stool), vomiting of blood or substance resembling coffee grounds, blood in the urine, coughing up of blood, bruising, or other bleeding.

**Recommendation:** Except under exceptional circumstances, it is best to avoid taking any NSAID while taking an oral anticoagulant because of the increased risk of bleeding.

Tolmetin **(Tolectin®)**

Anticoagulants (oral), such as dicumarol and warfarin **(Coumadin®, Panwarfin®)**

[for the prevention of blood clots]

Three potential problems may arise: (1) all nonsteroidal anti-inflammatory drugs (NSAIDs), a group of drugs including tolmetin, can increase the risk of bleeding in your stomach lining (usually minor, but occasionally will cause severe bleeding); (2) all NSAIDs can interfere with the action of platelets (small substances in the blood that help stop bleeding); (3) some NSAIDs (especially phenylbutazone) can increase the blood-thinning effect of oral anticoagulants.

If bleeding occurs, it may show up as black stool (or red blood in stool), vomiting of blood or substance resembling coffee grounds, blood in the urine, coughing up of blood, bruising, or other bleeding.

**Recommendation:** Except under exceptional circumstances, it is best to avoid taking any NSAID while taking an oral anticoagulant because of the increased risk of bleeding.

## CHAPTER 2

# DRUGS FOR INFECTION

Virtually every organ and tissue in your body is susceptible to infection, a condition in which microorganisms invade and multiply in the body. Some infections go totally unnoticed, as your body successfully rids itself of the intruders. Other infections may be mild, causing only swelling and tenderness at one location for a day or two. Yet other infections can inflict severe illness, which may be fatal.

All infections are caused by microorganisms, such as bacteria, viruses, fungi, protozoa, and others. Not all microorganisms cause disease—some of them are even beneficial to humans, such as certain intestinal bacteria that manufacture vitamin K, a vital nutrient necessary for normal blood clotting. The microorganisms that do cause disease are called *pathogens.* Many microorganisms do not ordinarily cause disease, but under certain conditions—as when a person's immune system is deficient—will bring on an *opportunistic* infection. For example, individuals with acquired immunodeficiency syndrome (AIDS) are more likely to suffer from opportunistic infections than healthy persons. Generally, opportunistic diseases tend to strike people already weakened by another disease.

One microorganism may be responsible for several conditions. For example, pneumonia, an infection of the air sacs of the lungs, may be caused by a bacterium known as *Streptococcus pneumonia,* but this bacterium may also cause infection of the ear, pneumococcal meningitis (an inflammation of the membranes that surround the brain and spinal cord), sinusitis (an inflammation of the sinuses), and other conditions. Furthermore, pneumonia may be caused by several different microorganisms, not just bacteria but also viruses, mycoplasmas, rickettsiae, or fungi.

## Pneumonia

According to the National Foundation for Infectious Diseases, about half of the cases of pneumonia are caused by bacteria, and 60 to 90 percent of these are caused by *Streptococcus pneumoniae.*[1] This type of pneumonia—called pneumococcal pneumonia—has been estimated to cause illness in 500,000 Americans each year and 25,000 deaths. As a group, all types of pneumonia are the sixth leading cause of death in the United States.[2] More than three fourths of those who die are over age sixty-five.

# Ear Infections

Ear infections may involve the outer ear canal or the middle ear. An outer ear infection, often called swimmer's ear, results when water-carrying bacteria or fungi get trapped in the ear canal. The microorganisms multiply and lead to ear infection. The ear becomes very sensitive, especially when touched, and often secretes a milky liquid. Doctors often treat this condition with ear drops containing an antibiotic.

Whereas swimmer's ear primarily affects adults, another type of ear infection affects mainly children. This is the classic children's ear infection, or more precisely a middle ear infection (technically known as otitis media). Such infections result when the air passage (eustachian tube) that drains the middle ear into the throat becomes inflamed, swollen, and obstructed, trapping bacteria in the middle ear. Pain results as the fluid in the ear accumulates.

Although not all ear pain is the result of an infection, it's important not to neglect ear pain because if infection is present and left untreated, hearing loss may result. Furthermore, the fluid accumulation associated with ear infections may in some cases lead to a ruptured eardrum. Therefore, it's best to check with your doctor. Signs of ear infection may include fever, poor appetite, fussiness, and trouble hearing. Infants may show signs of a problem by crying, tugging or trying to tug at their ears, or increasing the amount or intensity of their crying when lying down (the pain may be more severe in the lying position).

# "Strep" Infection

Some infections are self-limiting; that is, they'll typically go away by themselves even without medications. However, other infections tend to linger on; some may progress into far more serious conditions (that's why if you suspect an infection, you should contact your doctor). One infection not to leave unchecked is a *Streptococcus,* or "strep," infection.

There are more than eighty known types of Group A *Streptococcus.* As its name implies, these microorganisms can cause strep throat, an extremely painful sore throat. Left untreated, the infection may trigger an immunological reaction that may damage the heart, joints, and brain (acute rheumatic fever) or the kidneys (glomerulonephritis).

# A Word about Haemophilus Influenzae

By its name, one would think that bacteria known as *Haemophilus influenzae* are related to influenza (the flu). Actually, this bacterium was so named because when it was first identified, it was *erroneously* believed to cause influenza (which is actually caused by a virus). *Haemophilus influenzae* is the most common cause of bacterial meningitis in the United States. Since one particular strain of this bug (type b) is the causative agent, it is often known as "Hib," for *Haemophilus influenzae* type b. Hib can also cause other infections, such as pneumonia.

When caused by bacteria (meningitis may also be caused by viruses), meningitis is potentially fatal. The neurological effects of bacterial meningitis may persist after the infection has ended; aftereffects may include hearing loss, mental retardation, and recurrent convulsions. These problems are especially devastating in children, who are affected by meningitis more frequently than adults; nearly one half of the approximately 3,000 annual cases of meningitis in the United States involve children and teens, and one fourth of all cases involve preschool children. Whenever meningitis is suspected—in children or adults—the person should be rushed to the nearest hospital. Symptoms of bacterial meningitis include high fever, headache, stiff neck, confusion, and lethargy.

# Viral Infections

Viruses consist of a core of genetic material surrounded by a protein coat. A virus cannot multiply on its own; it uses a host's (i.e., a person's) own cells—and the biological machinery within the cells—to reproduce. Because a virus is dependent on the host, scientists have had a difficult time developing drugs that destroy the virus without harming human cells as well.

Some examples of illness caused by viruses include the common cold, the flu (influenza), measles, chicken pox, mumps, rabies, infectious mononucleosis, shingles, and yellow fever. Certain conditions may be caused by bacteria or viruses, such as pneumonia, bronchitis, or meningitis. Warts are also caused by a virus.

# Medications for Viral Infections

For reasons mentioned earlier, the development of antiviral medications has not been nearly as successful as that of antibacterial drugs. It is important to note that antibiotics are *not* effective for treating viral infections. Nevertheless, several medications are useful in the treatment of viral conditions. Furthermore, immunization has been used successfully to prevent viral infections by stimulating the body's defense mechanisms.

Some antiviral drugs include acyclovir (Zovirax®), amantadine (Symmetrel®), cytarabine (Cytosar-U®), idoxuridine (Herplex®, Stoxil®), inteferon (Alferon-N®, Intron A®, Roferon-A®), ribavirin (Virazole®), trifluridine (Viroptic®), vidarabine (Vira-A®), and zidovudine (Retrovir®).

42

# Fungal Infections

Like bacterial infections, fungal infections range in severity from self-limiting (they go away by themselves) to severe, even fatal, illness. Again like bacterial infections, fungi may infect virtually any organ in the body. One fungal infection, typically not severe, that may be seen in otherwise healthy infants and in elderly persons (especially those in poor health) is oral thrush, which leaves a white substance covering the tongue, inner cheeks, and palate. Oral thrush may or may not be painful, but, in infants, treatment may be necessary to prevent the infection from spreading to other sites. Oral thrush may also occur in persons taking antibiotics. Other fungi may cause lung infection (such as a severe type of pneumonia) or meningitis.

Many fungi breed on and infect the skin. These skin infections typically occur on warm parts of the body where sweat may gather, such as between the toes or in the groin area. Athlete's foot is a common fungal infection of the foot, usually between the toes. The skin there becomes dry and cracked, leading to pain. Fungus may also infect the scalp, trunk, or nails.

The key in preventing fungal infections of the skin is to stay dry. After a bath or a swim, thoroughly towel off. Use talcum powder to help absorb moisture. Wear footwear that "breathes" and is not confining. Avoid plastic or vinyl shoes, which tend to trap moisture around your feet.

Prescription medications used to treat fungal infections include amphotericin B (Fungizone®), ciclopirox olamine (Loprox®), fluconazole (Diflucan®), flucytosine (Ancobon®), griseofulvin (Fulvicin® P/G, Grisactin®, and Gris-PEG®), haloprogin (Halotex®), ketoconazole (Nizoral®), nystatin (Mycolog®II, Mycostatin®), and others. Nonprescription medications to combat fungal infection include clioquinol (Vioform®), miconazole (Micatin®), povidone-iodine (Betadine®), tolnaftate (Aftate®, Tinactin®), undecylenic acid (Cruex®, Desenex®), and others. Some medications, such as clotrimazole (Gyne-Lotrimin®, Lotrimin®, Mycelex®) are available in both prescription and nonprescription forms.

# Medications for Bacterial Infection

Although anti-infective medications include drugs used to treat bacterial, viral, yeast, parasitic, and other types of infection, this chapter will focus primarily on antibiotic medications, which are used to treat bacterial infections. Antibiotics are substances derived from mold or bacteria (or synthetically produced), and are used to retard the growth of or to kill other bacteria. Generally, antibiotics are not effective against viruses, parasites, or fungi.

# Penicillin

The world's first antibiotic—penicillin—was discovered by British scientist Alexander Fleming in 1928. Since Fleming's time, scientists have been able to manipulate the basic structure of the penicillin compound so that today more than twenty different types of penicillins are available. Penicillin, which is no longer one drug but a class of drugs, is used to treat many different types of infections, including infections of the ear, nose, throat, respiratory tract, urinary tract, and prostate, as well as certain sexually transmitted diseases.

Penicillins work by attacking a bacterium's cell wall. Every cell in a human is surrounded by a thin cell membrane. In addition to a cell membrane, bacteria have a rigid cell wall, which surrounds the organism. Penicillins interfere with the building—and promote the destruction—of this cell wall. Because humans lack cell walls, the destructive capability of penicillin is directed selectively at the invading bacteria.

Penicillin derived directly from the fungus *Penicillium* is called *natural* penicillin. Natural penicillins include penicillin G (Pentids®, Pfizerpen®, Bicillin®, and others) and penicillin V (Ledercillin VK®, Pen-Vee K®, V-Cillin K®, Veetids®, and others). Scientists have been able to develop many other penicillins—semisynthetic ones—by altering the basic nucleus of natural penicillin.

One group of semisynthetic penicillins—dubbed aminopenicillins—include ampicillin (Amcill®, Omnipen®, Polycillin®, Principen®, Unasyn®), amoxicillin (Amoxil®, Larotid®, Polymox®, Trimox®, Utimox®, Wymox®), bacampicillin (Spectrobid®), and cyclacillin (Cyclapen-W®). Some of these aminopenicillins have likely become almost household words, particularly in homes with young children prone to ear infections. Other penicillins your doctor may use for specific types of infection include azlocillin (Azlin®), carbenicillin (Geocillin®, Geopen®), cloxacillin (Cloxapen®, Tegopen®), dicloxacillin (Dycill, Dynapen, Pathocil), methicillin (Staphcillin®), mezlocillin (Mezlin®), nafcillin (Nafcil®, Nallpen®, Unipen®), oxacillin (Bactocill®, Prostaphlin®), piperacillin (Pipracil®), ticarcillin (Ticar®), and others, including combination products.

Because penicillins can change the results of some medical tests, tell laboratory personnel if you are taking penicillin. Some types of penicillin may cause false test results on some urine sugar tests.[3] Women on an estrogen-containing oral contraceptive should use an additional method of birth control when taking any penicillin because the effect of the oral contraceptive may be diminished.

# Cephalosporins

Another group of antibiotics structurally related to the penicillins is the cephalosporins. Certain cephalosporins can be used to treat urinary tract infections, pharyngitis (throat inflammation), pneumonia, bronchitis, ear infections, skin infections, and many other types of infection. Cephalosporins are also used to prevent infections following surgery. Cephalosporins are typically classified as first, second, or third "generation"; with a few exceptions, each successive generation has broader activity—the ability to kill or halt the growth of more types of microorganisms—than the previous generation. However, second- and third-generation cephalosporins are more expensive, and should be used for bacteria not covered by first-generation agents.

First-generation cephalosporins include cefadroxil (Duricef®, Ultracef®), cephalexin (Keflet®, Keflex®), cephalothin (Keflin®), cefazolin (Ancef®, Kefzol®), cephradine (Anspor®, Velosef®), and others. Second-generation cephalosporins include cefaclor (Ceclor®), cefamandole (Mandol®), cefmetazole (Zefazone®), cefonicid (Monocid®), ceforanide (Precef®), cefotetan (Cefotan®), cefoxitin (Mefoxin®), cefuroxime (Zinacef®), cefuroxime axetil (Ceftin®), and others. Third-generation cephalosporins include cefixime (Suprax®), cefoperazone (Cefobid®), cefotaxime (Claforan®), ceftazidime (Fortaz®, Tazicef®, Tazidime®), ceftriaxone (Rocephin®), moxalactam (Moxam®), and others.

# Erythromycin

Erythromycin is used to treat several conditions, such as diphtheria, Legionnaire's disease, pneumonia, pertussis (whooping cough), conjunctivitis, and others. Erythromycin is a good "backup" medication for certain conditions normally treated with penicillin for those individuals who either cannot tolerate penicillin or who are allergic to it. For example, erythromycin is used to treat syphilis in persons who are allergic to penicillin.

Erythromycin has one important characteristic that makes it predisposed to drug interactions; it can inhibit the ability of your liver to inactivate certain other drugs. So before taking erythromycin, it's a good idea to make sure medications that you are currently taking do not interact with erythromycin.

Various forms of erythromycin are available. Trade names include E.E.S.®, E-Mycin®, E-Base®, ERYC®, Ery-Tab®, Erythrocin®, Ery-Ped®, Ilosone®, Ilotycin®, Pediamycin®, Pediazole®, Robimycin®, Wyamycin® S, and others. Recently, some new erythromycin-like agents have been released. Clarithromycin (Biaxin®), like erythromycin, may reduce drug metabolism in the liver, while azithromycin (Zithromax®) does not appear to do so.

# Tetracyclines

Tetracyclines are a class of broad-spectrum antibiotics prescribed for acne, bacterial infections of the mouth, Rocky Mountain spotted fever (and other conditions caused by bacteria that are carried by ticks), respiratory system infections, gonorrhea, and other infections.

The "family" of tetracyclines includes demeclocycline (Declomycin®), doxycycline (Doryx®, Doxy®, Vibramycin®, Vibra-Tabs®), methacycline (Rondomycin®), minocycline (Minocin®), oxytetracycline (Terramycin®), tetracycline (Achromycin®, Panmycin®, Robitet®, Sumycin®), and others.

One important caveat about taking tetracycline is to avoid dairy products within two hours of any dose of tetracycline. Combining dairy products with tetracycline may greatly reduce the amount of drug that is absorbed into the blood; as result, the infection-fighting ability of this antibiotic may be substantially diminished. Other nutrients—calcium, magnesium, aluminum, and iron—can also reduce the absorption of tetracycline. As a result, do not take multivitamin supplements together with tetracycline (separate the doses as far as possible). Laxatives may also contain aluminum or magnesium. When taking tetracycline, either avoid aluminum- or magnesium-containing laxatives or take them two hours before or after taking tetracycline. Talk to your doctor or pharmacist about these interactions.

All antibiotics, regardless of class, should be taken for the full time prescribed by your doctor—even if symptoms are no longer present—to ensure that the infection does not recur (an exception to this rule is if side effects occur, in which case you should contact your doctor).

Amantadine
(**Symmetrel**®)

Anticholinergic drugs:

- atropine
- belladonna
- benztropine (**Cogentin**®)
- biperiden (**Akineton**®)
- clidinium (**Quarzan**®) dicyclomine (**Bentyl**®) ethopropazine (**Parsidol**®)
- glycopyrrolate (**Robinul**®)
- hexocyclium (**Tral**®)
- isopropamide (**Darbid**®)
- methantheline (**Banthine**®)
- methscopolamine (**Pamine**®)
- orphenadrine (**Disipal**®)
- oxyphencyclimine (**Daricon**®)
- propantheline (**Pro-Banthine**®)
- trihexyphenidyl (**Artane**®)

[used for gastrointestinal diseases, Parkinson's disease, and other disorders]

If you are taking large doses of anticholinergic drugs, concurrent use of amantadine may increase the risk of unwanted symptoms such as confusion and hallucinations. The degree to which other anticholinergic drugs can produce a similar effect with amantadine is not known, but the possibility should be considered.

Aminoglycosides:
- amikacin (**Amikin**®)
- gentamicin (**Garamycin**®)
- kanamycin (**Kantrex**®)
- netilmicin (**Netromycin**®)
- tobramycin (**Nebcin**®)

Amphotericin B
(**Fungizone**®)

[used to treat certain fungal infections]

The risk of kidney damage may be increased if gentamicin and amphotericin B are taken concurrently. This may also occur when amphotericin B is combined with other aminoglycosides (see list at left).

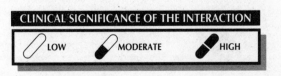

**CLINICAL SIGNIFICANCE OF THE INTERACTION**

LOW   MODERATE   HIGH

| ANTI-INFECTION DRUG | INTERACTING DRUG | RESULT |
|---|---|---|

Aminoglycosides:

- amikacin (**Amikin**®)
- gentamicin (**Garamycin**®)
- kanamycin (**Kantrex**®)
- netilmicin (**Netromycin**®)
- tobramycin (**Nebcin**®)

Bumetanide (**Bumex**®)

[used to reduce high blood pressure and fluid accumulation]

Damage to hearing (ototoxicity) may result when aminoglycosides are used with potent diuretics such as bumetanide.

---

Aminoglycosides:

- amikacin (**Amikin**®)
- gentamicin (**Garamycin**®)
- kanamycin (**Kantrex**®)
- netilmicin (**Netromycin**®)
- tobramycin (**Nebcin**®)

Cisplatin (**Platinol**®)

[used in the management of ovarian, testicular, and bladder cancer]

Preliminary evidence suggests that the risk of kidney damage may be increased.

Your doctor may want to monitor your kidney function more closely if you are on this combination.

---

Aminoglycosides:

- amikacin (**Amikin**®)
- gentamicin

Cyclosporine (**Sandimmune**®)

[for immune suppression, which is needed after organ transplantation to prevent rejection of the transplanted organ]

The risk of kidney damage may be increased.

Your doctor may want to monitor your kidney function more closely if you are on this combination.

| ANTI-INFECTION DRUG | INTERACTING DRUG | RESULT |
|---|---|---|

*(cont.)*
Aminoglycosides:

**(Garamycin®)**
- kanamycin **(Kantrex®)**
- netilmicin **(Netromycin®)**
- tobramycin **(Nebcin®)**

Cyclosporine

---

Aminoglycosides (oral):

- kanamycin **(Kantrex®)**
- neomycin **(Mycifradin®)**
- paromomycin **(Humatin®)**

Digoxin **(Lanoxin®)**

[for heart failure and heart abnormalities, such as atrial fibrillation and atrial flutter]

Neomycin (and probably other oral aminoglycosides) may inhibit the absorption of oral digoxin, thus reducing digoxin effect.

**Recommendation:** Since separating the doses of the digoxin from the aminoglycoside may not prevent this interaction, your doctor may need to monitor your blood digoxin level to make sure it is high enough.

---

Aminoglycosides:

- amikacin **(Amikin®)**
- gentamicin **(Garamycin®)**
- kanamycin **(Kantrex®)**
- netilmicin **(Netromycin®)**
- tobramycin **(Nebcin®)**

Ethacrynic acid **(Edecrin®)**

[used to reduce high blood pressure and fluid accumulation]

Aminoglycosides alone can cause hearing loss, and the concurrent use of ethacrynic acid markedly increases the risk (especially if the person has poor kidney function).

**Recommendation:** Combined use of aminoglycosides and ethacrynic acid should generally be avoided. If the combination is used, it should be done only with extreme caution and with careful monitoring for hearing loss.

Furosemide (Lasix®), another diuretic (i.e., medication used to reduce high blood pressure and fluid accumulation), appears to be less likely to interact with aminoglycosides than ethacrynic acid.

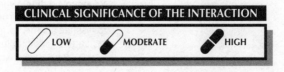

CLINICAL SIGNIFICANCE OF THE INTERACTION

LOW    MODERATE    HIGH

| | | |
|---|---|---|
| Aminoglycosides:<br><br>• amikacin (**Amikin**®)<br>• gentamicin (**Garamycin**®)<br>• kanamycin (**Kantrex**®)<br>• netilmicin (**Netromycin**®)<br>• tobramycin (**Nebcin**®) | Penicillins (antipseudomonal)<br><br>• azlocillin (**Azlin**®)<br>• carbenicillin (**Geopen**®, **Geocillin**®)<br>• mezlocillin (**Mezlin**®)<br>• piperacillin (**Pipracil**®)<br>• ticarcillin (**Ticar**®)<br><br>[used to treat various bacterial infections] | These penicillins may inactivate aminoglycosides in patients with severe kidney disease, but in many people the combination does not interact. |

| | | |
|---|---|---|
| Aminoglycosides (oral):<br><br>• kanamycin (**Kantrex**®)<br>• neomycin (**Mycifradin**®)<br>• paromomycin (**Humatin**®) | Penicillin V (**Ledercillin VK**®, **Pen-Vee K**®, **V-Cillin K**®, **Veetids**®, and others)<br><br>[used to treat various bacterial infections] | Neomycin (and probably other oral aminoglycosides) may inhibit the absorption of penicillin V, thus reducing the effect of the penicillin. It is possible that other oral penicillins may also be affected in this way.<br><br>**Recommendation:** Since separating the doses of the drugs may not prevent this interaction, your doctor may decide to use a larger than normal dose or oral penicillin if you are receiving an oral aminoglycoside. |

| | | |
|---|---|---|
| Amoxicillin (**Amoxil**®, **Larotid**®, and others)<br><br> | Estrogen-containing oral contraceptives such as **Brevicon**®, **Demulen**®, **Enovid**®, **Lo/Ovral**®, **Norinyl**®, **Ortho Novum**®, **Ovcon**®, **Ovral**®, **Tri-Norinyl**®, **Triphasil**®, and many others<br><br>[for prevention of pregnancy] | Although aminopenicillins (such as amoxicillin) may increase the risk of pregnancy in women taking oral contraceptives, this result is probably rare. Menstrual irregularities, such as spotting or breakthrough bleeding, may be a sign that this interaction is occurring. Other types of penicillins and other oral antibiotics in general may produce similar effects.<br><br>**Recommendation:** Women wishing to avoid pregnancy would be prudent to institute another form of contraception—in addition to use of their oral contraceptive—while taking |

50

| ANTI-INFECTION DRUG | INTERACTING DRUG | RESULT |
|---|---|---|

*(cont.)*
**Amoxicillin**

Estrogen-containing oral contraceptives

amoxicillin or other penicillins in this class (i.e., aminopenicillins).

---

**Amphotericin B (Fungizone®)**

Corticosteroids:

- cortisone (**Cortone®**)
- hydrocortisone (**Cortef®, Hydrocortone®, Solu-Cortef®**)
- methylprednisolone (**Medrol®, Depo-Medrol®, Solu-Medrol®**)
- prednisolone (**Delta-Cortef®, Hydeltrasol®, Pediapred®, Prelone®**)
- prednisone (**Deltasone®, Liquid-Pred®, Meticorten®**)

[for relieving inflammation and suppressing allergic reactions]

Decreased amount of potassium in the body, which may lead to muscle problems (such as weakness, twitching, and pain), nocturia (need to urinate at night), and abnormal sensations, such as feelings of numbness, tingling, or burning.

Corticosteroids can produce potassium depletion if they are given by injection or orally (especially with large doses), but other routes of administration (e.g., inhalation or topical application on the skin or in the eye, ear, etc.) generally have little effect on potassium.

Cortisone and hydrocortisone are more likely than other corticosteroids to lead to these effects.

---

**Amphotericin B (Fungizone®)**

Cyclosporine (**Sandimmune®**)

[for immune suppression, which is needed after organ transplantation to prevent rejection of the transplanted organ]

May increase the risk of kidney damage.

Your doctor may want to monitor your kidney function more closely if you are on this combination.

---

**Amphotericin B (Fungizone®)**

Digitoxin (**Crystodigin®**)

[for heart failure and other heart abnormalities]

The potassium loss resulting from amphotericin B may increase the risk of digitoxin toxicity. Symptoms of digitoxin toxicity include nausea, vomiting, poor appetite, weakness, lethargy, visual abnormalities, and irregular heartbeat.

---

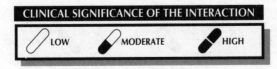

**CLINICAL SIGNIFICANCE OF THE INTERACTION**

LOW    MODERATE    HIGH

| ANTI-INFECTION DRUG | INTERACTING DRUG | RESULT |
|---|---|---|
| Amphotericin B (**Fungizone**®)  | Digoxin (**Lanoxin**®) [for heart failure and other heart abnormalities] | The potassium loss resulting from amphotericin B may increase the risk of digoxin toxicity. Symptoms of digoxin toxicity include nausea, vomiting, poor appetite, weakness, lethargy, visual abnormalities, and irregular heartbeat. |
| Ampicillin (**Amcill**®, **Omnipen**®, **Polycillin**®, **Principen**®, **Unasyn**®)  | Allopurinol (**Zyloprim**®, **Lopurin**®) [for treatment of gout] | Persons receiving allopurinol may be more likely to develop an ampicillin rash. |
| Ampicillin (**Amcil**®, **Omnipen**®, **Polycillin**®, **Principen**®, **Unasyn**®) | Atenolol (**Tenormin**®) [used for the treatment of high blood pressure] | Ampicillin may reduce the effect of the atenolol, particularly when ampicillin is used in high doses. **Recommendation:** Your doctor may want to check your blood pressure if he or she starts, stops, or changes the dosage of ampicillin. |

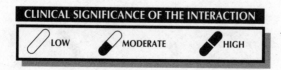

CLINICAL SIGNIFICANCE OF THE INTERACTION

LOW     MODERATE     HIGH

| ANTI-INFECTION DRUG | INTERACTING DRUG | RESULT |
|---|---|---|

Ampicillin **(Amcil®, Omnipen®, Polycillin®, Principen®, Unasyn®)**

Estrogen-containing oral contraceptives such as **Brevicon®, Demulen®, Enovid®, Lo/Ovral®, Norinyl®, Ortho Novum®, Ovcon®, Ovral®, Tri-Norinyl®, Triphasil®**, and many others

[for prevention of pregnancy]

Although aminopenicillins (such as ampicillin) may increase the risk of pregnancy in women taking oral contraceptives, this result is probably rare. Menstrual irregularities, such as spotting or breakthrough bleeding, may be a sign that this interaction is occurring. Other types of penicillins and other oral antibiotics in general may produce similar effects.

**Recommendation:** Women wishing to avoid pregnancy would be prudent to institute another form of contraception—in addition to use of their oral contraceptive—while taking ampicillin or other penicillins in this class (i.e., aminopenicillins).

---

Bacampicillin **(Spectrobid®)**

Estrogen-containing oral contraceptives such as **Brevicon®, Demulen®, Enovid®, Lo/Ovral®, Norinyl®, Ortho Novum®, Ovcon®, Ovral®, Tri-Norinyl®, Triphasil®**, and many others

[for prevention of pregnancy]

Although aminopenicillins (such as bacampicillin) may increase the risk of pregnancy in women taking oral contraceptives, this result is probably rare. Menstrual irregularities, such as spotting or breakthrough bleeding, may be a sign that this interaction is occurring. Other types of penicillins and other oral antibiotics in general may produce similar effects.

**Recommendation:** Women wishing to avoid pregnancy would be prudent to institute another form of contraception—in addition to use of their oral contraceptive—while taking ampicillin or other penicillins in this class (i.e., aminopenicillins).

---

Cefamandole **(Mandol®)**

Alcohol

Persons taking cefamandole may develop symptoms such as flushing, nausea, headache, and rapid heart rate if they drink alcoholic beverages.

**Recommendation:** Avoid alcohol while you are taking cefamandole.

| ANTI-INFECTION DRUG | INTERACTING DRUG | RESULT |
|---|---|---|

Cefoperazone
**(Cefobid®)**

Alcohol

Persons taking cefoperazone may develop symptoms such as flushing, nausea, headache, and rapid heart rate if they drink alcoholic beverages.

**Recommendation:** Avoid alcohol while you are taking cefoperazone.

---

Cefotetan
**(Cefotan®)**

Alcohol

Persons taking cefotetan may develop symptoms such as flushing, nausea, headache, and rapid heart rate if they drink alcoholic beverages.

**Recommendation:** Avoid alcohol while you are taking cefotetan.

---

Cefpodoxime proxetil

Antacids

[for acid indigestion or heartburn]

Aluminum hydroxide and sodium bicarbonate (and probably other antacids) may reduce the absorption of cefpodoxime proxetil, which may decrease its ability to fight infection. This effect seems to be due to a reduction in stomach acid, so it is likely that the effect occurs with antacids in general.

**Recommendation:** Do not take cefpodoxime proxetil and antacids simultaneously. Avoid taking antacids four hours before and two hours after cefpodoxime proxetil.

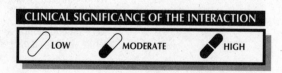

CLINICAL SIGNIFICANCE OF THE INTERACTION

LOW        MODERATE        HIGH

| ANTI-INFECTION DRUG | INTERACTING DRUG | RESULT |
|---|---|---|
| Cefpodoxime proxetil | Ranitidine (**Zantac**®)<br><br>[for relief of stomach and intestinal ulcers] | Ranitidine reduces the absorption of cefpodoxime proxetil. Other antiulcer drugs—cimetidine (Tagamet®), famotidine (Pepcid®), and nizatidine (Axid®)—probably have the same effect.<br><br>The effect of these antiulcer drugs on other cephalosporins (the class of antibiotic to which cefpodoxime proxetil belongs) is not known. |
| Ceftazidime (**Fortaz**®) | Chloramphenicol (**Chloromycetin**®)<br><br>[for treatment of various bacterial infections] | Some evidence suggests that chloramphenicol inhibits the antibiotic effect of ceftazidime. It is possible that other cephalosporin antibiotics would be similarly affected by chloramphenicol, but little information is available. |
| Cefuroxime axetil (**Ceftin**®) | Antacids<br><br>[for acid indigestion or heartburn] | Aluminum hydroxide and sodium bicarbonate (and probably other antacids) may reduce the absorption of cefuroxime axetil (Ceftin®), which may decrease its ability to fight infection. This effect seems to be due to reduction in stomach acid, so it is likely that the effect occurs with antacids in general.<br><br>**Recommendation:** Do not take cefuroxime axetil and antacids simultaneously. Avoid taking antacids four hours before and two hours after cefuroxime axetil. |
| Cefuroxime axetil (**Ceftin**®) | Ranitidine (**Zantac**®)<br><br>[for relief of stomach and intestinal ulcers] | Ranitidine reduces the absorption of cefuroxime. Other antiulcer drugs—cimetidine (Tagamet®), famotidine (Pepcid®), and nizatidine (Axid®)—probably have the same effect.<br><br>The effect of these antiulcer drugs on other cephalosporins (the class of antibiotic to which cefuroxime belongs) is not known.<br><br>**Recommendation:** Separation of the doses may not prevent this interaction, so be on the lookout for signs that the antibiotic is not working. |

Chloramphenicol **(Chloromycetin®)**

Barbiturates:

- amobarbital **(Amytal®)**
- butabarbital **(Butisol®)**
- butalbital
- pentobarbital **(Nembutal®)**
- phenobarbital **(Luminal®, Solfoton®)**
- primidone **(Mysoline®)**
- secobarbital **(Seconal®)**,
  and others

[used to treat insomnia and anxiety; certain barbiturates are used to prevent seizures]

May elevate the amount of barbiturate in the blood, increasing the risk of adverse effects (such as enhanced sedation).

In addition, barbiturates may reduce the amount of chloramphenicol in the blood, possibly decreasing the bacteria-fighting ability of chloramphenicol.

---

Chloramphenicol **(Chloromycetin®)**

Chlorpropamide **(Diabinese®)**

[for treatment of diabetes mellitus, a condition that results in excessively high amounts of sugar in the blood and urine]

Chloramphenicol enhances the effect of chlorpropamide, resulting in excessively low blood sugar levels. Symptoms of an excessive drop in blood sugar levels include increased heart rate, cold sweats, trembling, nausea, hunger, mental confusion, and, in severe cases, coma.

Your doctor may need to reduce the dose of chlorpropamide when you are taking chloramphenicol simultaneously.

**Recommendation:** Diabetics should be especially careful when checking their blood sugar levels if they are taking both chloramphenicol and chlorpropamide.

---

Chloramphenicol **(Chloromycetin®)**

Cyclophosphamide **(Cytoxan®)**

[used to treat a variety of cancers, such as cancer of the ovary, testicles, breast, and lung]

Chloramphenicol may slow the ability of the liver to metabolize cyclophosphamide, but the importance of this effect is not established.

**Recommendation:** Your doctor may wish to carefully monitor the effect of cyclophosphamide if chloramphenicol is started or stopped.

| ANTI-INFECTION DRUG | INTERACTING DRUG | RESULT |
|---|---|---|
| Chloramphenicol **(Chloromycetin®)**  | Iron [needed for normal development of red blood cells and other biological functions] | Chloramphenicol may inhibit the ability of iron to correct iron-deficiency anemia. |
| Chloramphenicol **(Chloromycetin®)** | Rifampin **(Rifadin®, Rimactane®)** [used in combination with at least one other drug, rifampin is used to treat tuberculosis; also used in the treatment of individuals who are carriers of meningitis] | Rifampin can reduce the amount of chloramphenicol in the blood, possibly reducing the bacteria-fighting ability of chloramphenicol. |
| Chloramphenicol **(Chloromycetin®)** | Tolbutamide **(Orinase®)** [for treatment of diabetes mellitus, a condition that results in excessively high amounts of sugar in the blood and urine] | Chloramphenicol enhances the effect of tolbutamide, possibly resulting in excessively low blood sugar levels. Symptoms of low blood sugar levels include increased heart rate, cold sweats, trembling, nausea, hunger, mental confusion, and, in severe cases, coma. Your doctor may need to reduce the dose of tolbutamide when you are taking chloramphenicol simultaneously. **Recommendation:** Diabetics should be especially careful when checking their blood sugar levels if they are taking both chloramphenicol and tolbutamide. |
| Chloramphenicol **(Chloromycetin®)**  | Vitamin $B_{12}$ [used to treat pernicious anemia; vitamin $B_{12}$ is needed for several functions, such as healthy blood and nerves] | Patients with pernicious anemia may not respond adequately to vitamin $B_{12}$ if they are also receiving chloramphenicol. |

| ANTI-INFECTION DRUG | INTERACTING DRUG | RESULT |
|---|---|---|

**Chloroquine (Aralen®)**

**Cimetidine (Tagamet®)**
[for relief of stomach and intestinal ulcers]

Cimetidine may increase blood chloroquine concentrations, which may increase the risk of chloroquine toxicity. Symptoms of chloroquine toxicity can include blurred vision, lightheadedness, fainting, hearing loss, and muscle weakness. If any of these occur, see your doctor.

**Recommendation:** Your doctor may wish to substitute famotidine (Pepcid®), rantidine (Zantac®), or nizatidine (Axid®) in place of cimetidine, since they may be less likely to interact with chloroquine.

---

**Ciprofloxacin (Cipro®)**

Antacids (containing aluminum or magnesium)
[for acid indigestion or heartburn]

Antacids containing aluminum or magnesium (e.g., Gaviscon®, Maalox®, Mylanta®) bind with ciprofloxacin and may markedly reduce its absorption, possibly leading to decreased antibiotic effect. Calcium antacids (e.g., Tums®) also bind with ciprofloxacin, but not as tightly so they do not reduce the antibiotic effect as much as aluminum or magnesium antacids.

**Recommendation:** Do not take ciprofloxacin and antacids simultaneously. Ciprofloxacin should be taken at least two hours before or six hours after antacids.

---

**Ciprofloxacin (Cipro®)**

Caffeine (found in caffeinated coffee, tea, certain carbonated beverages, and in other beverages, foods, and certain medications)

Ciprofloxacin can substantially increase the amount of caffeine in the blood. Symptoms of elevated blood caffeine levels include fast heartbeat, shaking, or tremors.

**Recommendation:** It is probably a good idea to reduce your consumption of coffee and other sources of caffeine while taking ciprofloxacin. A related antibiotic, ofloxacin (Floxin®), does not appear to increase the amount of caffeine in the blood.

**CLINICAL SIGNIFICANCE OF THE INTERACTION**

LOW    MODERATE    HIGH

Ciprofloxacin
(**Cipro**®)

Cyclosporine
(**Sandimmune**®)

[for immune suppression, which is needed after organ transplantation to prevent rejection of the transplanted organ]

Although evidence is limited, some reports indicate that ciprofloxacin may increase the amount of cyclosporine in the blood, possibly increasing the risk of kidney damage.

**Recommendation:** Ofloxacin (Floxin®), an antibiotic in the same class as ciprofloxacin, does not appear to affect blood levels of cyclosporine and may be a good alternative antibiotic if problems develop with ciprofloxacin.

Ciprofloxacin
(**Cipro**®)

Iron

[a mineral necessary for normal development of red blood cells and other biological functions]

Iron preparations may substantially reduce the absorption of ciprofloxacin. As a result, the effect of ciprofloxacin may be markedly reduced.

**Recommendation:** Do not take ciprofloxacin and iron preparations (such as iron-containing vitamin supplements) simultaneously. Ciprofloxacin should be taken at least two hours before or six hours after taking iron to minimize the occurrence of this interaction.

Ciprofloxacin
(**Cipro**®)

Sucralfate (**Carafate**®)

[used to treat duodenal ulcers]

When taken together, sucralfate may markedly reduce the absorption of ciprofloxacin. As a result, this antibiotic may not work as effectively when taken with sucralfate.

**Recommendation:** Do not take ciprofloxacin and sucralfate simultaneously. Ciprofloxacin should be taken at least two hours before or at least six hours after taking sucralfate.

| | | |
|---|---|---|
| Ciprofloxacin **(Cipro®)**  | Theophylline **(Primatene® Tablets, Slo-bid®, Theo-Dur®, Theo-24®, Uniphyl®,** and others) [for relief of asthma and bronchospasm] | Increased amount of theophylline in the blood, possibly leading to theophylline toxicity; signs of such toxicity include nausea, vomiting, diarrhea, headache, irritability, nervousness, rapid heartbeat, insomnia, and tremor. In serious cases, seizure can occur. **Recommendation:** Ofloxacin (Floxin®) is unlikely to affect theophylline; your doctor may wish to use this drug in place of ciprofloxacin. If ciprofloxacin is used, your doctor may need to adjust the dose of your theophylline when ciprofloxacin is started or stopped. |
| Ciprofloxacin **(Cipro®)**  | Zinc [a nutrient necessary for normal growth and development] | Zinc (found in many multivitamin supplements) may cause a modest reduction in the amount of ciprofloxacin in the blood, possibly reducing the effectiveness of the antibiotic. **Recommendation:** Do not take ciprofloxacin and zinc simultaneously. Ciprofloxacin should be taken at least two hours before or six hours after taking zinc to minimize the occurrence of this interaction. |
| Cyclacillin **(Cyclapen-W®)**  | Estrogen-containing oral contraceptives such as **Brevicon®, Demulen®, Enovid®, Lo/Ovral®, Norinyl®, Ortho Novum®, Ovcon®, Ovral®, Tri-Norinyl®, Triphasil®,** and many others [for prevention of pregnancy] | Although aminopenicillins (such as cyclacillin) may increase the risk of pregnancy in women taking oral contraceptives, this result is probably rare. Menstrual irregularities, such as spotting or breakthrough bleeding, may be a sign that this interaction is occurring. Other types of penicillins and other oral antibiotics in general may produce similar effects. **Recommendation:** Women wishing to avoid pregnancy would be prudent to institute another form of contraception—in addition to use of their oral contraceptive—while taking cyclacillin or other penicillins in this class (i.e., aminopenicillins). |

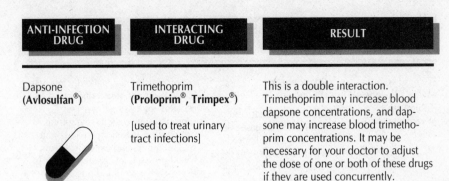

**Dapsone (Avlosulfan®)**

Trimethoprim **(Proloprim®, Trimpex®)**

[used to treat urinary tract infections]

This is a double interaction. Trimethoprim may increase blood dapsone concentrations, and dapsone may increase blood trimethoprim concentrations. It may be necessary for your doctor to adjust the dose of one or both of these drugs if they are used concurrently.

---

Doxycycline **(Vibramycin®)**

Calcium (found in milk, dairy products, calcium supplements, calcium-containing multivitamins)

[a mineral needed for the heart, muscles, and nerves to function properly; also needed for strong bones and teeth]

Calcium supplements, calcium-fortified vitamins, and foods containing calcium may reduce the absorption of doxycycline, thereby diminishing the effect of doxycycline.

Foods with moderate to high amounts of calcium include milk, yogurt, cheese, sardines, salmon, soybeans, tofu, broccoli, turnip greens, and other foods.

**Recommendation:** Do not take doxycycline and calcium products simultaneously. Take doxycycline at least two hours before or at least four hours after eating dairy products or calcium-containing vitamins.

---

Doxycycline **(Vibramycin®)**

Carbamazepine **(Tegretol®)**

[for epilepsy, trigeminal neuralgia (spasms of pain in the face), and other disorders]

Carbamazepine reduces blood concentrations of doxycycline, and may inhibit its antibiotic effect.

**Recommendation:** Your doctor may wish to use an antibiotic other than doxycycline. If the combination is used, be alert to reduced antibiotic effect.

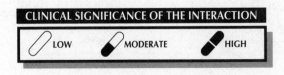

CLINICAL SIGNIFICANCE OF THE INTERACTION

LOW    MODERATE    HIGH

| ANTI-INFECTION DRUG | INTERACTING DRUG | RESULT |
|---|---|---|

Erythromycin (**E-Mycin®, Ilosone®, Robimycin®, Wyamycin® S,** and others)

Bromocriptine (**Parlodel®**)

[used in the treatment of Parkinson's disease; also used to stop milk production in mothers who do not wish to breast-feed]

Erythromycin may markedly increase blood bromocriptine concentrations, possibly increasing the risk of bromocriptine toxicity. Symptoms of bromocriptine toxicity include nausea, vomiting, and excessively low blood pressure levels (symptoms of excessively low blood pressure include lightheadedness and fainting).

---

Erythromycin (**E-Mycin®, Ilosone®, Robimycin®, Wyamycin® S,** and others)

Cyclosporine (**Sandimmune®**)

[for immune suppression, which is needed after organ transplantation to prevent rejection of the transplanted organ]

Erythromycin markedly increases the amount of cyclosporine in the blood, and may increase the risk of cyclosporine-induced kidney damage.

**Recommendation:** Erythromycin should be avoided if possible in persons taking cyclosporine. If the combination is given, your doctor will probably want to monitor your cyclosporine blood concentrations carefully during and after treatment with erythromycin.

---

Erythromycin (**E-Mycin®, Ilosone®, Robimycin®, Wyamycin® S,** and others)

Digoxin (**Lanoxin®**)

[for heart failure and heart abnormalities, such as atrial fibrillation and atrial flutter]

In about 10 percent of the population, erythromycin may increase blood digoxin concentrations, possibly increasing the risk of digoxin toxicity. Symptoms of digoxin toxicity include nausea, vomiting, poor appetite, weakness, lethargy, visual abnormalities, and irregular heartbeat.

It is possible that some other antibiotics (e.g., tetracyclines) may produce a similar effect.

---

Erythromycin (**E-Mycin®, Ilosone®, Robimycin®, Wyamycin® S,** and others)

Lovastatin (**Mevacor®**)

[used to lower blood cholesterol levels]

Erythromycin may increase the risk of lovastatin-induced muscle damage.

**Recommendation:** If possible, erythromycin should be avoided in persons taking lovastatin. If the combination is used, you should promptly report any muscle pain or muscle weakness to your doctor.

| ANTI-INFECTION DRUG | INTERACTING DRUG | RESULT |
|---|---|---|

Erythromycin **(E-Mycin®, Erythrocin®, Ilosone®, Robimycin®, Wyamycin® S,** and others)

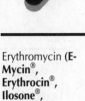

Terfenadine **(Seldane®)**

[nonsedating antihistamine, used to treat hay fever and other allergic disorders]

May lead to higher levels of terfenadine, which could result in terfenadine toxicity. Symptoms may include lightheadedness, fainting, and palpitations; serious disturbances of heart rhythms have also occurred. Clarithromycin **(Biaxin®)** may also cause terfenadine toxicity.

**Recommendation:** Do not take erythromycin and terfenadine concurrently.

---

Erythromycin **(E-Mycin®, Erythrocin®, Ilosone®, Robimycin®, Wyamycin® S,** and others)

Theophylline **(Primatene® Tablets, Slo-bid®, Theo-Dur®, Theo-24®, Uniphyl®,** and others)

[for relief of asthma and bronchospasm]

Erythromycin may increase the amount of theophylline in the blood. Although most people do not seem to have much trouble with this interaction, some develop theophylline toxicity. Symptoms of theophylline toxicity include nausea, vomiting, diarrhea, headache, irritability, nervousness, rapid heartbeat, insomnia, and tremor. In serious cases, seizure can occur. Clarithromycin **(Biaxin®)** may also increase theophylline blood levels.

The effect is usually delayed so that theophylline concentrations start to rise after five to seven days of treatment with erythromycin.

Furthermore, theophylline may cause reduced blood levels of erythromycin, possibly leading to diminished effect of erythromycin.

**Recommendation:** Some doctors prefer to avoid giving erythromycin to people taking theophylline, while others advise their patients to watch for symptoms of theophylline toxicity. Those who advise the latter should probably monitor theophylline blood levels.

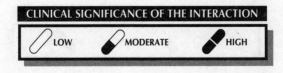

CLINICAL SIGNIFICANCE OF THE INTERACTION

LOW    MODERATE    HIGH

| ANTI-INFECTION DRUG | INTERACTING DRUG | RESULT |
|---|---|---|

Erythromycin (**E-Mycin**®, **Erythrocin**®, **Ilosone**®, **Robimycin**®, **Wyamycin**® **S,** and others)

Triazolam (**Halcion**®)

[used in the treatment of insomnia, or difficulty falling or staying asleep]

Can lead to a substantial increase in the concentration of triazolam in the blood, possibly increasing its sedative effect, which could lead to drowsiness, impaired ability to concentrate, and forgetfulness.

**Recommendation:** Your doctor may need to reduce your dose of triazolam when erythromycin is taken concurrently. (Of course, *never* alter the dosage of any medication without your doctor's consent and supervision.)

---

Fluconazole (**Diflucan**®)

Cyclosporine (**Sandimmune**®)

[for immune suppression, which is needed after organ transplantation to prevent rejection of the transplanted organ]

Fluconazole (especially in doses of 200 milligrams a day or more) may substantially increase blood concentrations of cyclosporine, which increases the risk of cyclosporine toxicity. Increased blood levels of cyclosporine have been associated with kidney damage.

**Recommendation:** Your doctor may need to monitor carefully the amount of cyclosporine in your blood if fluconazole is taken concurrently.

---

Furazolidone (**Furoxone**®)

Alcohol

A limited amount of evidence suggests that persons taking furazolidone may develop symptoms such as flushing, nausea, and sweating if they drink alcoholic beverages.

**Recommendation:** It would be best to avoid alcohol while you are taking furazolidone; if you do drink, be alert for the symptoms described above.

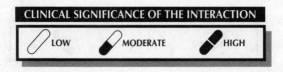

CLINICAL SIGNIFICANCE OF THE INTERACTION

LOW    MODERATE    HIGH

| ANTI-INFECTION DRUG | INTERACTING DRUG | RESULT |
|---|---|---|

Furazolidone
(**Furoxone**®)

Amphetamines:

- benzphetamine
  (**Didrex**®)
- dextroamphetamine
  (**Dexedrine**®)
- fenfluramine
  (**Pondimin**®)
- mazindol (**Sanorex**®)
- methylphenidate
  (**Ritalin**®)
- pemoline (**Cylert**®)
- phenmetrazine
  (**Preludin**®)
  and others

[various amphetamines
have different uses, such
as the management of
abnormal and uncontrol-
lable sleeping during the
day; another use is to
help suppress appetite;
methylphenidate is used
to treat attention-deficit
disorders]

Taking amphetamines may result in
an acute increase in blood pressure
in people taking furazolidone.

**Recommendation:** People taking furazolidone should avoid taking amphetamines.

Griseofulvin
(**Fulvicin**® P/G,
**Grisactin**®, and
**Gris-PEG**®)

Estrogen-containing oral
contraceptives such as
**Brevicon**®, **Demulen**®,
**Enovid**®, **Lo/Ovral**®,
**Norinyl**®, **Ortho
Novum**®, **Ovcon**®,
**Ovral**®, **Tri-Norinyl**®,
**Triphasil**®, and many
others

[for prevention of
pregnancy]

Some evidence suggests that griseofulvin may decrease the effectiveness
of the oral contraceptive, resulting in
unintended pregnancy or menstrual
irregularities (such as spotting, breakthrough bleeding, or absence or abnormal stopping of the menses).

**Recommendation:** Women taking
griseofulvin who wish to avoid becoming pregnant should check with
their doctor. Another method of contraception instead of or in addition to
an oral contraceptive may be necessary. Or, your doctor may need to
adjust the dose of the oral contraceptive in order to overcome the effect
of the griseofulvin. Of course, only
your doctor should make such a
dosage adjustment.

| ANTI-INFECTION DRUG | INTERACTING DRUG | RESULT |
|---|---|---|
| Griseofulvin (**Fulvicin® P/G, Grisactin®**, and **Gris-PEG®**) | Phenobarbital (**Luminal®, Solfoton®**)<br><br>[used to prevent seizures] | Phenobarbital may reduce blood concentrations of griseofulvin, but it is not known how much this reduction inhibits the antifungal effect of griseofulvin. Not much is known about the effect of other barbiturates (e.g., amobarbital, pentobarbital, secobarbital) on griseofulvin, but they might have the same effect.<br><br>**Recommendation:** Your doctor may decide to use larger doses of griseofulvin if you are taking phenobarbital. (Do *not* change the dosage of either drug yourself; only your doctor should do this.) |
| Hydroxychloroquine (**Plaquenil®**) | Digoxin (**Lanoxin®**)<br><br>[for heart failure and heart abnormalities, such as atrial fibrillation and atrial flutter] | Hydroxychloroquine may increase blood digoxin levels, possibly increasing the risk of digoxin toxicity. Symptoms of digoxin toxicity include nausea, vomiting, poor appetite, weakness, lethargy, visual abnormalities, and irregular heartbeat. |
| Isoniazid (**INH®**) | Alcohol | Alcoholics appear to have a higher incidence of isoniazid-induced liver damage than nonalcoholics.<br><br>**Recommendation:** Persons taking isoniazid should try to avoid drinking large amounts of alcohol. |
| Isoniazid (**INH®**) | Antacids<br><br>[for acid indigestion or heartburn] | Antacids may reduce the absorption of isoniazid, possibly inhibiting the effect of isoniazid (i.e., diminished tuberculosis-fighting ability of isoniazid).<br><br>**Recommendation:** Take isoniazid two hours before or four hours after taking the antacid to minimize this interaction. |

## CLINICAL SIGNIFICANCE OF THE INTERACTION

LOW    MODERATE    HIGH

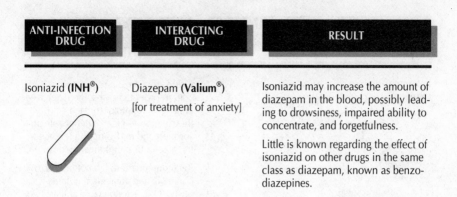

| ANTI-INFECTION DRUG | INTERACTING DRUG | RESULT |
|---|---|---|
| Isoniazid **(INH®)**  | Diazepam **(Valium®)** [for treatment of anxiety] | Isoniazid may increase the amount of diazepam in the blood, possibly leading to drowsiness, impaired ability to concentrate, and forgetfulness. Little is known regarding the effect of isoniazid on other drugs in the same class as diazepam, known as benzodiazepines. |
| Isoniazid **(INH®)**  | Disulfiram **(Antabuse®)** [used to help alcoholics abstain from drinking alcohol] | Persons receiving isoniazid and disulfiram have developed behavioral changes and coordination difficulties |
| Isoniazid **(INH®)** | Theophylline **(Primatene® Tablets, Slo-bid®, Theo-Dur®, Theo-24®, Uniphyl®,** and others) [for relief of asthma and bronchospasm] | May cause an increase in the amount of theophylline in the blood, possibly leading to theophylline toxicity; signs of such toxicity include nausea, vomiting, diarrhea, headache, irritability, nervousness, rapid heart beat, insomnia, tremor, and seizure. **Recommendation:** Your doctor may need to adjust your theophylline dose if isoniazid is started or stopped. |
| Isoniazid **(INH®)**  | Triazolam **(Halcion®)** [used in the treatment of insomnia, or difficulty falling or staying asleep] | Isoniazid may increase the amount of triazolam in the blood, possibly leading to drowsiness, impaired ability to concentrate, and forgetfulness. Little is known regarding the effect of isoniazid on other drugs in the same class as triazolam, known as benzodiazepines. |

Ketoconazole **(Nizoral®)** ·

Antacids

[for acid indigestion or heartburn]

Oral ketoconazole requires stomach acid in order to be absorbed; because antacids neutralize stomach acid, they tend to reduce ketoconazole absorption and may diminish the effectiveness of this antifungal medication.

**Recommendation:** Do not take ketoconazole and antacids simultaneously. Take ketoconazole at least two hours before or four hours after taking antacids.

---

Ketoconazole **(Nizoral®)**

Chlordiazepoxide **(Librium®)**

[used to treat anxiety]

Ketoconazole may increase the amount of chlordiazepoxide in the blood, possibly enhancing the sedative effect of chlordiazepoxide. This enhanced effect could lead to decreased alertness, an impaired ability to concentrate, forgetfulness, and drowsiness.

---

Ketoconazole **(Nizoral®)**

Cimetidine **(Tagamet®)**

[for relief of stomach and intestinal ulcers]

Stomach acid is needed for the proper absorption (and thus effectiveness) of oral ketoconazole. Since cimetidine reduces the secretion of stomach acid, cimetidine tends to reduce the absorption of ketoconazole.

**Recommendation:** Your doctor may need to adjust the dosing times of these drugs so that the ketoconazole is given when the effect of cimetidine is low. Alternatively, the manufacturer of ketoconazole describes a method of dissolving the ketoconazole in a very mild acid before administration. Your doctor or pharmacist may help you with this.

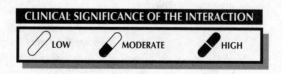

CLINICAL SIGNIFICANCE OF THE INTERACTION

LOW    MODERATE    HIGH

Ketoconazole
(**Nizoral**®)

Cyclosporine
(**Sandimmune**®)

[for immune suppression, which is needed after organ transplantation to prevent rejection of the transplanted organ]

Ketoconazole may markedly increase the amount of cyclosporine in the blood, possibly increasing the risk of cyclosporine-induced kidney damage.

**Recommendation:** Your doctor may need to adjust your cyclosporine dosage if you start or stop taking ketoconazole.

---

Ketoconazole
(**Nizoral**®)

Famotidine (**Pepcid**®)

[for relief of stomach and intestinal ulcers]

Stomach acid is needed for the proper absorption (and thus effectiveness) of oral ketoconazole. Since famotidine reduces the secretion of stomach acid, famotidine is likely to reduce the absorption of ketoconazole.

**Recommendation:** Your doctor may need to adjust the dosing times of these drugs so that the ketoconazole is given when the effect of famotidine is low. Alternatively, the manufacturer of ketoconazole describes a method of dissolving the ketoconazole in a very mild acid before administration. Your doctor or pharmacist may help you with this.

---

Ketoconazole
(**Nizoral**®)

Methylprednisolone
(**Medrol**®)

[for relieving inflammation and suppressing allergic reactions]

Ketoconazole may increase the amount of methylprednisolone in the blood, possibly leading to methylprednisolone toxicity. Symptoms of methylprednisolone toxicity include increased blood pressure, increased blood sugar, thinning of the bones (osteoporosis), muscle weakness, insomnia, stomach ulcers, and infection.

Methylprednisolone is a corticosteroid. The effect of ketoconazole on other corticosteroids is not well established. One other corticosteroid, in particular, prednisolone, may not be affected by ketoconazole.

| ANTI-INFECTION DRUG | INTERACTING DRUG | RESULT |
|---|---|---|
| Ketoconazole (**Nizoral**®) | Nizatidine (**Axid**®) [for relief of stomach and intestinal ulcers] | Stomach acid is needed for the proper absorption (and thus effectiveness) of oral ketoconazole. Since nizatidine reduces the secretion of stomach acid, nizatidine is likely to reduce the absorption of ketoconazole. **Recommendation:** Your doctor may need to adjust the dosing times of these drugs so that the ketoconazole is given when the effect of nizatidine is low. Alternatively, the manufacturer of ketoconazole describes a method of dissolving the ketoconazole in a very mild acid before administration. Your doctor or pharmacist may help you with this. |
| Ketoconazole (**Nizoral**®) | Omeprazole (**Prilosec**®) [for relief of stomach and intestinal ulcers] | Stomach acid is needed for the proper absorption (and thus effectiveness) of oral ketoconazole. Since omeprazole reduces the secretion of stomach acid, omeprazole is likely to reduce the absorption of ketoconazole. **Recommendation:** The manufacturer of ketoconazole describes a method of dissolving the ketoconazole in a very mild acid before administration. Your doctor or pharmacist may help you with this. |
| Ketoconazole (**Nizoral**®) | Ranitidine (**Zantac**®) [for relief of stomach and intestinal ulcers] | Stomach acid is needed for the proper absorption (and thus effectiveness) of oral ketoconazole. Since ranitidine reduces the secretion of stomach acid, ranitidine is likely to reduce the absorption of ketoconazole. **Recommendation:** Your doctor may need to adjust the dosing times of these drugs so that the ketoconazole is given when the effect of ranitidine is low. Alternatively, the manufacturer of ketoconazole describes a method of dissolving the ketoconazole in a very mild acid before administration. Your doctor or pharmacist may help you with this. |

Ketoconazole **(Nizoral®)**

Rifampin **(Rifadin®, Rimactane®)**

[used in combination with at least one other drug, rifampin is used to treat tuberculosis; also used in the treatment of individuals who are carriers of meningitis]

A complicated interaction that tends to lower the amount of both drugs—ketoconazole and rifampin—in the blood. As a result, the effect of both drugs may be diminished.

**Recommendation:** Separation of the doses of ketoconazole from the rifampin by twelve hours appears to prevent the lowering of rifampin blood levels, but it is not clear that this will prevent the lowering of ketoconazole levels. Your doctor will need to monitor your response and make any needed adjustments in your doses or dosing times.

Ketoconazole **(Nizoral®)**

Terfenadine **(Seldane®)**

[nonsedating antihistamine, used to treat hay fever and other allergic disorders]

May lead to higher levels of terfenadine, which could result in terfenadine toxicity. Symptoms of terfenadine toxicity may include lightheadedness, fainting, and palpitations; serious disturbances of heart rhythms have also occurred.

**Recommendation:** Do not take ketoconazole and terfenadine together. Other related antifungal drugs such as fluconazole (Diflucan®) and itraconazole (Sporanox®) should also be avoided if you are taking terfenadine (until we have evidence that they are safe).

Lincomycin **(Lincocin®)**

Kaolin-Pectin **(Donnagel-PG®)**

[used to relieve diarrhea]

Kaolin-pectin mixtures markedly inhibit the absorption of lincomycin.

**Recommendation:** Take kaolin-pectin two hours before or four hours after the lincomycin. Note: This recommendation is different from most recommendations for interactions of this type; usually, the binding agent (i.e., antacid or kaolin-pectin) should be taken four hours before or two hours after the affected drug.

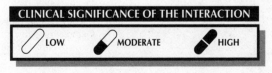

CLINICAL SIGNIFICANCE OF THE INTERACTION

LOW    MODERATE    HIGH

| ANTI-INFECTION DRUG | INTERACTING DRUG | RESULT |
|---|---|---|
| Methenamine hippurate (**Hiprex®, Urex®**) 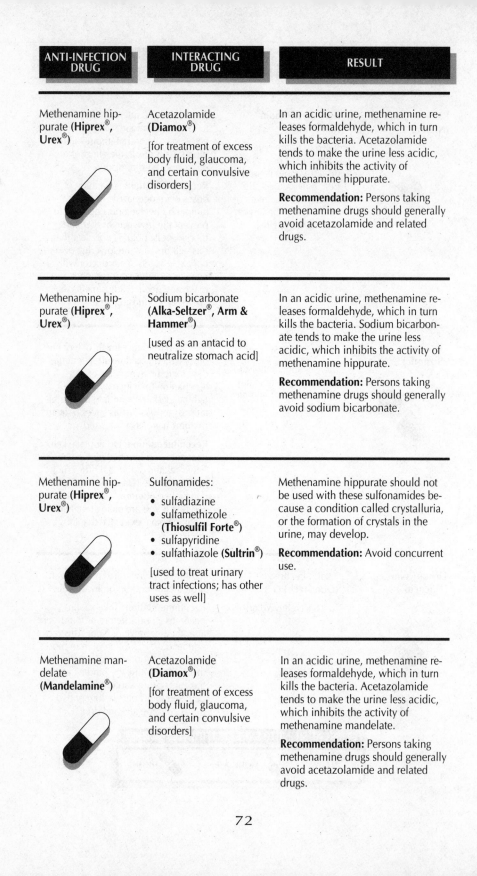 | Acetazolamide (**Diamox®**) [for treatment of excess body fluid, glaucoma, and certain convulsive disorders] | In an acidic urine, methenamine releases formaldehyde, which in turn kills the bacteria. Acetazolamide tends to make the urine less acidic, which inhibits the activity of methenamine hippurate. **Recommendation:** Persons taking methenamine drugs should generally avoid acetazolamide and related drugs. |
| Methenamine hippurate (**Hiprex®, Urex®**) | Sodium bicarbonate (**Alka-Seltzer®, Arm & Hammer®**) [used as an antacid to neutralize stomach acid] | In an acidic urine, methenamine releases formaldehyde, which in turn kills the bacteria. Sodium bicarbonate tends to make the urine less acidic, which inhibits the activity of methenamine hippurate. **Recommendation:** Persons taking methenamine drugs should generally avoid sodium bicarbonate. |
| Methenamine hippurate (**Hiprex®, Urex®**) | Sulfonamides: • sulfadiazine • sulfamethizole (**Thiosulfil Forte®**) • sulfapyridine • sulfathiazole (**Sultrin®**) [used to treat urinary tract infections; has other uses as well] | Methenamine hippurate should not be used with these sulfonamides because a condition called crystalluria, or the formation of crystals in the urine, may develop. **Recommendation:** Avoid concurrent use. |
| Methenamine mandelate (**Mandelamine®**) | Acetazolamide (**Diamox®**) [for treatment of excess body fluid, glaucoma, and certain convulsive disorders] | In an acidic urine, methenamine releases formaldehyde, which in turn kills the bacteria. Acetazolamide tends to make the urine less acidic, which inhibits the activity of methenamine mandelate. **Recommendation:** Persons taking methenamine drugs should generally avoid acetazolamide and related drugs. |

| ANTI-INFECTION DRUG | INTERACTING DRUG | RESULT |
| --- | --- | --- |
| Methenamine mandelate (**Mandelamine**®) | Sodium bicarbonate (**Alka-Seltzer**®, **Arm & Hammer**®)<br><br>[used as an antacid to neutralize stomach acid] | In an acidic urine, methenamine releases formaldehyde, which in turn kills the bacteria. Sodium bicarbonate tends to make the urine less acidic, which inhibits the activity of methenamine mandelate.<br><br>**Recommendation:** Persons taking methenamine drugs should generally avoid sodium bicarbonate. |
| Methenamine mandelate (**Mandelamine**®) | Sulfonamides:<br>• sulfadiazine<br>• sulfamethizole (**Thiosulfil Forte**®)<br>• sulfapyridine<br>• sulfathiazole (**Sultrin**®)<br><br>[used to treat urinary tract infections; has other uses as well] | Methenamine mandelate should not be used with these sulfonamides because a condition called crystalluria, or the formation of crystals in the urine, may develop.<br><br>**Recommendation:** Avoid concurrent use. |
| Metronidazole (**Flagyl**®, **Metric 21**®, **Protostat**®) | Alcohol | Some people taking metronidazole develop a reaction with symptoms such as flushing, nausea, vomiting, and headache.<br><br>**Recommendation:** Although the reaction does not occur in everyone, it would be best to avoid alcohol while you are taking metronidazole. |
| Metronidazole (**Flagyl**®, **Metric 21**®, **Protostat**®) | Cimetidine (**Tagamet**®)<br><br>[for relief of stomach and intestinal ulcers] | Especially when the metronidazole is given orally or intravenously, this combination could lead to increased serum levels of metronidazole, which could cause dizziness, vertigo (a sensation in which you feel as if you are revolving in space or your surroundings are revolving around you), nausea, numbness, and tingling. |

## CLINICAL SIGNIFICANCE OF THE INTERACTION

LOW    MODERATE    HIGH

| ANTI-INFECTION DRUG | INTERACTING DRUG | RESULT |
|---|---|---|
| Metronidazole (**Flagyl®, Metric 21®, Protostat®**) | Disulfiram (**Antabuse®**) [used to help alcoholics abstain from drinking alcohol] | Some people taking this combination have developed confusion and psychotic episodes. **Recommendation:** Although this interaction is not well documented, it would be best to avoid taking this combination of drugs. |
| Metronidazole (**Flagyl®, Metric 21®, Protostat®**) | Trimethoprim and sulfamethoxazole (**Bactrim®, Septra®**) [used to treat various bacterial infections] | The intravenous form of trimethoprim and sulfamethoxazole contains 10 percent alcohol, which can cause a reaction in people taking metronidazole. The usual symptoms include flushing, nausea, vomiting, and headache. **Recommendation:** If possible, persons taking metronidazole should take oral—rather than intravenous—trimethoprim and sulfamethoxazole. |
| Minocycline (**Minocin®**) | Calcium (found in milk, dairy products, calcium supplements, calcium-containing multivitamins) [a mineral needed for the heart, muscles, and nerves to function properly; also needed for strong bones and teeth] | Calcium supplements, calcium-fortified vitamins, and foods containing calcium may reduce the absorption of minocycline, thereby diminishing its effect. Foods with moderate to high amounts of calcium include milk, yogurt, cheese, sardines, salmon, soybeans, tofu, broccoli, turnip greens, and other foods. **Recommendation:** Do not take minocycline and calcium products simultaneously. Take minocycline at least two hours before or at least four hours after eating dairy products or calcium-containing vitamins. |
| Moxalactam (**Moxam®**) | Alcohol | Persons taking moxalactam may develop symptoms such as flushing, nausea, headache, and rapid heart rate if they drink alcoholic beverages. **Recommendation:** Avoid alcohol while you are taking moxalactam. |

Norfloxacin
**(Noroxin®)**

Antacids **(Maalox®, Mylanta®**, and others)

[for relief of acid indigestion and heartburn]

Antacids containing aluminum or magnesium (e.g., Maalox®, Mylanta®) bind with norfloxacin and may markedly reduce its absorption, possibly leading to decreased antibiotic effect. Calcium antacids (e.g., Tums®) also bind with norfloxacin, but not as tightly so they do not reduce the antibiotic effect as much as aluminum or magnesium antacids.

**Recommendation:** Do not take norfloxacin and antacids simultaneously. Norfloxacin should be taken at least two hours before or six hours after antacids.

---

Norfloxacin
**(Noroxin®)**

Caffeine (found in caffeinated coffee, tea, certain carbonated beverages, and in other beverages, foods, and some medications)

Norfloxacin may increase slightly the amount of caffeine in the blood. Symptoms of elevated blood caffeine levels include fast heartbeat, shaking, or tremors. These symptoms, however, most likely will not occur because norfloxacin increases blood caffeine levels only slightly (as opposed to a related antibiotic, ciprofloxacin, which raises blood caffeine levels substantially).

**Recommendation:** You may wish to reduce your consumption of coffee and other sources of caffeine while taking norfloxacin. A related antibiotic, ofloxacin (Floxin®), does not appear to increase the amount of caffeine in the blood.

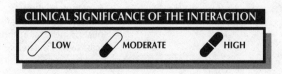

CLINICAL SIGNIFICANCE OF THE INTERACTION

LOW    MODERATE    HIGH

| | | |
| --- | --- | --- |
| Norfloxacin **(Noroxin®)**  | Cyclosporine **(Sandimmune®)** [for immune suppression, which is needed after organ transplantation to prevent rejection of the transplanted organ] | Although evidence is limited, some reports indicate that norfloxacin may increase the amount of cyclosporine in the blood, possibly increasing the risk of kidney damage. **Recommendation:** Ofloxacin (Floxin®), an antibiotic in the same class as norfloxacin, does not appear to affect blood levels of cyclosporine and may be a good alternative antibiotic if problems develop with norfloxacin. |
| Norfloxacin **(Noroxin®)**  | Iron (found in many multivitamin/mineral supplements) [a mineral needed for normal development of red blood cells and other biological functions] | Iron preparations may substantially reduce the absorption of norfloxacin. As a result, the effect of norfloxacin may be markedly reduced. **Recommendation**: Do not take norfloxacin and iron preparations (such as iron-containing vitamin supplements) simultaneously. Norfloxacin should be taken at least two hours before or six hours after taking iron to minimize the occurrence of this interaction. |
| Norfloxacin **(Noroxin®)**  | Sucralfate **(Carafate®)** [used to treat duodenal ulcers] | When taken together, sucralfate is highly likely to markedly reduce the absorption and effectiveness of norfloxacin. **Recommendation**: Do not take norfloxacin and sucralfate simultaneously. Norfloxacin should be taken at least two hours before or at least six hours after taking sucralfate. |

| ANTI-INFECTION DRUG | INTERACTING DRUG | RESULT |
|---|---|---|

Norfloxacin **(Noroxin®)**

Zinc (found in many multivitamin mineral supplements)

[a mineral essential for various metabolic reactions in the body, including the normal production of genetic material]

Zinc may cause a modest reduction in the amount of norfloxacin in the blood, possibly reducing the effectiveness of the antibiotic.

**Recommendation:** Do not take norfloxacin and zinc simultaneously. Norfloxacin should be taken at least two hours before or six hours after taking zinc to minimize the occurrence of this interaction.

---

Ofloxacin **(Floxin®)**

Antacids **(Maalox®, Mylanta®, and others)**

[for relief of acid indigestion and heartburn]

Antacids containing aluminum or magnesium (e.g., Maalox®, Mylanta®) bind with ofloxacin and may markedly reduce its absorption, possibly leading to decreased antibiotic effect.

**Recommendation:** Do not take ofloxacin and antacids simultaneously. Ofloxacin should be taken at least two hours before or six hours after taking antacids.

---

Ofloxacin **(Floxin®)**

Iron (found in many multivitamin/mineral supplements)

[a mineral needed for normal development of red blood cells and other biological functions]

Iron preparations may substantially reduce the absorption of ofloxacin. As a result, the effect of ofloxacin may be markedly reduced.

**Recommendation:** Ofloxacin should be taken at least two hours before or six hours after taking iron preparations (such as iron-containing vitamin supplements) to minimize the occurrence of this interaction.

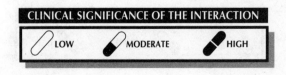

CLINICAL SIGNIFICANCE OF THE INTERACTION

LOW     MODERATE     HIGH

| ANTI-INFECTION DRUG | INTERACTING DRUG | RESULT |
| --- | --- | --- |

Ofloxacin **(Floxin®)**

Zinc (found in many multivitamin/mineral supplements)

[a mineral essential for various metabolic reactions in the body, including the normal production of genetic material]

Zinc may cause a modest reduction in the amount of ofloxacin in the blood, possibly reducing the effectiveness of the antibiotic.

**Recommendation:** Do not take ofloxacin and zinc simultaneously. Ofloxacin should be taken at least two hours before or six hours after taking zinc to minimize the occurrence of this interaction.

Penicillins

Methotrexate **(Mexate®)**

[for treatment of certain cancers, such as breast, lung, and certain forms of leukemia; also used for treatment of psoriasis and rheumatoid arthritis]

Carbenicillin and perhaps other penicillins taken in large amounts (intravenously) may increase the amount of methotrexate in the blood, possibly to toxic levels. Symptoms of methotrexate toxicity include fever, sores in the mouth and on the skin, bleeding, vomiting, diarrhea, and severe reduction in the number of white blood cells produced by the bone marrow.

It's important to note that the risk of toxicity from this interaction is much greater when methotrexate is given in high doses, such as for the treatment of cancer. Low-dose methotrexate therapy—which is used to treat arthritis and psoriasis—poses a smaller risk of inducing methotrexate toxicity. However, caution is still warranted.

**Recommendation:** Your doctor may need to adjust your methotrexate dose if these penicillins are used.

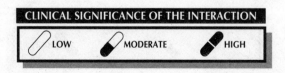

CLINICAL SIGNIFICANCE OF THE INTERACTION

LOW     MODERATE     HIGH

Penicillins

Probenecid **(Benemid®, Proban®)**

[for reduction of uric acid levels in the body to prevent gout and gouty arthritis; also used to increase the effectiveness of certain antibiotics]

Probenecid was designed to inhibit the elimination of penicillins by the kidneys; as a result of this action, the amount of penicillin in the blood will increase. This is usually a favorable interaction and is often used intentionally.

---

Penicillins

Tetracyclines:

- doxycycline **(Doryx®, Vibramycin®, Vibra-Tabs®)**
- methacycline **(Rondomycin®)**
- minocycline **(Minocin®)**
- oxytetracycline **(Terramycin®)**
- tetracycline **(Achromycin®, Panmycin®, Robitet®, Sumycin®)**

[used to treat various bacterial infections]

For certain infections, tetracyclines may inhibit the antibiotic effect of penicillins, but experts disagree on the importance of this effect.

**Recommendation:** It is not common to require both a pencillin and a tetracycline to treat an infection. If you do need both, ask your doctor if there is any problem with inhibition of the penicillin effect.

---

Penicillin V **(Ledercillin VI®, Pen-Vee K®, V-Cillin K®, Veetids®)**

Estrogen-containing oral contraceptives such as **Brevicon®, Demulen®, Enovid®, Lo/Ovral®, Norinyl®, Ortho Novum®, Ovcon®, Ovral®, Tri-Norinyl®, Triphasil®**, and many others

[for prevention of pregnancy]

Although penicillin V may increase the risk of pregnancy in women taking oral contraceptives, this result is probably rare. Menstrual irregularities, such as spotting or breakthrough bleeding, may be a sign that his interaction is occurring. Other types of penicillins and other oral antibiotics in general may produce similar effects.

**Recommendation:** Women wishing to avoid pregnancy would be prudent to use another form of contraception—in addition to use of their oral contraceptive—while taking penicillin V or other penicillins.

| ANTI-INFECTION DRUG | INTERACTING DRUG | RESULT |
|---|---|---|

Pyrimethamine **(Daraprim®)**

Folic acid

[a vitamin essential for healthy development]

Folic acid may inhibit the effect of pyrimethamine when pyrimethamine is used to treat toxoplasmosis infections, and may worsen leukemia when it is used to treat infections associated with leukemia.

---

Rifampin **(Rifadin®, Rimactane®)**

Clorazepate **(Tranxene®)**

[for treatment of anxiety]

Rifampin may decrease the effect of clorazepate (i.e., inadequately control anxiety).

---

Rifampin **(Rifadin®, Rimactane®)**

Corticosteroids:

• betamethasone **(Celestone®, Diprolene®, Diprosone®, Valisone®)**
• cortisone **(Cortone®)**
• dexamethasone **(Decadron®, Hexadrol®)**
• hydrocortisone **(Cortef®, Hydrocortone®, Solu-Cortef®)**
• methylprednisolone **(Medrol®, Depo-Medrol®, Solu-Medrol®)**
• prednisolone **®, Delta-Cortef®, Hydeltrasol®)**
• prednisone **(Deltasone®, Liquid Pred®, Prednicen-M®)** and others

[for relieving inflammation and suppressing allergic reaction]

Rifampin may substantially reduce the effectiveness of corticosteroids in some persons.

**Recommendation:** Watch for inadequate control of the condition being treated by the corticosteroid (e.g., asthma, arthritis, etc.). Your doctor may need to use higher than normal doses of corticosteroids during rifampin therapy. (Do *not* change the dosage of either drug yourself; only your doctor should do this.)

| ANTI-INFECTION DRUG | INTERACTING DRUG | RESULT |
|---|---|---|
| Rifampin (**Rifadin®, Rimactane®**) | Cyclosporine (**Sandimmune®**) [for immune suppression, which is needed after organ transplantation to prevent rejection of the transplanted organ] | Rifampin may reduce the amount of cyclosporine in the blood, possibly leading to a reduced effect of cyclosporine. **Recommendation:** Your doctor may need to increase the amount of cyclosporine that you are receiving if you are taking rifampin concurrently. (Of course, *never* alter the dosage of cyclosporine or rifampin without your doctor's consent and supervision.) |
| Rifampin (**Rifadin®, Rimactane®**) | Diazepam (**Valium®**) [for treatment of anxiety] | Rifampin may lower the concentration of diazepam in the body, possibly leading to a decreased effect (i.e., inadequate control of anxiety). The same result may occur when using rifampin with similar drugs, such as clorazepate (Tranxene®), halazepam (Paxipam®), and prazepam (Centrax®). |
| Rifampin (**Rifadin®, Rimactane®**) | Digitoxin (**Crystodigin®**) [for heart failure and other heart abnormalities] | Rifampin may substantially reduce the amount of digitoxin in the blood, diminishing the effect of the digitoxin. |
| Rifampin (**Rifadin®, Rimactane®**) | Digoxin (**Lanoxin®**) [for heart failure and heart abnormalities, such as atrial fibrillation and atrial flutter] | Rifampin may reduce the amount of digoxin in the blood; in some persons, this reduction may be large enough to diminish the effect of the digoxin. |

CLINICAL SIGNIFICANCE OF THE INTERACTION

LOW    MODERATE    HIGH

| ANTI-INFECTION DRUG | INTERACTING DRUG | RESULT |
|---|---|---|

Rifampin (**Rifadin®, Rimactane®**)

Estrogen-containing oral contraceptives such as **Brevicon®, Demulen®, Enovid®, Lo/Ovral®, Norinyl®, Ortho Novum®, Ovcon®, Ovral®, Tri-Norinyl®, Triphasil®**, and many others

[for prevention of pregnancy]

Rifampin significantly increases the likelihood of becoming pregnant while taking an oral contraceptive. Menstrual irregularities—such as spotting, breakthrough bleeding, or absence or abnormal stopping of the menses—may occur while taking these two medications concomitantly.

**Recommendation:** You could use contraceptive methods other than oral contraceptives to avoid this interaction. If the combination is used, your doctor may need to increase the strength of your oral contraceptive. You may also wish to use an additional form of contraception while taking—and for one cycle after finishing—rifampin.

---

Rifampin (**Rifadin®, Rimactane®**)

Halazepam (**Paxipam®**)

[for treatment of anxiety]

Rifampin may decrease the effect of halazepam (i.e., inadequately control anxiety).

---

Rifampin (**Rifadin®, Rimactane®**)

Methadone (**Dolophine®**)

[used to treat severe pain; also used to treat narcotic addiction]

Rifampin may cause the concentration of methadone in the blood to drop, leading to a decreased effect of the methadone and sometimes to symptoms of methadone withdrawal.

---

Rifampin (**Rifadin®, Rimactane®**)

Prazepam (**Centrax®**)

[for treatment of anxiety]

Rifampin may decrease the effect of prazepam (i.e., inadequately control anxiety).

Rifampin **(Rifadin®, Rimactane®)**

Tolbutamide **(Orinase®)**

[for treatment of diabetes mellitus, a condition that results in excessively high amounts of sugar in the blood and urine]

Rifampin reduces the amount of tolbutamide in the body and may reduce the sugar-lowering effect of tolbutamide. The result may be an unexpected increase in the amount of sugar in the blood.

**Recommendation:** It may be necessary for your doctor to adjust the dose of tolbutamide if rifampin is started, stopped, or changed in dosage. (Of course, only your doctor should change medication dosages, when appropriate.)

---

Rifampin **(Rifadin®, Rimactane®)** .

Verapamil **(Calan®, Isoptin®, Verelan®)**

[for treatment of high blood pressure and angina]

This interaction may cause a large decrease in verapamil plasma levels, possibly leading to a decreased effect (i.e., inadequate control of hypertension or angina). This interaction occurs with oral verapamil, but is unlikely with intravenous verapamil.

**Recommendation:** It may be necessary for your doctor to adjust the dose of verapamil if rifampin is started, stopped, or changed in dosage. (Of course, only your doctor should change medication dosages, when appropriate.)

---

Rifampin **(Rifadin®, Rimactane®)**

Theophylline **(Primatene® Tablets, Slo-bid®, Theo-Dur®, Theo-24®, Uniphyl®,** and others)

[for relief of asthma]

Decreased amount of theophylline in the blood, possibly leading to a decreased effect (i.e., inadequate control of asthma).

**Recommendation:** Your doctor may need to adjust your theophylline dose if rifampin is started or stopped.

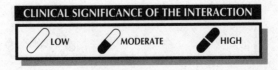

CLINICAL SIGNIFICANCE OF THE INTERACTION

LOW    MODERATE    HIGH

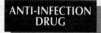

| ANTI-INFECTION DRUG | INTERACTING DRUG | RESULT |
|---|---|---|

Sulfasalazine (**Azulfidine®**)

Digoxin (**Lanoxin®**)

[for heart failure and heart abnormalities, such as atrial fibrillation and atrial flutter]

Sulfasalazine taken together with digoxin may decrease the absorption and effectiveness of digoxin.

**Recommendation:** Your doctor should monitor the amount of digoxin in your blood when adding sulfasalazine therapy.

---

Sulfonamides:

- sulfamethizole (**Thiosulfil®**)
- sulfamethoxazole (**Gantanol®**)
- sulfisoxazole (**Gantrisin®**)
- trimethoprim and sulfamethoxazole (**Bactrim®, Septra®**), and others

Antidiabetic drugs:

- acetohexamide (**Dymelor®**)
- chlorpropamide (**Diabinese®**)
- glipizide (**Glucotrol®**)
- glyburide (**DiaBeta®, Micronase®**)
- tolazamide (**Tolinase®**)
- tolbutamide (**Orinase®**), and others

[for treatment of diabetes mellitus, a condition that results in excessively high amounts of sugar in the blood and urine]

Some sulfonamides enhance the effect of oral antidiabetic drugs, which may lead to excessively low levels of blood sugar. Symptoms of excessively low blood sugar levels include increased heart rate, cold sweats, trembling, nausea, hunger, mental confusion, and, in severe cases, coma.

**Recommendation:** Diabetics should be particularly careful when checking their blood sugar levels if a sulfonamide medication is started or stopped, or if it undergoes a change in dosage.

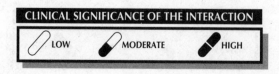

CLINICAL SIGNIFICANCE OF THE INTERACTION

LOW    MODERATE    HIGH

| | | |
|---|---|---|
| Tetracyclines:<br><br>• doxycycline **(Doryx®, Vibramycin®, Vibra-Tabs®)**<br>• methacycline **(Rondomycin®)**<br>• minocycline **(Minocin®)**<br>• oxytetracycline **(Terramycin®)**<br>• tetracycline **(Achromycin®, Panmycin®, Robitet®, Sumycin®)** | Antacids **(Maalox®, Mylanta®** and others)<br><br>[for acid indigestion or heartburn] | Antacids containing aluminum, magnesium, or calcium (e.g., Maalox®, Mylanta®, Tums®) substantially reduce the absorption of tetracycline, thereby diminishing its effect.<br><br>**Recommendation:** Take tetracyclines at least two hours before or at least four hours after taking antacids. |

| | | |
|---|---|---|
| Tetracyclines:<br><br>• doxycycline **(Doryx®, Vibramycin®, Vibra-Tabs®)** methacycline **(Rondomycin®)**<br>• minocycline **(Minocin®)**<br>• oxytetracycline **(Terramycin®)**<br>• tetracycline **(Achromycin®, Panmycin®, Robitet®, Sumycin®)** | Bismuth subsalicylate **(Pepto-Bismol®)**<br><br>[used to relieve indigestion and diarrhea] | Bismuth subsalicylate may markedly reduce the absorption of tetracyclines, possibly reducing their antibacterial effect.<br><br>**Recommendation:** Take tetracyclines at least two hours before or at least four hours after taking bismuth subsalicylate. |

Tetracyclines
(**Achromycin**®,
**Panmycin**®,
**Robitet**®, **Sumycin**®)

Calcium (found in milk, dairy products, calcium supplements, calcium-containing multivitamins)

[a mineral needed for the heart, muscles, and nerves to function properly; also needed for strong bones and teeth]

Calcium supplements, calcium-fortified vitamins, and foods containing calcium may substantially reduce the absorption of tetracycline, thereby diminishing its effect. The absorption of related compounds (i.e., doxycycline, minocycline) when taken with calcium is also reduced, but to a lesser extent than with tetracycline. Foods with moderate to high amounts of calcium include milk, yogurt, cheese, sardines, salmon, soybeans, tofu, broccoli, turnip greens, and other foods.

**Recommendation:** Do not take tetracycline and calcium products simultaneously. Take tetracyclines at least two hours before or at least four hours after eating dairy products or calcium-containing vitamins.

---

Tetracyclines:

- doxycycline (**Doryx**®, **Vibramycin**®, **Vibra-Tabs**®)
- methacycline (**Rondomycin**®)
- minocycline (**Minocin**®)
- oxytetracycline (**Terramycin**®)
- tetracycline (**Achromycin**®, **Panmycin**®, **Robitet**®, **Sumycin**®)

Estrogen-containing oral contraceptives such as **Brevicon**®, **Demulen**®, **Enovid**®, **Lo/Ovral**®, **Norinyl**®, **Ortho Novum**®, **Ovcon**®, **Ovral**®, **Tri-Norinyl**®, **Triphasil**®, and many others

[for prevention of pregnancy]

Tetracyclines may reduce the effectiveness of oral contraceptives, resulting in unintended pregnancy (probably rare) and menstrual irregularities (such as spotting, breakthrough bleeding, or absence or abnormal stopping of the menses).

**Recommendation:** While taking tetracyclines, additional forms of contraception are advised for women who are taking an oral contraceptive to prevent pregnancy.

**Note**: No oral antibiotic has been proven *not* to affect oral contraceptives, so precautions are warranted even if a different antibiotic is used.

| ANTI-INFECTION DRUG | INTERACTING DRUG | RESULT |
|---|---|---|

Tetracyclines:

- doxycycline (**Doryx®, Vibramycin®, Vibra-Tabs®**)
- methacycline (**Rondomycin®**)
- minocycline (**Minocin®**)
- oxytetracycline (**Terramycin®**)
- tetracycline (**Achromycin®, Panmycin®, Robitet®, Sumycin®**)

Iron (found in many multivitamin/mineral supplements)

[a mineral needed for normal development of red blood cells and other biological functions]

Iron reduces the absorption of tetracycline, possibly leading to its decreased effectiveness.

Iron is found in beef, lamb, poultry, liver, tuna, eggs, enriched grains, broccoli, peas, beans, and other foods.

**Recommendation:** Do not take tetracycline and iron (including iron-rich foods) simultaneously. Take tetracyclines at least two hours before or at least four hours after taking iron.

Tetracyclines (**Achromycin®, Panmycin®, Robitet®, Sumycin®**)

Magnesium (found in many multivitamin/mineral supplements)

[a mineral essential for the proper functioning of muscles, nerves, and various cellular reactions]

Magnesium reduces the absorption of tetracyclines, possibly leading to their decreased effectiveness.

Magnesium is found in oatmeal, whole grain cereals, broccoli, corn, peas, beets, milk, bananas, oranges, prunes, pineapples, and other foods.

**Recommendation:** Do not take tetracyclines and magnesium (including magnesium-rich foods) simultaneously. Take tetracyclines at least two hours before or at least four hours after taking magnesium.

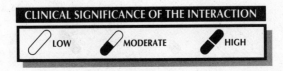

CLINICAL SIGNIFICANCE OF THE INTERACTION

LOW    MODERATE    HIGH

| ANTI-INFECTION DRUG | INTERACTING DRUG | RESULT |
|---|---|---|

Tetracyclines **(Achromycin®, Panmycin®, Robitet®, Sumycin®)**

Zinc (found in many multivitamin/mineral supplements)

[a mineral essential for various metabolic reactions in the body, including the normal production of genetic material]

Zinc reduces the absorption of tetracyclines, possibly leading to their decreased effectiveness.

Zinc is found in beef, lamb, poultry, wheat bran, enriched bread and crackers, eggs, and other foods.

**Recommendation:** Do not take tetracyclines and zinc (including zinc-rich foods) simultaneously. Take tetracyclines at least two hours before or at least four hours after taking zinc.

---

Trimethoprim and sulfamethoxazole **(Bactrim®, Septra®)**

Cyclosporine **(Sandimmune®)**

[for immune suppression, which is needed after organ transplantation to prevent rejection of the transplanted organ]

Trimethoprim and sulfamethoxazole may affect your response to cyclosporine.

**Recommendation:** Your doctor may need to monitor you even more closely if you are taking cyclosporine and trimethoprim and sulfamethoxazole is started or stopped.

---

Trimethoprim **(Proloprim®, Bactrim®** and **Septra®** contain trimethoprim combined with sulfamethoxazole)

Procainamide **(Procan SR®, Pronestyl®)**

[for treatment of irregular heartbeat and heart rhythm]

May lead to a substantial increase in the amount of procainamide in the body, possibly leading to toxicity. Signs of procainamide toxicity include nausea, vomiting, malaise, weakness, and lightheadedness.

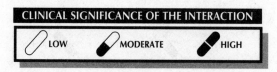

**CLINICAL SIGNIFICANCE OF THE INTERACTION**

LOW    MODERATE    HIGH

| ANTI-INFECTION DRUG | INTERACTING DRUG | RESULT |
|---|---|---|

Troleandomycin **(TAO®)**

Methylprednisolone **(Medrol®)**

[for relieving inflammation and suppressing allergic reactions]

Troleandomycin significantly enhances the effect of methylprednisolone, possibly leading to methylprednisolone toxicity. Symptoms of methylprednisolone toxicity include increased blood pressure, increased blood sugar, thinning of the bones (osteoporosis), muscle weakness, insomnia, stomach ulcers, and infection (symptoms of infection include sore throat and fever).

---

Troleandomycin **(TAO®)**

Terfenadine **(Seldane®)**

[nonsedating antihistamine, used to treat hay fever and other allergic disorders]

May lead to higher levels of terfenadine, which could result in terfenadine toxicity. Symptoms of terfenadine toxicity may include lightheadedness, fainting, and palpitations; serious disturbances of heart rhythms have also occurred.

**Recommendation:** Do not take troleandomycin and terfenadine concurrently.

---

Troleandomycin **(TAO®)**

Theophylline **(Primatene® Tablets, Slo-bid®, Theo-Dur®, Theo-24®, Uniphyl®, and others)**

[for relief of asthma and bronchospasm]

Increased amount of theophylline in the blood, possibly leading to theophylline toxicity. Symptoms of theophylline toxicity include nausea, vomiting, diarrhea, headache, irritability, nervousness, rapid heartbeat, insomnia, tremor, and seizure.

**Recommendation:** Your doctor may need to adjust your theophylline dose if troleandomycin is started or stopped.

---

Trolenadomycin **(TAO®)**

Triazolam **(Halcion®)**

[used in the treatment of insomnia, or difficulty falling or staying asleep]

Taking triazolam together with troleandomycin can result in a substantial increase in the concentration of triazolam in the body, leading to drowsiness, impaired ability to concentrate, and forgetfulness.

## CHAPTER 3

# DRUGS FOR ALLERGY, COLD, AND COUGH

Although allergy and the common cold are distinct conditions, both of them often produce similar symptoms: sneezing, runny nose, and congestion. For this reason, both conditions are discussed in this chapter. A cough may be caused by a variety of respiratory illnesses—such as asthma or bronchitis (see Chapter 4 for more details)—or by physical or chemical irritation to the airway. Postnasal drip, which often accompanies a cold and certain allergies, may lead to a cough as well.

## Allergy

Allergy is an overreaction of the body's immune system. Items that set off an allergic reaction are typically inhaled—such as pollen, molds, house dust, animal dander—or consumed, such as certain foods or medications. The first time you are exposed to the allergen (the substance that triggers an allergic reaction), your immune system calls into action your body's natural defense mechanisms. One of these mechanisms is the production of a group of proteins, called antibodies, whose purpose is to neutralize foreign substances (such as the allergen) in your body. The next time you come in contact with this allergen, a particular antibody—known an immunoglobulin E, or IgE for short—stimulates the release of several chemicals, one of which is histamine. These chemicals trigger several allergic responses, such as sneezing, runny nose, congestion, wheezing, and itchy skin.

Hay fever is one of the most commonly experienced nasal allergies. (The name "hay fever" is misleading because hay rarely brings on the allergic reaction, and fever is not associated with this allergy.) The allergen comes from pollens produced by certain weeds, trees, and grasses. Medical experts call hay fever by its more technical name: seasonal allergic rhinitis; it's seasonal in the sense that this allergy lasts for distinct seasons, which start when the number of pollen grains in the air begin to climb and end when the amount of pollen declines.

Perennial allergic rhinitis is a nasal allergy that is experienced year round. Common triggers are spores from molds (which are found in soil and on decaying organic matter), animal dander, and dust.

# Medications Used to Treat Allergy

The largest group of the drugs used to treat allergy is the *antihistamines,* which work by blocking the released histamine from reaching its destination—such as histamine receptors in the lining membrane of the nose—where it can cause a problem. A commonly used over-the-counter antihistamine is chlorpheniramine maleate (Chlor-Trimeton®). Several brand name chlorpheniramine-containing antihistamine/decongestant combination products are available, such as Allerest® Allergy Tablets, Comtrex® Multi-Symptom Cold Reliever, Contac® Continuous Action Nasal Decongestant/Antihistamine Capsules, Coricidin® Tablets, Dristan® Decongestant/Antihistamine/Analgesic Coated Tablets, Naldecon®, PediaCare® Cough-Cold Formula, Sinarest®, Sine-Off®, Sinutab®, Triaminicol® Multi-Symptom Cold Tablets, Tylenol® Cold Medication, Vicks Formula 44® Cough Medicine, and many others.

An antihistamine similar to chlorpheniramine maleate is brompheniramine maleate. Trade names include Dimetane®, Dimetapp®, Drixoral® Antihistamine/Nasal Decongestant Syrup, and others. Other antihistamines of different chemical classes include clemastine (Tavist®), diphenhydramine hydrochloride (Benadryl®, Benylin®, Caladryl® Cream and Lotion, and Dermarest®); doxylamine succinate (Contac® Nighttime Cold Medicine, Vicks Nyquil® Nighttime Colds Medicine); and triprolidine hydrochloride (Actidil®, Actifed®, AllerAct®).

Some commonly used prescription antihistamines and antihistamine/decongestant combination medications include Atrohist®, Bromfed®, Deconamine®, Extendryl®, Fedahist®, Ornade®, Rondec®, Ru-Tuss®, and Rynatan®.

One of the most common side effects of the antihistamines is drowsiness. The intensity of this side effect varies according to the *class* of antihistamine. Two antihistamines in particular—diphenhydramine hydrochloride and doxylamine succinate—are highly sedating. If you become very drowsy in response to an antihistamine, you may develop some tolerance to this side effect over time (i.e., after a while, the drug won't make you as tired). If tolerance does not develop, your doctor or pharmacist should be able to recommend another class of drug that is less sedating.

Certain prescription antihistamines have recently become available that rarely cause drowsiness. One is terfenadine (Seldane®); another is astemizole (Hismanal®).

A group of drugs used either for moderate to severe allergic reactions or when antihistamines are insufficient is a group of hormones known as adrenal corticosteroids. Corticosteroids taken orally for a long period of time have been associated with unwanted side effects, such as weight gain, puffiness in the face, insomnia, increased blood sugar, thinning of the bones, high blood pressure, cataracts, and others. Corticosteroid nasal sprays, however, are much less likely to cause these side effects. Because these nasal sprays are used topically, far less of the drug is absorbed into the bloodstream; as a result, the nasal sprays are much less likely to cause the same unwanted side effects that may appear with oral corticosteroids. Corticosteroid nasal sprays used to relieve symptoms of hay fever include beclomethasone (Beconase®, Vancenase®), flunisolide (Nasalide®), and triamcinolone (Nasacort®).

A nonhormonal nasal spray used to prevent and treat symptoms of hay fever is cromolyn sodium (Nasalcrom®). Although decongestants (oral and nasal) also reduce nasal swelling and congestion in allergic and nonallergic conditions, these medications are discussed later in this chapter because they are often used to relieve symptoms of the common cold.

## Symptomatic Relief of the Common Cold

Treatment of the common cold typically refers to *symptomatic* treatment. In other words, medications alleviate symptoms such as runny or stuffy nose, congestion, sneezing, and headache, but do not treat the underlying cause, which is viral. Generally, drugs have not been effective in destroying cold-producing viruses because these viruses use many of the body's normal processes to keep themselves alive. As a result, drugs that harm the virus also harm the person. However, one drug, interferon, a virus-fighting substance that occurs naturally in the body, has shown promise. Some evidence has indicated that a nasal spray form of interferon can reduce the spread of colds by approximately 40 percent.[1]

Drug therapy for the common cold is typically limited to use of analgesics (see Chapter 1) to relieve minor aches and pains and nasal decongestants. Dozens of nasal decongestants are available; many of them come combined with other medications, such as an analgesic, expectorant (which promotes the thinning and coughing up of mucus), an antitussive (which suppresses a cough), or an antihistamine. Although numerous cold products contain an antihistamine, little evidence supports the beneficial effect of the antihistamine ingredient; histamine is released during an allergic response, not during a cold caused by rhinoviruses, a major group of viruses that can cause a cold.[2]

When treating the symptoms of a cold, many physicians recommend taking a medication that is specific to your symptoms, rather than a "shot-gun approach," which combines several different types of medications in one product. In other words, if you suffer from stuffiness, take a decongestant; if your major problem is a headache, take a pain reliever. Always check with your doctor before taking any of these medications, especially if you suffer from kidney or liver disease.

# Decongestants

The three most common decongestant ingredients are phenylephrine, phenyl-propanolamine, and pseudoephedrine. Phenylephrine is found in nonprescription medications such as Congestpirin®, Dimetane® Decongestant, Dristan® Decongestant, 4-Way® Fast Acting Nasal Spray, Neo-Synephrine®, Pediacof® Cough Syrup, Phenergan® VC, Robitussin® Night Relief, and many others. Prescription products containing phenylephrine include Atrohist®, Extendryl®, Naldecon®, Ru-Tuss®, Rynatan®, and others.

Nonprescription phenylpropanolamine is found in Allerest®, Comtrex® Multi-Symptom Cold Reliever, Contac® Continuous Action Decongestant, Coricidin "D"®, Dexatrim®, Dimetapp®, Propagest®, Sinarest® Regular and Extra Strength, Triaminic®, and many others. Phenylpropanolamine is also used as an appetite suppressant (e.g., Acutrim®, Dexatrim®). Prescription medications containing phenylpropanolamine include Entex® LA, Naldecon®, Ornade®, Ru-Tuss®, Tavist-D®, and others.

Over-the-counter pseudoephedrine is found in products such as Actifed®, Benadryl® Decongestant, CoAdvil®, Contac® Nighttime Cold Medicine, Novahistine® DMX, Robitussin-DAC®, Sine-Aid®, Sine-Off®, Sinutab®, Sudafed®, Tylenol® Cold Medication, Vicks Formula 44D®, Vicks Nyquil®, and many others. Prescription pseudoephedrine is found in products such as Atrohist® L.A., Bromfed®, Deconamine®, Deconsal® L.A., Fedahist®, Guaifed®, and others.

One especially dangerous drug interaction occurs with all three deconges-tants—phenylephrine, phenylpropanolamine, and pseudoephedrine. These de-congestants can interact with monoamine oxidase inhibitors, a family of medications used to treat depression. This combination can lead to a sudden—and potentially harmful—rise in blood pressure.

Phenylephrine, phenylpropanolamine, and pseudoephedrine should also be used with caution in persons with high blood pressure because these deconges-tants may worsen this condition. These decongestants can cause blood vessels to narrow or prevent their dilation. Since many antihypertensive drugs lower blood pressure by relaxing or dilating blood vessels, these decongestants could interfere with the effectiveness of the antihypertensive medication (see Chapter 7 for more information).

Because so many allergy and cold medications (particularly nonprescription ones) contain the analgesic aspirin or acetaminophen to help relieve minor aches and pains associated with these conditions, we've included these analgesic inter-actions in this chapter. (For more information on these products and how they work, see Chapter 1.) It's important to note that these pain relievers may be useful if the cold is associated with a fever or aching muscles; however, analgesics do not relieve nasal congestion. On the contrary, a recent study indicated that aspirin and acetaminophen may aggrevate nasal swelling and stuffiness.[3] Therefore, if a stuffed nose is your worst symptom, a single-ingredient decongestant may be your best bet. Decongestants that contain only phenylephrine include Alconefrin®, Neo-Synephrine®, and Nostril®. Decongestants that contain only phenyl-propanolamine include Prolamine® and Propagest®. Decongestants that contain only pseudoephedrine include Novafed®, Sudafed®, and Afrinol®.

# Cough

Coughing serves a protective function: it removes secretions, irritants, or foreign objects from our air passages so that breathing is unobstructed. It's important to distinguish between a "productive" cough and an unproductive one: a productive cough helps to remove excess phlegm from the lungs and air passages, whereas an unproductive one does not. The dry, unproductive cough just irritates the respiratory tract (which can lead to further coughing) and often interrupts sleep, making you feel even worse.

Since the productive cough helps remove accumulated phlegm, you do not want to suppress it. Rather, one way to help the productive cough is to drink plenty of liquids. Water, in particular, is helpful in thinning excess mucus that collects in your respiratory tract.

A nonproductive cough, on the other hand, may be treated with an *antitussive* (cough suppressant). These include codeine, a narcotic drug, and dextromethor-phan, a nonnarcotic cough suppressant. If you wish to suppress only the cough (rather than buying a product with other ingredients, such as a decongestant), several nonprescription medications are available that contain only dextromethor-phan, such as Benylin® DM, Delsym®, and Sucrets® Cough Control Lozenges.

If, on the other hand, you wish to take a medication that not only suppresses the cough but also relieves cold or allergy symptoms, many combination-type products are available. Combination cough medications containing codeine include Novahistine® DH, Nucofed®, Phenergan® VC, Robitussin®-DAC, and others. Combination cough medications containing dextromethorphan include Cheracol D®, Dimacol®, Novahistine DMX®, PediaCare® Cough-Cold Formula, Phenergan®, Triaminicol® Multi-Symptom Relief, Vicks® Formula 44 Cough Medicine (as well as several other Vicks® products), and many others.

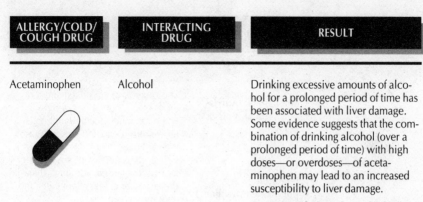

Acetaminophen

Alcohol

Drinking excessive amounts of alcohol for a prolonged period of time has been associated with liver damage. Some evidence suggests that the combination of drinking alcohol (over a prolonged period of time) with high doses—or overdoses—of acetaminophen may lead to an increased susceptibility to liver damage.

**Recommendation:** If you drink a lot of alcohol (i.e., several drinks a day), it would be good idea to avoid taking acetaminophen regularly unless advised to do so by your doctor.

Acetaminophen

Anticoagulants (oral), such as dicumarol and warfarin (**Coumadin®, Panwarfin®**)

[for the prevention of blood clots]

Acetaminophen usually does not cause problems in persons taking oral anticoagulants, but a few cases of increased anticoagulant effect have been reported.

**Recommendation:** Although acetaminophen is often recommended as a pain reliever in people taking oral anticoagulants and usually causes no problems, it would be prudent to take acetaminophen only when you really need it and make sure you do not exceed the recommended doses. Aspirin is much more likely to interact with oral anticoagulants than acetaminophen; thus, aspirin is not a good alternative.

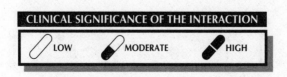

CLINICAL SIGNIFICANCE OF THE INTERACTION

LOW     MODERATE     HIGH

Acetaminophen

Barbiturates:

- amobarbital (**Amytal**®)
- butabarbital (**Butisol**®)
- butalbital
- pentobarbital (**Nembutal**®)
- phenobarbital (**Solfoton**®)
- primidone (**Mysoline**®)
- secobarbital (**Seconal**®)
and others

[used to treat insominia and anxiety; certain barbiturates are used to prevent seizures]

Persons who regularly take barbiturates may have a reduced effect of the acetaminophen. In addition, when too much acetaminophen is taken, this interaction may increase the likelihood of toxicity and the risk of liver damage. Symptoms of toxicity include nausea, vomiting, diarrhea, sweating, loss of appetite, and abdominal pain.

**Recommendation:** If you are taking barbiturates, be sure not to take more than the recommended amount of acetaminophen per day. It would also be wise to avoid taking acetaminophen for prolonged periods unless your doctor has advised you to do so.

---

Acetaminophen

Charcoal

[for relief of gas]

Large amounts of activated charcoal may reduce serum acetaminophen concentrations in the body by reducing the amount of acetaminophen that is absorbed into the blood.

**Recommendation:** If you are taking an activated charcoal preparation, take it at least two hours before or after taking acetaminophen.

---

Acetaminophen

Cholestyramine (**Questran**®)

[for treatment of high cholesterol levels]

Cholestyramine markedly reduces plasma concentrations of acetaminophen, thereby reducing the effect of the acetaminophen.

**Recommendation:** Take acetaminophen one hour before or several hours after taking cholestyramine.

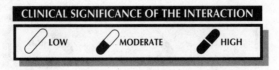

CLINICAL SIGNIFICANCE OF THE INTERACTION

LOW          MODERATE          HIGH

| | | |
|---|---|---|
| Aspirin | ACE inhibitors:<br><br>• benazepril **(Lotensin®)**<br>• captopril **(Capoten®)**<br>• enalapril **(Vasotec®)**<br>• fosinopril **(Monopril®)**<br>• lisinopril **(Prinivil®, Zestril®)**<br>• ramipril **(Altace®)**, and others<br><br>[for treatment of high blood pressure and congestive heart failure] | Repeated doses of aspirin decrease the antihypertensive effect of captopril (and probably other ACE inhibitors) in certain persons. Occasional doses of aspirin do not affect captopril.<br><br>**Recommendation:** If aspirin is used often, however, blood pressure should be checked frequently to ensure the aspirin is not interfering with the antihypertensive effect of the ACE inhibitor prescribed for you. |

| | | |
|---|---|---|
| Aspirin | Acetazolamide **(Diamox®)**<br><br>[for treatment of excess body fluid, glaucoma, and certain convulsive disorders] | Aspirin may increase the concentration of acetazolamide in the body, possibly leading to central nervous system toxicity. Symptoms of central nervous system toxicity include lethargy, confusion, sleepiness, anorexia (an abnormal and persistent loss of appetite), and ringing or a clicking sound in the ears. |

| | | |
|---|---|---|
| Aspirin | Alcohol | Alcohol may enhance two of the adverse side effects that are related to aspirin use: (1) damage to the lining of the stomach, particularly minor bleeding of the stomach lining; and (2) increased time for blood to clot.<br><br>**Recommendation:** Whenever possible, avoid aspirin use within eight to ten hours of moderate to heavy alcohol consumption. |

| ALLERGY/COLD/ COUGH DRUG | INTERACTING DRUG | RESULT |
| --- | --- | --- |

Aspirin

Antacids that contain aluminum or magnesium, such as **Gaviscon®, Gelusil®, Maalox®, Mylanta®, Phillips' Milk of Magnesia®**, and others

[for relief of acid indigestion, heartburn, and abdominal pain caused by too much acid in the stomach]

With large doses of aspirin (3,000 milligrams a day or more in an adult), this interaction could result in a reduced concentration of aspirin in the body, which could lead to a decreased effect of the aspirin.

Aspirin is in a chemical class known as salicylates. When these salicylates are taken in large doses with antacids, this interaction could result in a reduced effect of the salicylate. Some salicylate medications include choline salicylate (Arthropan®), magnesium salicylate (Magsal®), sodium salicylate (Pabalate®), and salsalate (Disalcid®).

Aspirin

Anticoagulants (oral), such as dicumarol and warfarin **(Coumadin®, Panwarfin®)**

[for the prevention of blood clots]

Use of aspirin in persons taking an oral anticoagulant increases the risk of bleeding. Such bleeding is evidenced by blood in the urine, coughing up of blood, black stool (or red blood in stool), vomiting of blood or substance resembling coffee grounds, bruising, or other bleeding.

In doses of even 75 milligrams a day, aspirin has been shown to impair the body's ability to stop bleeding. Combined with an anticoagulant—which inactivates certain substances in the blood, leading to the prevention of blood clotting—use of aspirin exacerbates the impairment of the body's ability to clot blood. As a result, abnormal bleeding may result, particularly in the stomach because aspirin can irritate the stomach's lining.

**Recommendation:** Avoid using aspirin-containing products when taking an oral anticoagulant, unless specifically instructed to do so by the

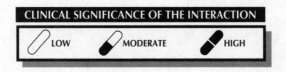

CLINICAL SIGNIFICANCE OF THE INTERACTION

LOW    MODERATE    HIGH

| ALLERGY/COLD/ COUGH DRUG | INTERACTING DRUG | RESULT |
|---|---|---|

*(cont.)*
Aspirin

Anticoagulants (oral)

physician who prescribed the anticoagulant. If a mild pain reliever is needed, acetaminophen may be preferable to aspirin. (Of course, discuss your personal medical condition with your doctor.)

**Note**: Occasionally doctors prescribe aspirin and warfarin together intentionally, but only when they feel that the increased risk of bleeding is outweighed by the stronger anticoagulant effect.

---

Aspirin

Antidiabetic agents:

- acetohexamide (**Dymelor**®)
- chlorpropamide (**Diabinese**®)
- glipizide (**Glucotrol**®)
- glyburide (**DiaBeta**®, **Micronase**®)
- insulin (**Humulin**®, **Lente**®, **Novolin**®, and others
- tolazamide (**Tolinase**®)
- tolbutamide (**Orinase**®) and others

[for treatment of diabetes mellitus, a condition that results in excessively high amounts of sugar in the blood and urine]

Aspirin may increase the blood sugar–lowering (hypoglycemic) effect of antidiabetic drugs. Symptoms of an excessively low amount of sugar in the blood include cold sweats, trembling, and an increased heart rate.

Occasional use of aspirin probably has little effect on antidiabetic drugs with the possible exception of chlorpropamide.

---

Aspirin

Corticosteroids:

- betamethasone (**Celestone**®, **Diprolene**®, **Diprosone**®, **Valisone**®)
- cortisone (**Cortone**®)
- dexamethasone (**Decadron**®)

Corticosteroids (especially when taken orally or by injection) may reduce the concentration of aspirin in the blood, leading to a decrease in the effectiveness of the aspirin.

This interaction may be important in persons taking large amounts of aspirin, such as arthritis sufferers.

| ALLERGY/COLD/ COUGH DRUG | INTERACTING DRUG | RESULT |
|---|---|---|

*(cont.)*
Aspirin

Corticosteroids:

- hydrocortisone (**Hytone®, Vytone®**)
- prednisone (**Deltasone®, Liquid Pred®, Prednicen-M®**), and others

[For relieving inflammation and suppressing allergic reactions]

Aspirin toxicity could result if persons taking moderate to high doses of aspirin suddenly discontinue corticosteroid therapy. Signs of aspirin toxicity include hearing loss, ringing in the ears, rapid breathing, rapid heart rate, nausea, vomiting, agitation, slurred speech, hallucinations, disorientation, and seizures.

**Recommendation:** If you are taking moderate to high doses of aspirin (3,000 milligrams per day or more in an adult) for a prolonged period of time (more than a week), check with your doctor if oral or injected corticosteroids are started, stopped, or changed in dosage. Your aspirin blood level is likely to be affected.

Aspirin

Heparin (**Calciparine®, Liquaemin®**)

[for the prevention and control of blood clots]

Use of aspirin by persons taking heparin increases the risk of bleeding. Such bleeding is evidenced by blood in the urine, coughing up of blood, black stool (or red blood in stool), vomiting of blood or substance resembling coffee grounds, bruising, or other bleeding.

**Recommendation:** Avoid using aspirin-containing products when taking heparin unless specifically advised to do so by the physician who prescribed the heparin. Acetaminophen is often an adequate substitute for aspirin to relieve pain or reduce fever.

Aspirin

Methotrexate (**Mexate®**)

[for treatment of certain cancers, such as breast, lung, and certain forms of leukemia; also used for treatment of psoriasis and rheumatoid arthritis]

Increased effect of the methotrexate, possibly leading to methotrexate toxicity. Symptoms of toxicity include fever, sores in the mouth and on the skin, bleeding, vomiting, diarrhea, and severe reduction in the number of white blood cells produced by the bone marrow.

| ALLERGY/COLD/ COUGH DRUG | INTERACTING DRUG | RESULT |
|---|---|---|

*(cont.)*
Aspirin | Methotrexate | It's important to note that the risk of toxicity from this interaction is much greater when methotrexate is given in high doses, such as for the treatment of cancer. Low-dose methotrexate therapy—which is used to treat arthritis and psoriasis—poses a smaller risk of inducing methotrexate toxicity. However, caution is still warranted.

**Recommendation:** Avoid taking aspirin and aspirin-containing products while taking methotrexate unless the doctor who prescribed the methotrexate specifically advises you to do so. (Make sure *all* of your doctors are aware of *all* of the drugs you are taking.)

Aspirin | Nitroglycerin **(Deponit®, Minitran®, Nitro-Bid®, Nitrodisc®, Nitro-Dur®, Nitrogard®, Nitrong®, Nitrostat®)**

[used to relieve the pain of an angina attack] | The effect of the nitroglycerin is enhanced. Nitroglycerin dilates blood vessels by causing the muscles that surround them to relax. This interaction may result in excessive dilation of blood vessels, which may lead to headaches and low blood pressure. The low blood pressure may cause dizziness and/or fainting.

This result is based on the interaction of aspirin with nitroglycerin taken under the tongue. The effect of aspirin on an oral form of nitroglycerin is not known.

Aspirin | Phenytoin **(Dilantin®)**

[for the prevention of seizures] | Large doses of aspirin (i.e., more than 2,000 milligrams a day) could lead to phenytoin intoxication in some people, symptoms of which include double vision, incoordination, uncontrolled eye movements, and mental impairment.

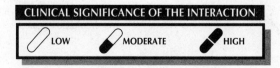

CLINICAL SIGNIFICANCE OF THE INTERACTION

LOW     MODERATE     HIGH

101

| ALLERGY/COLD/COUGH DRUG | INTERACTING DRUG | RESULT |
|---|---|---|
| Aspirin  | Probenecid **(Benemid®)**<br><br>[for reduction of uric acid levels in the body to prevent gout and gouty arthritis; also used to increase the effectiveness of certain antibiotics] | Large amounts of aspirin can reduce the effectiveness of probenecid in ridding the body of excess uric acid.<br><br>Taking a small dose of aspirin, however—such as an occasional one or two aspirins—probably does not influence the effectiveness of probenecid. |
| Aspirin  | Sulfinpyrazone **(Anturane®)**<br><br>[for the treatment—particularly prevention—of gout] | Large amounts of aspirin can reduce the effectiveness of sulfinpyrazone in ridding the body of excess uric acid.<br><br>Taking a small dose of aspirin, however—such as an occasional one or two aspirins—probably does not influence the effectiveness of sulfinpyrazone. |
| Aspirin  | Valproic acid **(Depakene®)**<br><br>[for the treatment of seizures] | When more than a few doses of aspirin are taken, an increase in the concentration of valproic acid—possibly leading to toxicity—has been noted. Symptoms of valproic toxicity include drowsiness, nausea, vomiting, confusion, excessive weight gain, hair loss, and tremor. |
| Codeine-containing cough medicine  | Alcohol | The effects of these two drugs may be addictive, leading to excessive sedation and greatly reduced alertness.<br><br>**Recommendation:** This combination should be avoided. |

| ALLERGY/COLD/ COUGH DRUG | INTERACTING DRUG | RESULT |
|---|---|---|

Dextromethorphan (found in several cough medicines)

Monoamine oxidase inhibitors:

- isocarboxazid (**Marplan**®)
- phenelzine (**Nardil**®)
- tranylcypromine (**Parnate**®), and others

[used to treat depression]

Preliminary data indicate that this combination may be serious, possibly leading to dizziness, nausea, tremor, fever, and coma.

**Recommendation:** Until more is known about this possible interaction, people taking monoamine oxidase inhibitors should avoid taking dextromethorphan.

---

Phenylephrine (**Congespirin**®, **Dimetane**® **Decongestant, Dristan**® **Decongestant, 4-Way**® **Fast Acting Nasal Spray, Naldecon**®**, Neo-Synephrine**®**, Pediacof**® **Cough Syrup, Phenergan**® **VC, Robitussin**® **Night Relief, Ru-Tuss**®**, Rynatan**®**, and others)

Guanethidine (**Ismelin**®)

[for the treatment of high blood pressure]

Phenylephrine may inhibit the ability of guanethidine to lower the blood pressure. As a result, blood pressure levels may increase.

**Recommendation:** Phenylephrine (and other decongestants) should probably be avoided in persons taking guanethidine.

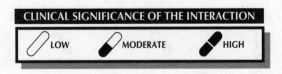

CLINICAL SIGNIFICANCE OF THE INTERACTION

LOW    MODERATE    HIGH

Phenylephrine (**Neo-Synephrine**® Injection)

Imipramine (**Janimine**®, **Tofranil**®)

[used to treat depression]

Imipraine, when taken with phenylephrine that is in an intravenous form, may lead to an increase in blood pressure and the force with which the heart contracts. Symptoms that may be associated with an acute increase in blood pressure include headache, nausea, vomiting, sleepiness, irritability, confusion, visual disturbances, and chest pain.

This interaction is based on phenylephrine given intravenously; it is not known whether this result occurs when phenylephrine is taken orally. However, one should be alert to the reactions mentioned above when an oral form of phenylephrine is taken with imipramine and other drugs in the same class as imipramine (known as tricyclic antidepressants). Oral forms of phenylephrine include Dristan®, Neo-Synephrine® Nasal Spray, Dimetane®, Novahistine® Elixir, Robitussin® Night Relief, and others.

Although this interaction has been shown to occur with imipramine, other tricyclic antidepressants are expected to act similarly when combined with phenylephrine. These include amitriptyline (Elavil®; Endep®), amoxapine (Asendin®), desipramine (Pertofrane®, Norpramin®), doxepin (Adapin®, Sinequan®), nortriptyline (Aventyl®, Pamelor®), protriptyline (Vivactil®), and trimipramine (Surmontil®).

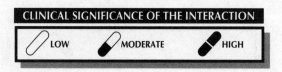

CLINICAL SIGNIFICANCE OF THE INTERACTION

LOW    MODERATE    HIGH

104

| | | |
|---|---|---|
| Phenylephrine (**Congespirin®**, **Dimetane® Decongestant, Dristan® Decongestant, 4-Way® Fast Acting Nasal Spray, Naldecon®, Neo-Synephrine®, Pediacof® Cough Syrup, Phenergan® VC, Robitussin® Night Relief, Ru-Tuss®, Rynatan®,** and others) | Monoamine oxidase inhibitors:<br><br>• isocarboxazid (**Marplan®**)<br>• phenelzine (**Nardil®**)<br>• tranylcypromine (**Parnate®**), and others<br><br>[used to treat depression] | Oral phenylephrine taken with antidepressants in the monoamine oxidase inhibitor family can cause an increase in blood pressure levels, rapid heartbeat, and hypertensive reaction, symptoms of which include headache, palpitations, visual disturbances, and chest pain.<br><br>The effect of phenylephrine-containing nasal sprays in persons receiving MAO inhibitors is not established, but such nasal sprays should probably be avoided until more is known about this interaction.<br><br>**Recommendation:** Phenylephrine should not be taken by persons who are using an antidepressant in the monoamine oxidase inhibitor family, or within two weeks after stopping an MAO inhibitor. |

| | | |
|---|---|---|
| Phenylpropanolamine (**Acutrim®, Allerest®, Comtrex® Multi-Symptom Cold Reliever, Contac® Continuous Action Decongestant, Coricidin "D"®, Dexatrim®, Dimetapp®, Naldecon®, Ornade®, Ru-Tuss®, Sinarest® Regular and Extra Strength, Tavist-D®, Triaminic®,** and others) | Monoamine oxidase inhibitors:<br><br>• isocarboxazid (**Marplan®**)<br>• phenelzine (**Nardil®**)<br>• tranylcypromine (**Parnate®**), and others<br><br>[used to treat depression] | Can result in severe hypertensive reactions, which include symptoms such as elevated blood pressure levels, flushing of the face, pounding of the heart, and lightheadedness. Persons taking medications containing phenylpropanolamine with a monoamine oxidase inhibitor have reported other symptoms, such as headache, vomiting, and irregularities of the heartbeat and heart rhythm.<br><br>**Recommendation:** Phenylpropanolamine should not be taken by persons who are using an antidepressant in the monoamine oxidase inhibitor family, or within two weeks after stopping an MAO inhibitor. |

Pseudoephedrine (**Actifed**®, **Benadryl**®, **Bromfed**®, **Contac**® **Nighttime Cold Medicine, Deconamine**®, **Deconsal**® **L.A., Fedashist**®, **Novahistine**® **DMX, Robitussin-DAC**®, **Sine-Aid**®, **Sine-Off**®, **Sinutab**®, **Sudafed**®, **Tylenol**® **Cold Medication, Vicks Formula 44D**®, **Vicks Nyquil**®, and others)

Monoamine oxidase inhibitors:

- isocarboxazid (**Marplan**®)
- phenelzine (**Nardil**®)
- tranylcypromine (**Parnate**®), and others

[used to treat depression]

Severe high blood pressure may result when taking medications that contain pseudoephedrine with an antidepressant in the monoamine oxidase inhibitor class. Symptoms may include headache, palpitations, visual disturbances, and chest pain.

**Recommendation:** Persons taking an antidepressant that is in the monoamine oxidase inhibitor family (or who have taken such a drug in the past two weeks) should avoid taking pseudoephedrine and medications containing pseudoephedrine.

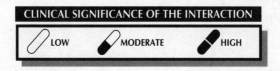

CLINICAL SIGNIFICANCE OF THE INTERACTION

LOW     MODERATE     HIGH

| ALLERGY/COLD/ COUGH DRUG | INTERACTING DRUG | RESULT |
|---|---|---|
| Pseudoephedrine (**Actifed®**, **Benadryl®**, **Bromfed®**, **Contac® Nighttime Cold Medicine**, **Deconamine®**, **Deconsal® L.A.**, **Fedahist®**, **Novashistine® DMX, Robitussin-DAC®**, **Sine-Aid®**, **Sine-Off®**, **Sinutab®**, **Sudafed®**, **Tylenol® Cold Medication**, **Vicks Formula 44D®**, **Vicks Nyquil®**, and others) | Sodium bicarbonate **Alka-Seltzer®, Arm & Hammer®)** [antacid used to relieve heartburn and acid indigestion] | Combined with pseudoephedrine, sodium bicarbonate—taken in large amounts—can result in an increased effect of pseudoephedrine, possibly leading to anxiety, tremor, palpitations, and mood changes. |

| | | |
|---|---|---|
| Terfenadine (**Seldane®**)  | Ketoconazole (**Nizoral®**) [for treatment of various fungus infections] | May lead to higher levels of terfenadine, which could result in terfenadine toxicity. Symptoms of terfenadine toxicity may include lightheadedness, fainting, and palpitations; serious disturbances of heart rhythms have also occurred. **Recommendation:** Do not take terfenadine and ketoconazole together. Other related antifungal drugs such as fluconazole (Diflucan®) and itraconazole (Sporanox®) should also be avoided if you are taking terfenadine (until we have evidence that they are safe). |

## CHAPTER 4

# DRUGS FOR ASTHMA AND OTHER BREATHING DISORDERS

About 12 million adults and 25 million children in the United States suffer from asthma, a condition—often allergic—leaving the sufferer struggling to obtain a full, satisfying breath. To gain a better understanding of asthma, and other breathing disorders, a very basic description of the respiratory tract is necessary.

## Basic Breathing

Air is inhaled through the nose or mouth and is channeled down the *trachea* or windpipe. The trachea divides into two branches, called *bronchi,* each one supplying air to each lung. Each bronchus further divides into many smaller branches called *bronchioles* (to visualize this, think of the pattern of veins in a leaf or a tree hanging upside down). These bronchioles end in clusters of small air sacs, known as *alveoli.* These alveoli must remain elastic to work properly (so air can be forced into and out of them); as we'll see momentarily, certain diseases of the lung involve a loss of elasticity of these sacs.

## What Is Asthma?

Asthma is a predominately allergic reaction in which the trachea and bronchi become overly sensitive due to various stimuli. These stimuli may be environmental—such as molds, feathers, or animal dander—which trigger allergic asthma, or may be occupational stimuli, such as certain chemicals at the worksite (or home, as is the case with certain paints and cleaning agents). Respiratory viral infection (such as the common cold) often aggravates asthma. Air pollution, weather changes, exercise (especially in cold weather), emotional stress or excitement, certain medications, and other factors have been known to trigger an attack in some asthmatics.

Asthma has traditionally been considered a disease that primarily involved bronchoconstriction: a narrowing of the bronchi and bronchioles. The muscular band that surrounds the bronchi and bronchioles normally contracts to carry on necessary functions of the lung; however, in an asthmatic, these muscles contract excessively—presumably in response to one or more asthma-triggering stimuli—narrowing the air passageways. Furthermore, the bronchioles often become clogged with mucus, which exacerbates the problem.

More recent evidence, however—as suggested by a panel of experts convened by the National Heart, Lung, and Blood Institute's National Asthma Education Program—indicates that *inflammation* is the predominant feature in asthma.[1] The inflammation may worsen the bronchoconstriction. As a result, when treating asthma, these experts recommend methods to reduce and prevent inflammation rather than just reversing bronchoconstriction.

Symptoms of asthma include coughing, shortness of breath, labored breathing, wheezing (a whistling sound when you exhale), and a tightness in the chest. These symptoms can range from mild, in which case medication is needed only to combat an individual asthma attack, to severe enough to warrant daily use of medication. Severe asthma is dangerous because breathing becomes so difficult that respiratory failure (suffocation) may follow.

# Drugs Used to Treat Asthma

Medications to treat asthma are primarily in two groups: (1) bronchodilators, or medications that relax the muscles surrounding the bronchioles, and (2) medications that reduce or prevent inflammation. The muscle-relaxing medications, or bronchodilators as they're called, consist of theophylline (Primatene® Tablets, Slo-bid®, Theo-Dur®, Theo-24®, Uniphyl®, and others), epinephrine, and derivatives of epinephrine called beta-2-agonists.

One of the earliest beta-2-agonists available was isoproternol (Isuprel®). Epinephrine and isoproterenol are unavailable in oral form because they are degraded by the corrosive digestive juices of the stomach and intestine. As a result, these medications are available only by inhalation or injection. Several other beta-2 agonists are available as both an inhaled form as well as an oral preparation.

The inhaled form of certain asthma-treating medications is available as a "metered-dose" inhaler, which is a small aerosol pump. These inhalers, which have been tremendously helpful to asthmatics, are held near the open mouth or pressed against the lips; when you squeeze the inhaler, a measured amount of the drug is released. You take a breath as the drug is released so that the aerosolized drug can be delivered to the air passageways. Some commonly used metered-dose inhalers include albuterol (Proventil®, Ventolin®), bitolterol (Tornalate®), isoetharine (Bronkometer®), isoproterenol (Duo-Medihaler®, Isuprel®, Medihaler-Iso®), metaproterenol (Alupent®, Metaprel®), pirbuterol (Maxair®), and terbutaline (Brethaire®, Bricanyl®).

Inhaled epinephrine is widely available as a nonprescription medication. Some trade names include AsthmaHaler®, AsthmaNefrin®, Bronkaid® Mist, Medihaler-Epi®, Primatene® Mist, and others. Consumers should note that epinephrine (as well as isoproterenol) may be associated with heart and blood pressure complications (such as increased heart rate and blood pressure, and palpitations) and should be used with caution by anyone with heart disease. (Remember, always keep all of your doctors fully informed of your medical conditions and tell them all of the medications you are taking.)

When using a metered-dose inhaler to deliver an asthma medication, ask your doctor about a device known as a spacer. This device attaches to the inhaler, increasing the likelihood that the medication will reach your lungs, where it's needed, rather than being deposited on your tongue, cheeks, or throat. Spacers can double the amount of medication tht actually reaches the small airways.

Cromolyn (Intal®) is a drug used only for prevention of asthma. It seems to stabilize the cells of the body that release the chemicals causing the narrowing of the airways. It may take several days to weeks after starting cromolyn before the favorable effects are seen, so it is normally given on a daily basis. Cromolyn may also help to block asthma arising from exercise or exposure to a pet or allergen (i.e., anything that triggers an allergic reaction), if used just prior to that exposure. Cromolyn has very few side effects, and is especially popular for children.

Corticosteroid drugs also are used for symptomatic treatment and prevention of asthma. These drugs are similar to cortisone, a hormone occurring naturally in the body. Corticosteroids are potent anti-inflammatory agents, and the reduced inflammation helps to relieve obstructed airways. Corticosteroids are typically used when occasional use of bronchodilators or daily use of cromolyn does not provide relief. They are available in oral, inhaled, or injectable forms. Prednisone (Deltasone®) and prednisolone (Delta-Cortef®) are typical corticosteroids that are used for a short time to relieve symptoms. Other corticosteroids include betamethasone (Celestone®), dexamethasone (Decadron®), methylprednisolone (Medrol®), and triamcinolone (Artistocort®, Kenacort®).

Oral or injected corticosteroids can be given for up to two weeks with little risk of serious toxicity. Taken for longer periods, however, oral corticosteroid drugs do have side effects including weight gain, puffiness in the face, insomnia, increased blood sugar, thinning of the bones, high blood pressure, cataracts, and others. These toxic effects can be largely avoided, however, if the asthmatic can use corticosteroids in metered-dose inhalers instead of oral or injected forms.

Because inhaled corticosteroids go directly to the lungs, only small doses are needed, thus minimizing the adverse effects. Inhaled corticosteroids are used primarily to prevent asthma attacks rather than to relieve one that has already begun. Examples of inhaled corticosteroids include beclomethasone (Beclovent®, Vanceril®), flunisolide (AeroBid®), and triamcinolone (Azmacort®).

# Chronic Bronchitis and Emphysema

Two other disorders involving impaired breathing are chronic bronchitis and emphysema. These conditions can lead to a general term known as chronic obstructive pulmonary disease (COPD), the fifth leading cause of death in the United States according to the U.S. Public Health Service.[2] We'll briefly discuss each disorder.

Chronic bronchitis may develop after years of exposure to one or more irritants, such as cigarette smoke, organic chemicals, or air pollution. It's important not to confuse *chronic* bronchitis with *acute* bronchitis. Chronic refers to the fact that the condition lasts a long time. Furthermore, this condition typically requires exposure to an irritant over a long period of time. In contrast, acute bronchitis is usually caused by a respiratory tract infection, typically viral. Acute bronchitis develops quickly and lasts from a few days to a few weeks.

Emphysema is a disease of the alveoli, or air sacs, in the lungs. These air sacs are normally elastic so that air can easily fill them. Blood vessels surround these sacs, allowing oxygen to leave the lungs and enter the blood (for circulation to various organs and tissues in the body). Carbon dioxide, a waste product, is also transferred from the blood, delivered to the alveoli, then exhaled.

With emphysema, the alveoli become enlarged and lose their elasticity. As a result, "stale" air accumulates in the sacs (leading to their enlargement) because they do not empty entirely. Efficient exchange of gases (oxygen from the lungs into the bloodstream and carbon dioxide from the bloodstream into, and then exhaled out of, the lungs) is often impaired, thus increasing the work necessary to breathe.

We would be remiss in our discussion of COPD if we did not point out that over the last quarter of a century an increasing amount of evidence has accumulated to link cigarette smoking to the development of chronic bronchitis and emphysema. In fact, a 1989 report of the Surgeon General stated that 80 to 85 percent of deaths from COPD are attributed to cigarette smoking.[3] Furthermore, it has been estimated that the risk of death from chronic bronchitis or emphysema is thirty times greater for heavy smokers (i.e., more than twenty-five cigarettes a day) than for nonsmokers.[4]

Medications used to treat chronic bronchitis and emphysema include bronchodilators, long-term administration of oxygen, corticosteroids, and antibiotics (to clear up an infection). Many of the bronchodilators are the same ones that are used to relieve the bronchospasm of asthmatics (e.g., albuterol [Proventil®, Ventolin®], bitolterol [Tornalate®], metaproterenol [Alupent®], and others). Ipratropium (Atrovent®) is a bronchodilator used to relieve the symptoms of chronic bronchitis and emphysema, but it is also used in some persons with asthma. Smoking cessation and rehabilitative programs (such as breathing retraining and graded physical exercise) are also extremely helpful in alleviating symptoms and slowing down any further lung disease.

Corticosteroids:

- betamethasone **(Celestone®)**
- cortisone **(Cortone®)**
- dexamethasone **(Decadron®, Dalalone®)**
- hydrocortisone **(Cortef®, Hydrocortone®, Solu-Cortef®)**
- methylpred-nisolone **(Medrol®, Depo-Medrol®, Solu-Medrol®)**
- paramethasone **(Haldrone®)**
- prednisolone **(Delta-Cortef®, Hydeltrasol®, Pedilapred®, Prelone®)**
- prednisone **(Deltasone®, Liquid Pred®, Meticorten®)**
- triamcinolone **(Aristocort®, Kenacort®, Kenalog®)**

Aminoglutethimide **(Cytadren®)**

[used to suppress adrenal function in certain persons with Cushing's syndrome]

Reduced effect of dexamethasone and probably other corticosteroids. This may result in a worsening of the condition being treated by the corticosteroid (e.g., asthma, arthritis, organ transplantation, etc.). This interaction is not likely to be a problem if the corticosteroid is inhaled of applied locally to the skin, eye, ear, etc.

**Recommendation:** Your doctor may need to adjust the dose of your corticosteroid if aminoglutethimide is started or stopped.

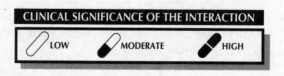

CLINICAL SIGNIFICANCE OF THE INTERACTION

LOW    MODERATE    HIGH

| ASTHMA DRUG | INTERACTING DRUG | RESULT |
| --- | --- | --- |
| Corticosteroids:<br><br>• cortisone **(Cortone®)**<br>• hydrocortisone **(Cortef®, Hydrocortone®, Solu-cortef®)**<br>• methylpred-nisolone **(Medrol®, Depo-Medrol®, Solu-Medrol®)**<br>• prednisolone **(Delta-Cortef®, Hydeltrasol®, Pediapred®, Prelone®)**<br>• prednisone **(Deltasone®, Liquid Pred®, Metlcorten®)**<br><br> | Amphotericin B **(Fungizone®)**<br><br>[for treatment of various fungal infections] | Decreased amount of potassium in the body, which may lead to muscle problems (such as weakness, twitching, and pain), nocturia (need to urinate at night), and abnormal sensations, such as feelings of numbness, tingling, or burning.<br><br>Corticosteroids can produce potassium depletion if they are given by injection or orally (especially with large doses), but other routes of administration (e.g., inhalation or topical application on the skin or in the eye, ear, etc.) generally have little effect on potassium.<br><br>Cortisone and hydrocortisone are more likely than other corticosteroids to lead to these effects. |
| Corticosteroids:<br><br>• bethamethasone **(Celestone®)**<br>• cortisone **(Cortone®)**<br>• dexamethasone **(Decadrone®), Dalalone®)**<br>• hydrocortisone **(Cortef®, Hydrocortone®, Solu-Cortef®)**<br>• methylpred-nisolone **(Medrol®, Depo-Medrol®, Solu-Medrol®)**<br>• paramethasone **(Haldrone®)**<br>• prednisolone **(Delta-Cortef®, Hydeltrasol®, Pediapred®, Prelone®)** | Antidiabetic drugs:<br><br>• acetohexamide **(Dymelor®)**<br>• chlorpropamide **(Diabinese®)**<br>• glipizide **(Glucotrol®)**<br>• glyburide **(DiaBeta®, Micronase®)**<br>• insulin **(Humulin®, Lente®, Novolin®,** and others<br>• tolazamide **(Tolinase®)**<br>• tolbutamide **(Orinase®),** and others<br><br>[for treatment of diabetes mellitus, a condition that results in excessively high amounts of sugar in the blood and urine] | Corticosteroids may increase the amount of sugar in the blood (i.e., hyperglycemic effect). This is most likely to occur when the corticosteroid is taken orally or injected. Other routes of administration (e.g., inhalation, or topical application on the skin, eye, ear, etc.) usually have little effect on blood sugar.<br><br>**Recommendation:** Diabetics should be particularly careful when checking their blood sugar levels if a corticosteroid drug is started or stopped, or if its dosage is changed. |

| ASTHMA DRUG | INTERACTING DRUG | RESULT |
|---|---|---|

*(cont.)*

**Corticosteroids:**                Antidiabetic

- prednisone **(Deltasone®, Liquid Pred®, Meticorten®)**
- triamcinolone **(Aristocort®, Kenacort®, Kenalog®)**

---

**Corticosteroids:**

- bethamethasone **(Celestone®)**
- cortisone **(Cortone®)**
- dexamethasone **(Decadrone®), Dalalone®)**
- hydrocortisone **(Cortef®, Hydrocortone®, Solu-Cortef®)**
- methyprednisolone **(Medrol®, Depo-Medrol®, Solu-Medrol®)**
- paramethasone **(Haldrone®)**
- prednisolone **(Delta-Cortef®,**
- **Hydeltrasol®, Pediapred®, Prelone®)**
- prednisone **(Deltasone®, Liquid Pred®, Meticorten®)**

Aspirin

[for relief of pain and reduction of fever; pain often relieved due to reduced inflammation]

Corticosteroids may reduce the concentration of aspirin in the blood, leading to a decrease in the effectiveness of the aspirin.

Aspirin toxicity could result if persons taking moderate to high doses of aspirin suddenly discontinued corticosteroid therapy; signs of aspirin toxicity include hearing loss, ringing in the ears, rapid breathing, rapid heart rate, nausea, vomiting, agitation, slurred speech, hallucinations, disorientation, and seizures.

**Recommendation:** If you are taking moderate to high doses of aspirin (3,000 milligrams per day or more in an adult) for a prolonged period of time (more than a week), check with your doctor if oral or injected corticosteroids are started, stopped, or changed in dosage. Your aspirin blood level is likely to be affected.

114

| ASTHMA DRUG | INTERACTING DRUG | RESULT |
|---|---|---|

*(cont.)*

Corticosteroids:

• triamcinolone
(**Aristocort®**,
**Kenacort®**,
**Kenalog®**)

Aspirin

---

Corticosteroids:

• bethamethasone
(**Celestone®**)
• cortisone
(**Cortone®**)
• dexamethasone
(**Decadron®**,
**Dalalone®**)
• hydrocortisone
(**Cortef®**,
**Hydrocortone®**,
**Solu-cortef®**)
• methylpred-
nisolone
(**Medrol®**, **Depo-
Medrol®**, **Solu-
Medrol®**)
• paramethasone
(**Haldrone®**)
• prednisolone
(**Delta-Cortef®**,
**Hydeltrasol®**,
**Pediapred®**,
**Prelone®**)
• prednisone
(**Deltasone®**,
**Liquid Pred®**,
**Meticorten®**)
• triamcinolone
(**Aristocort®**,
**Kenacort®**,
**Kenalog®**)

Barbiturates:

• amobarbital (**Amytal®**)
• butabarbital (**Butisol®**)
• butalbital
• pentobarbital
(**Nembutal®**)
• phenobarbital
(**Luminal®**, **Solfoton®**)
• primidone (**Mysoline®**)
• secobarbital
(**Seconal®**),
and others

[used to treat insomnia
and anxiety; certain bar-
biturates are used to prevent seizures]

May cause a reduced amount of corticosteroid in the body, possibly
leading to a decreased effect of the
corticosteroid. This interaction has
been shown to occur with the barbiturate phenobarbital (i.e., it decreases the effect of dexamethasone)
when the corticosteroid is injected or
taken orally. Other barbiturates and
other corticosteroid medications are
expected to act similarly.

This interaction is not likely to be a
problem if the corticosteroid is inhaled or applied locally to the skin,
eye, ear, etc.

**Recommendation:** Your doctor may
need to adjust the dose of your corticosteroid if a barbiturate is started or
stopped.

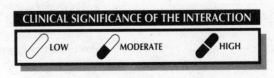

CLINICAL SIGNIFICANCE OF THE INTERACTION

LOW    MODERATE    HIGH

115

Corticosteroids:

- bethamethasone (**Celestone**®)
- cortisone (**Cortone**®)
- dexamethasone (**Decadron**®)
- hydrocortisone (**Cortef**®, **Hydrocortone**®, **Solu-Cortef**®)
- methylpred-nisolone (**Medrol**®, **Depo-Medrol**®, **Solu-Medrol**®)
- paramethasone (**Haldrone**®)
- prednisolone (**Delta-Cortef**®, **Hydeltrasol**® **Pediapred**® **Prelone**®)
- prednisone (**Deltasone**®, **Liquid Pred**® **Meticorton**®)
- triamcinolone (**Aristocort**®, **Kenacort**® **Kenalog**®)

Carbamazepine (**Tegretol**®)

[for epilepsy, trigeminal neuralgia (spasms of pain in the face), and other disorders]

Carbamazepine reduces the amount of dexamethasone or prednisolone in the body, leading to a decreased effect of the corticosteroid.

While this effect has been shown to occur with dexamethasone and pred-nisolone, this interaction is expected to occur with other corticosteroid drugs as well when the corticosteroid is injected or taken orally.

This interaction is not likely to be a problem if the corticosteroid is in-haled or applied locally to the skin, eye, ear, etc.

**Recommendation:** Your doctor may need to adjust the dose of your corti-costeroid if carbamazepine is started or stopped.

---

Corticosteroids:

- bethamethasone (**Celestone**®)
- cortisone (**Cortone**®)
- dexamethasone (**Decadron**®, **Dalalone**®)

Estrogen-containg oral contraceptives such as **Brevicon**®, **Demulen**®, **Enovid**®, **Lo/Ovral**®, **Norinyl**®, **Ortho Novum**®, **Ovcon**®, **Ovral**®, **Tri-Norinyl**®, **Triphasil**®, and many others

[for prevention of pregnancy]

Oral contraceptives—as well as es-trogens—may increase the effect of the corticosteroid and may increase the risk of corticosteroid toxicity. Corticosteroid toxicity can result in increased blood pressure, increased blood sugar, thinning of bone (osteo-porosis), muscle weakness, insomnia, stomach ulcers, and infections.

Although this interaction has been shown to occur with hydrocortisone and prednisolone, it is likely that other corticosteroids will react in a similar

(*cont.*)
Corticosteroids:

- hydrocortisone (**Cortef®, Hydrocortone®, Solu-Cortef®**)
- methylprednisolone (**Medrol®, Depo-Medrol®, Solu-Medrol®**)
- paramethasone (**Haldrone®**)
- prednisolone (**Delta-Cortef®, Hydeltrasol®, Pediapred®, Prelone®**)
- prednisone (**Deltasone®, Liquid Pred®, Meticorten®**)
- triamcinolone (**Aristocort®, Kenakort®, Kenalog®**)

Estrogen-containing oral contraceptives

manner when the corticosteroid is injected or taken orally.

This interaction is not likely to be a problem if the corticosteroid is inhaled or applied locally to the skin, eye, ear, etc.

**Recommendation:** Your doctor may need to adjust the dose of your corticosteroid if an oral contraceptive is started or stopped.

---

Corticosteroids:

- cortisone (**Cortone®**)
- hydrocortisone (**Cortef®, Hydrocortone®, Solu-Cortef®**)

Ethacrynic acid (**Edecrin®**)

[for the reduction of high blood pressure; also used to remove excess fluid from the body, as in congestive heart failure]

Decreased amount of potassium in the body, which may lead to muscle problems (such as weakness, twitching, and pain), nocturia (need to urinate at night), and abnormal sensations, such as feelings of numbness, tingling, or burning.

Corticosteroids can produce potassium depletion if they are given by injection or orally (especially with large doses), but other routes of administration (e.g., inhalation or topical application on the skin or in the eye, ear, etc.) generally have little effect on potassium.

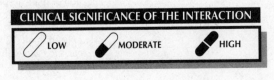

CLINICAL SIGNIFICANCE OF THE INTERACTION

LOW   MODERATE   HIGH

(*cont.*)

Corticosteroids:

- methylpred-
  nisolone
  (**Medrol**®, **Depo-
  Medrol**®, **Solu-
  Medrol**®)
- prednisolone
  (**Delta-Cortef**,®
  **Hydeltrasol**,®
  **Pediapred**,®
  **Prelone**®)
- prednisone
  (**Deltasone**,®
  **Liquid Pred**,®
  **Meticorten**®)
- cortisone
  (**Cortone**®)
- hydrocortisone
  (**Cortef**®,
  **Hydrocortone**®,
  **Solu-Cortef**®)
- methylpred-
  nisolone (**Medrol**®,
  **Solu-Medrol**®)
- prednisolone
  (**Delta-Cortef**®,
  **Hydeltrasol**®,
  **Pediapred**®,
  **Prelone**®)
- prednisone
  (**Deltasone**®,
  **Liquid Pred**®,
  **Melicorten**®)

Ethacrynic acid
(**Edecrin**®)

Cortisone and hydrocortisone are more likely than other corticosteroids to lead to these effects.

---

Corticosteroids:

- cortisone
  (**Cortone**®)
- hydrocortisone
  (**Cortef**®,
  **Hydrocortone**®,
  **Solu-Cortef**®)

Furosemide (**Lasix**®)

[for the reduction of high blood pressure; also used to remove excess fluid from the body, as in congestive heart failure]

Decreased amount of potassium in the body, which may lead to muscle problems (such as weakness, twitching, and pain), nocturia (need to urinate at night), and abnormal sensations, such as feelings of numbness, tingling, or burning.

Corticosteroids can produce potassium depletion if they are given by injection or orally (especially with large doses), but other routes of administration (e.g., inhalation or topical application on the skin or in the eye, ear, etc.) generally have little effect on potassium.

118

| ASTHMA DRUG | INTERACTING DRUG | RESULT |
|---|---|---|

*(cont.)*

**Corticosteroids:**

- methylpred-
nisolone
(**Medrol®, Solu-
Medrol®**)
- prednisolone
(**Delta-Cortef®,
Hydeltrasol®,
Pediapred®,
Prelone®**)
- prednisone
(**Deltasone®,
Liquid Pred®,
Melicorten®**)

Furosemide

Cortisone and hydrocortisone are more likely than other corticosteroids to lead to these effects.

---

**Corticosteroids:**

- bethamethasone
(**Celestone®**)
- cortisone
(**Cortone®**)
- dexamethasone
(**Decadron®,
Dalalone®**)
- hydrocortisone
(**Cortef®,
Hydrocortone®,
Solu-Cortef®**)
- methylpred-
nisolone
(**Medrol®, Depo-
Medrol®, Solu-
Medrol®**)
- paramethasone
(**Haldrone®**)

Phenytoin (**Dilantin®**)

[for the prevention of seizures]

Reduced effect of the corticosteroid, especially if it is injected or taken orally. This may result in a worsening of the condition being treated by the corticosteroid (e.g., asthma, arthritis, organ transplantation, etc.).

This interaction is not likely to be a problem if the corticosteroid is inhaled or applied locally to the skin, eye, ear, etc.

**Recommendation:** Your doctor may need to adjust the dose of your corticosteroid if phenytoin is started or stopped.

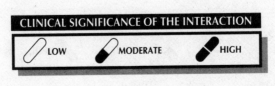

CLINICAL SIGNIFICANCE OF THE INTERACTION

LOW    MODERATE    HIGH

| ASTHMA DRUG | INTERACTING DRUG | RESULT |
| --- | --- | --- |

*(cont.)*

**Corticosteroids:**

- prednisolone **(Delta-Cortef®, Hydeltrasol®, Pediapred®, Prelone®)**
- prednisone **(Deltasone®, Liquid Pred®, Meticorten®)**
- triamcinolone **(Aristocort®, Kenacort®, Kenalog®)**

Phenytoin

---

**Corticosteroids:**

- bethamethasone **(Celestone®)**
- cortisone **(Cortone®)**
- dexamethasone **(Decadron®, Dalalone®)**
- hydrocortisone **(Cortef®, Hydrocortone®, Solu-Cortef®)**
- methylpred-nisolone **(Medrol®, Depo-Medrol®, Solu-Medrol®)**
- paramethasone **(Haldrone®)**

- prednisolone **(Delta-Cortef®, Hydeltrasol®, Pediapred®, Prelone®)**
- prednisone **(Deltasone®, Liquid Pred®, Meticorten®)**

Rifampin **(Rifadin®, Rifamate®, Rimactane®)**

[used in combination with at least one other drug, rifampin is used to treat tuberculosis; also used in the treatment of individuals who are carriers of meningitis]

Rifampin may substantially reduce the effectiveness of corticosteroids in some persons.

**Recommendation:** Watch for inadequate control of the condition being treated by the corticosteroid (e.g., asthma, arthritis, etc.). Your doctor may need to use higher than normal doses of corticosteroids during rifampin therapy. (Do *not* change the dosage of either drug yourself; only your doctor should do this.)

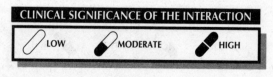

CLINICAL SIGNIFICANCE OF THE INTERACTION

LOW     MODERATE     HIGH

| ASTHMA DRUG | INTERACTING DRUG | RESULT |
|---|---|---|

(*cont.*)
Corticosteroids                Rifampin

- triamcinolone
  (**Aristocort®**,
  **Kenacort®**,
  **Kenalog®**)

---

Corticosteroids:

- cortisone
  (**Cortone®**)
- hydrocortisone
  (**Cortef®**,
  **Hydrocortone®**,
  **Solu-Cortef®**)
- methylpred-
  nisolone
  (**Medrol®, Depo-
  Medrol®, Solu-
  Medrol®**)
- prednisolone
  (**Delta-Cortef®**,
  **Hydeltrasol®**,
  **Pediapred®**,
  **Prelone®**)
- prednisone
  (**Deltasone®**,
  **Liquid Pred®**,
  **Meticorten®**)

Thiazide and thiazide-
like diuretics:

- Chlorothiazide
  (**Diuril®**)
- Chlorthalidone
  (**Hygroton®**)
- Hydrochlorothiazide
  (**Esidrix®**,
  **HydroDURIL®**,
  **Oretic®**, and others)
- Metolazone (**Diulo®**,
  **Zaroxolyn®**)

[for the reduction of high
blood pressure; also used
to remove excess fluid
from the body, as in con-
gestive heart failure]

Corticosteroids can produce potassium depletion if they are given by
injection or orally (especially with
large doses), but other routes of administration (e.g., inhalation or topical application on the skin or in the
eye, ear, etc.) generally have little effect on potassium.

Decreased amount of potassium in
the body, which may lead to muscle
problems (such as weakness, twitching, and pain), nocturia (need to urinate at night), and abnormal
sensations, such as feelings of numbness, tingling, or burning.

Cortisone and hydrocortisone are
more likely than other corticosteroids
to lead to these effects when used
with thiazide diuretics.

Ephedrine **(Primatene®, Broncholate®, Tedral®**, and others

Monoamine oxidase inhibitors:

- isocarboxazid **(Marplan®)**
- phenelzine **(Nardil®)**
- tranylcypromine **(Parnate®)** and others

[used to treat depression]

Can result in severe high blood pressure.

**Recommendation:** Avoid using these two medications together. Also, ephedrine should not be used within two weeks after stopping an MAO inhibitor.

---

Epinephrine **(Adrenalin®, Ana-Kit®, AsthmaHaler®, Bronkaid® Mist, EpiPen®, Primatene® Mist, Sus-Phrine®**, and others)

Antidiabetic drugs:

- acetohexamide **(Dymelor®)**
- chlorpropamide **(Diabinese®)**
- glipizide **(Glucotrol®)**
- glyburide **(DiaBeta®, Micronase®)**
- insulin **(Humulin®, Lente®, Novolin®**, and others)
- tolazamide **(Tolinase®)**
- tolbutamide **(Orinase®)**, and others

[for treatment of diabetes mellitus, a condition that results in excessively high amounts of sugar in the blood and urine]

Injections of epinephrine can lead to increased blood glucose (sugar) levels in the blood. Inhaled epinephrine is probably less likely to interact unless excessive amounts of epinephrine are used. The epinephrine found in local anesthetic injections would also be unlikely to interact unless large amounts are used.

**Recommendation:** Diabetics should watch for excessive blood sugar levels when epinephrine is being used.

---

Epinephrine **(Adrenalin®, Ana-Kit®, AsthmaHaler®, Bronkaid® Mist, Epi-Pen®, Primatene® Mist, Sus-Phrine®**, and others)

Carteolol **(Cartrol®)**

[for treatment of high blood pressure]

The outcome depends on the condition for which the patient is being treated, and on how the epinephrine is given.

**Persons with anaphylactic shock:** Some people develop a severe, possibly life-threatening allergic reaction (called anaphylactic shock) to insect stings or bites and cerain medications or foods. Symptoms of anaphylactic shock include hives, wheezing, difficulty breathing, abdominal pain, incontinence, fever, and loss of consciousness; death may also occur. Epinephrine injections help reverse

| ASTHMA DRUG | INTERACTING DRUG | RESULT |
|---|---|---|

(*cont.*)
Epinephrine

Carteolol

anaphylactic shock, but in persons taking a specific type of antihypertensive drug (i.e., nonselective beta blocker, such as carteolol), the epinephrine may not work very well and other measures often must be taken.

**Persons *not* in anaphylactic shock:** People taking carteolol who receive epinephrine for something other than anaphylactic shock are at risk of developing excessively high blood pressure levels. If the epinephrine is injected with the intention of systemic effects (i.e., reaching most of the tissues and organs in the body), the blood pressure may increase dramatically. If, however, the epinephrine is inhaled into the lungs, put in the eye, or injected for only local effects (e.g., by a dentist or dermatologist), the risk of a hypertensive reaction appears to be much less (unless a much larger than usual amount of epinephrine is used).

**Recommendation:** It is best for people who are at risk of anaphylactic shock (e.g., those allergic to bee stings) to avoid taking carteolol or other beta blockers.

Epinephrine (**Adrenalin®, Ana-Kit®, AsthmaHaler®,**

Nadolol (**Corgard®**)

[for treatment of high blood pressure and angina]

The outcome depends on the condition for which the patient is being treated, and on how the epinephrine is given.

**Persons with anaphylactic shock:** Some people develop a severe, possibly life-threatening, allergic reaction (called anaphylactic shock) to insect stings or bites and certain medications or foods.

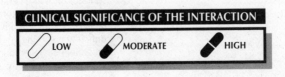

CLINICAL SIGNIFICANCE OF THE INTERACTION

LOW     MODERATE     HIGH

123

(*cont.*)
Epinephrine

**Bronkaid® Mist, Epi-Pen®, Primatene® Mist, Sus-Phrine®, and others)**

Nadolol

Symptoms of anaphylactic shock include hives, wheezing, difficulty breathing, abdominal pain, incontinence, fever, and loss of consciousness; death may also occur. Epinephrine injections help reverse anaphylactic shock, but in persons taking a specific type of antihypertensive drug (i.e., nonselective beta blocker, such as nadolol), the epinephrine may not work very well and other measures often must be taken.

**Persons *not* in anaphylactic shock:** People taking nadolol who receive epinephrine for something other than anaphylactic shock are at risk of developing excessively high blood pressure levels. If the epinephrine is injected with the intention of systemic effects (i.e., reaching most of the tissues and organs in the body), the blood pressure may increase dramatically. If, however, the epinephrine is inhaled into the lungs, put in the eye, or injected for only local effects (e.g., by a dentist or dermatologist), the risk of a hypertensive reaction appears to be much less (unless a much larger than usual amount of epinephrine is used).

**Recommendation:** It is best for people who are at risk of anaphylactic shock (e.g., those allergic to bee stings) to avoid taking nadolol or other beta blockers.

Epinephrine **(Adrenalin®, Ana-Kit®, AsthmaHaler®, Bronkaid® Mist, EpiPen®, Primatene® Mist, Sus-Phrine®, and others)**

Pindolol **(Visken®)**

[for treatment of high blood pressure]

The outcome depends on the condition for which the patient is being treated, and on how the epinephrine is given.

**Persons with anaphylactic shock:** Some people develop a severe, possibly life-threatening, allergic reaction (called anaphylactic shock) to insect stings or bites and certain medications or foods. Symptoms of anaphylactic shock include hives, wheezing, difficulty breathing, abdominal pain, incontinence, fever, and loss of consciousness; death may also occur.

| ASTHMA DRUG | INTERACTING DRUG | RESULT |
|---|---|---|

(*cont.*)
Epinephrine

Pindolol

Epinephrine injections help reverse anaphylactic shock, but in persons taking a specific type of antihypertensive drug (i.e., nonselective beta blocker, such as pindolol), the epinephrine may not work very well and other measures often must be taken.

**Persons *not* in anaphylactic shock:** People taking pindolol who receive epinephrine for something other than anaphylactic shock are at risk of developing excessively high blood pressure levels. If the epinephrine is injected with the intention of systemic effects (i.e., reaching most of the tissues and organs in the body), the blood pressure may increase dramatically. If, however, the epinephrine is inhaled into the lungs, put in the eye, or injected for only local effects (e.g., by a dentist or dermatologist), the risk of a hypertensive reaction appears to be much less (unless a much larger than usual amount of epinephrine is used).

**Recomendation:** It is best for people who are at risk of anaphylactic shock (e.g., those allergic to bee stings) to avoid taking pindolol or other beta blockers.

Epinephrine (**Adrenalin**®, **Ana-Kit**®, **AsthmaHaler**®, **Bronkaid**® **Mist**, **EpiPen**®, **Primatene**® **Mist,**

Propranolol (**Inderal**®)

[for treatment of high blood pressure and angina; also used to prevent migraine headaches]

The outcome depends on the condition for which the patient is being treated, and on how the epinephrine is given.

**Persons with anaphylatcic shock:** Some pepole develop a severe, possibly life-threatening, allergic reaction (called anaphylactic shock) to insect stings or bites and certain medications or foods. Symptoms of anaphylactic shock include hives, wheezing, difficulty breathing, abdominal pain,

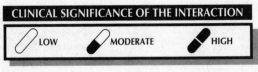

CLINICAL SIGNIFICANCE OF THE INTERACTION

LOW     MODERATE     HIGH

*(cont.)*
Epinephrine

**Sus-Phrine®, and others)**

Propranolol

incontinence, fever, and loss of consciousness; death may also occur. Epinephrine injections help reverse anaphylactic shock, but in persons taking a specific type of antihypertensive drug (i.e., nonselective beta blocker, such as propranolol), the epinephrine may not work very well and other measures often must be taken.

**Persons *not* in anaphylactic shock:** People taking propranolol who receive epinephrine for something other than anaphylactic shock are at risk of developing excessively high blood pressure levels. if the epinephrine is injected with the intention of systemic effects (i.e., reaching most of the tissues and organs in the body), the blood pressure may increase dramatically. If, however, the epinephrine is inhaled into the lungs, put in the eye, or injected for only local effects (e.g., by a dentist or dermatologist), the risk of a hypertensive reaction appears to be much less (unless a much larger than usual amount of epinephrine is used).

**Recommendation:** It is best for people who are at risk of anaphylactic shock (e.g., those allergic to bee stings) to avoid taking propranolol or other beta blockers.

---

Epinephrine
**(Adrenalin®, Ana-Kit®, AsthmaHaler®, Bronkaid® Mist, EpiPen®, Primatene® Mist, Sus-Phrine®, and others)**

Timolol **(Blocadren®)**

[for treatment of high blood pressure; in persons who have had a heart attack, this drug is used to reduce the likelihood of suffering from a second heart attack]

The outcome depends on the condition for which the patient is being treated, and on how the epinephrine is given.

**Persons with anaphylactic shock:** Some people develop a severe, possibly life-threatening, allergic reaction (called anaphylactic shock) to insect stings or bites and certain medications or foods. Symptoms of anaphylactic shock include hives, wheezing, difficulty breathing, abdominal pain, incontinence, fever, and loss of consciousness; death may also occur. Epinephrine injections help reverse

| ASTHMA DRUG | INTERACTING DRUG | RESULT |
|---|---|---|

*(cont.)*

**Epinephrine** — Timolol

anaphylactic shock, but in persons taking a specific type of antihypertensive drug (i.e., nonselective beta blocker, such as timolol), the epinephrine may not work very well and other measures often must be taken.

**Persons *not* in anaphylactic shock:** People taking timolol who receive epinephrine for something other than anaphylactic shock are at risk of developing excessively high blood pressure levels. If the epinephrine is injected with the intention of systemic effects (i.e., reaching most of the tissues and organs in the body), the blood pressure may increase dramatically. If, however, the epinephrine is inhaled into the lungs, put in the eye, or injected for only local effects (e.g., by a dentist or dermatologist), the risk of a hypertensive reaction appears to be much less (unless a much larger than usual amount of epinephrine is used).

**Recommendation:** It is best for people who are at risk of anaphylactic shock (e.g., those allergic to beestings) to avoid taking timolol or other beta blockers.

---

**Epinephrine (Adrenalin®, Ana-Kit®, AsthmaHaler®, Bronkaid® Mist, EpiPen®, Primatene® Mist, Sus-Phrine®, and others)**

Tricyclic antidepressants:

- amitriptyline **(Elavil®, Endep®)**
- amoxapine **(Asendin®)**
- desipramine **(Pertofrane®, Norpramin®)**
- doxepin **(Adapin®, Sinequan®)**
- imipramine **(Janimine®, Tofranil®)**

Can lead to excessively high blood pressure levels, rapid heartbeat, or irregular heartbeat if the epinephrine is injected. This effect may also occur when epinephrine is injected into the subcutaneous tissues (e.g., for severe allergic reactions). Epinephrine inhaled or taken as eye drops is probably less likely to interact unless excessive epinephrine doses are used.

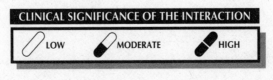

CLINICAL SIGNIFICANCE OF THE INTERACTION

LOW    MODERATE    HIGH

**(cont.)**
Epinephrine

Tricyclic antidepressants
- nortriptyline **(Aventyl®, Pamelor®)**
- protriptyline **(Vivactil®)**
- trimipramine **(Surmontil®)**

[for treatment of depression]

Although this interaction has been shown to occur with imipramine (Janimine®, Tofranil®), other tricyclic antidepressants (see list at left) are expected to act similarly when combined with epinephrine.

**Recommendation:** The benefit of using epinephrine may outweigh the risk of the interaction in some situations. Check with your doctor.

---

Hydrocortisone (oral) **(Cortef®, Hydrocortone®, Solu-Cortef®)**

Cholestyramine **(Questran®)**

[for the reduction of elevated cholestrol levels; also used to relieve severe itching associated with partial biliary obstruction]

Reduced effect of hydrocortisone due to reduced absorption of hydrocortisone into the body.

Although it has not been conclusively determined whether cholestyramine also reduces the effect of corticosteroids other than hydrocortisone, this should be considered a distinct possibility.

Colestipol (Colestid®) is similar to cholestyramine and might affect hydrocortisone in a similar way.

**Recommendation:** Take hydrocortisone at least two hours before or four hours after taking cholestyramine or colestipol.

---

Isoproterenol **(Isuprel®, Duo-Medihaler®,** and others)

Nadolol **(Corgard®)**

[for treatment of high blood pressure and angina]

Nadolol may reduce the bronchodilating effect of isoproterenol in asthmatic persons.

**Recommendation:** If possible, avoid the concurrent use of nadolol and isoproterenol.

Isoproterenol (**Isuprel®, Duo-Medihaler®,** and others)

Propranolol (**Inderal®**)

[for treatment of high blood pressure and angina; also used to prevent migraine headaches]

Propranolol may reduce the bronchodilating effect of isoproterenol in people with asthma. Other drugs in the same class as propranolol (known as beta blockers) may have a similar effect. Other beta blockers include acebutolol (Sectral®), atenolol (Tenormin®), betaxolol (Kerlone®), carteolol (Cartrol®), esmolol (Brevibloc®), labetalol (Normodyne®, Trandate®), metoprol (Lopressor®), nadolol (Corgard®), indolol (Visken®), and timolol (Blocadren®).

The nonselective beta blockers (i.e, Blocadren®, Cartrol®, Corgard®, Inderal®, and Visken®) are more likely to reduce the bronchodilating effect of isoproterenol than the selective beta blockers (i.e., Kerlone®, Lopressor®, Sectral®, or Tenormin®). Nonselective beta blockers tend to cause narrowing of the bronchi and should generally be avoided by persons with asthma.

Methylprednisolone (**Medrol®**)

Ketoconazole (**Nizoral®**)

[used to treat various fungal infections]

Ketoconazole may increase the amount of methylprednisolone in the blood, possibly leading to methylprednisolone toxicity. Symptoms of methylprednisolone toxicity include increased blood pressure, increased blood sugar, thinning of the bones (osteoporosis), muscle weakness, insomnia, stomach ulcers, and infection.

The effect of ketoconazole on other corticosteroids is not well established, but prednisolone may not be affected.

**CLINICAL SIGNIFICANCE OF THE INTERACTION**

 LOW   MODERATE   HIGH

| ASTHMA DRUG | INTERACTING DRUG | RESULT |
| --- | --- | --- |

Methylprednisolone **(Medrol®)**

Troleandomycin **(TAO®)**

[for treatment of upper and lower respiratory tract infections]

Troleandomycin significantly enhances the effect of methylprednisolone, possibly leading to methylprednisolone toxicity. Symptoms of methylprednisolone toxicity include increased blood pressure, increased blood sugar, thinning of the bones (osteoporosis), muscle weakness, insomnia, stomach ulcers, and infection (symptoms of infection include sore throat and fever).

---

Theophylline **(Primatene® Tablets, Slo-bid®, Theo-Dur®, Theo-24®, Uniphyl®, and others)**

Adenosine **(Adenocard®)**

[for treatment of certain types of arrhythmia (i.e, irregular heartbeat or heart rhythm)]

Theophylline may interfere with the effectiveness of adenosine to control arrhythmias. Your doctor may need to increase the dose of adenosine when these two drugs are taken together. (Do *not* change the dosage of either drug yourself; only your doctor should do this.)

---

Theophylline **(Primatene® Tablets, Slo-bid®, Theo-Dur®, Theo-24®, Uniphyl®, and others)**

Aminoglutethimide **(Cytadren®)**

[used to suppress adrenal function in certain persons with Cushing's syndrome]

May result in reduced amount of theophylline in the blood, possibly leading to a decreased effect (i.e., inadequate control of asthma).

**Recommendation:** Your doctor may need to adjust the dose of your theophylline if aminoglutethimide is started or stopped.

---

Theophylline

**Primatene® Tablets, Slo-bid®, Theo-Dur®, Theo-24®, Uniphyl®, and others**

Barbiturates:

- amobarbital **(Amytal®)**
- butabarbital **(Butisol®)**
- butalbital
- pentobarbital **(Nembutal®)**
- phenobarbital **(Luminal®, Solfoton®)**

Barbiturates may reduce the effectiveness of theophylline.

It may be necessary for your doctor to adjust the dose of theophylline if a barbiturate is started or stopped, or if its dosage is changed. (Of course, only your doctor should change medication dosages, when appropriate.)

| ASTHMA | INTERACTING DRUG | RESULT |
|---|---|---|

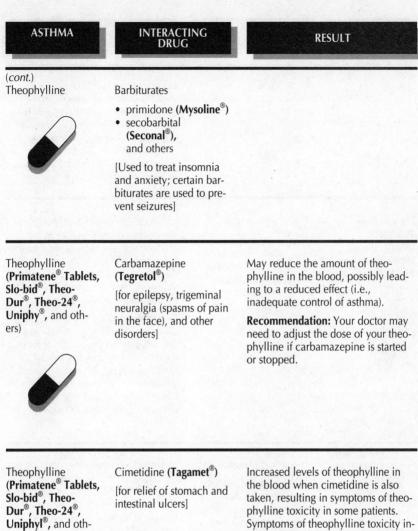

(*cont.*)
Theophylline

Barbiturates

- primidone (**Mysoline**®)
- secobarbital
  (**Seconal**®),
  and others

[Used to treat insomnia
and anxiety; certain bar-
biturates are used to prevent seizures]

---

Theophylline
(**Primatene**® **Tablets,
Slo-bid**®**, Theo-
Dur**®**, Theo-24**®**,
Uniphy**®**, and oth-
ers)

Carbamazepine
(**Tegretol**®)

[for epilepsy, trigeminal
neuralgia (spasms of pain
in the face), and other
disorders]

May reduce the amount of theophylline in the blood, possibly leading to a reduced effect (i.e.,
inadequate control of asthma).

**Recommendation:** Your doctor may
need to adjust the dose of your theophylline if carbamazepine is started
or stopped.

---

Theophylline
(**Primatene**® **Tablets,
Slo-bid**®**, Theo-
Dur**®**, Theo-24**®**,
Uniphyl**®**, and oth-
ers)

Cimetidine (**Tagamet**®)

[for relief of stomach and
intestinal ulcers]

Increased levels of theophylline in
the blood when cimetidine is also
taken, resulting in symptoms of theophylline toxicity in some patients.
Symptoms of theophylline toxicity include nausea, vomiting, diarrhea,
headache, irritability, restlessness,
nervousness, rapid heartbeat, insomnia, tremor, and seizure.

Your doctor may need to adjust the
amount of theophylline in your blood
if you begin or discontinue taking
cimetidine or if the dose of cimetidine changes. (Do *not* change the
dosage of either drug yourself; only
your doctor should do this.)

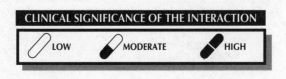

| CLINICAL SIGNIFICANCE OF THE INTERACTION | | |
|---|---|---|
| LOW | MODERATE | HIGH |

| ASTHMA DRUG | INTERACTING DRUG | RESULT |
|---|---|---|
| (cont.) Theophylline | Cimetidine | **Recommendation:** Your doctor should monitor the amount of theophylline in your blood after you have begun cimetidine therapy. You may wish to ask your doctor about similar drugs—ranitidine (Zantac®) or famotidine (Pepcid®)—which are less likely to interact with theophylline. |
| Theophylline (**Primatene® Tablets, Slo-bid®, Theo-Dur®, Theo-24®, Uniphyl®,** and others) | Ciprofloxacin (**Cipro®**) [for the treatment of various infections, including urinary tract and lower respiratory infections] | Increased amount of theophylline in the blood, possibly leading to theophylline toxicity; signs of such toxicity include nausea, vomiting, diarrhea, headache, irritability, nervousness, rapid heartbeat, insomnia, tremor, and seizure. **Recommendation:** A similar drug, ofloxacin (Floxin®)**,** is unlikely to affect theophylline; your doctor may wish to use this drug in place of ciprofloxacin. If ciprofloxacin is used, your doctor may need to adjust the dose of your theophylline when ciprofloxacin is started or stopped. |
| Theophylline (**Primatene® Tablets, Slo-bid®, Theo-Dur®, Theo-24®, Uniphyl®,** and others) | Disulfiram (**Antabuse®**) [used as an aid in the mangement of alcoholism for persons who want to remain sober] | Increased amount of theophylline in the blood, possibly leading to theophylline toxicity; signs of toxicity include nausea, vomiting, diarrhea, headache, irritability, nervousness, rapid heartbeat, insomnia, tremor, and seizure. **Recommendation:** Your doctor may need to adjust the theophylline dose when disulfiram is started or stopped. |
| Theophylline (**Primatene® Tablets, Slo-bid®,** | Erythromycin (**E-Mycin®, Ilosone®, Robimycin®, Wyamycin® S,** and others) [an antibiotic used to treat upper and lower respiratory infections, such as pneumonia and whooping cough; also | Erythromycin may increase the amount of theophylline in the blood. Although most people do not seem to have much trouble with this interaction, some develop theophylline toxicity. Symptoms of theophylline toxicity include nausea, vomiting, diarrhea, headache, irritability, nervousness, rapid heartbeat, insomnia, and tremor. |

(*cont.*)
Theophylline

**Theo-Dur®, Theo-24®, Uniphy®, and others)**

Erythromycin

[used to treat other infections, such as syphilis, in individuals allergic to penicillin]

In serious cases, seizure can occur.

The effect is usually delayed so that theophylline concentrations start to rise after five to seven days of treatment with erythromycin.

This is a *double* interaction, causing (1) an increased effect of the theophylline, with symptoms mentioned above, and (2) a decreased effect of the erythromycin.

**Recommendation:** Some doctors prefer to avoid giving erythromycin to people taking theophylline, while others advise their patients to watch for symptoms of theophylline toxicity. Those who advise the latter should probably monitor theophylline blood levels.

---

Theophylline **(Primatene® Tablets, Slo-bid®, Theo-Dur®, Theo-24®, Uniphyl®, and others)**

Isoniazid **(INH®, Laniazid®, Rifamate®)**

[for the prevention of tuberculosis; give in combination with other medications to treat tuberculosis]

May cause an increase in the amount of theophylline in the blood, possibly leading to theophylline toxicity; signs of such toxicity include nausea, vomiting, diarrhea, headache, irritability, nervousness, rapid heartbeat, insomnia, tremor, and seizure.

**Recommendation:** Your doctor may need to adjust your theophylline dose if isoniazid is started or stopped.

---

Theophylline

Lithium **(Cibalith-S®, Eskalith®, Lithane®, Lithobid®, and others)**

[for manic-depressive disorder]

Reduced effect of the lithium in some persons. In these individuals, your doctor may need to increase the dosage of your lithium. (Do *not* change the dosage of either drug yourself; only your doctor should do this.)

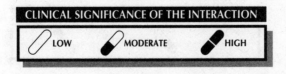

CLINICAL SIGNIFICANCE OF THE INTERACTION

LOW   MODERATE   HIGH

133

| ASTHMA DRUG | INTERACTING DRUG | RESULT |
|---|---|---|

(cont.)
Theophylline

(**Primatene® Tablets, Slo-bid®, Theo-Dur®, Theo-24®, Uniphyl®**, and others)

Lithium

This interaction is also important in individuals on long-term lithium therapy who intermittently use theophylline preparations.

---

Theophylline (**Primatene® Tablets, Slo-bid®, Theo-Dur®, Theo-24®, Uniphyl®**, and others)

Mexiletine (**Mexitil®**)

[used to correct irregular heartbeat]

Elevated amount of theophylline in the blood, possibly leading to theophylline toxicity. Signs of toxicity include nausea, vomiting, diarrhea, headache, irritability, rapid heart rate, insomnia, tremor, and seizure.

**Recommendation:** Your doctor may need to adjust your theophylline dose if mexiletine is started or stopped.

---

Theophylline (**Primatene® Tablets, Slo-bid®, Theo-Dur®, Theo-24®, Uniphyl®**, and others)

Phenytoin (**Dilantin®**)

[for the prevention of seizures]

Decreased amount of theophylline in the blood, possibly leading to a decreased effect of theophylline (i.e., inadequate control of asthma).

**Recommendation:** Your doctor may need to adjust your theophylline dose if phenytoin is started or stopped.

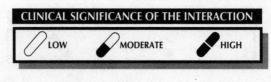

CLINICAL SIGNIFICANCE OF THE INTERACTION

LOW    MODERATE    HIGH

| ASTHMA DRUG | INTERACTING DRUG | RESULT |
| --- | --- | --- |
| Theophylline (**Primatene® Tablets, Slo-bid®, Theo-Dur®, Theo-24®, Uniphyl®**, and others)  | Propranolol (**Inderal®**) [for treatment of high blood pressure and angina; also used to prevent migraine headaches] | Increased amount of theophylline in the blood, possibly leading to toxicity. Symptoms of theophylline toxicity include nausea, vomiting, diarrhea, headache, irritability, nervousness, rapid heartbeat, insomnia, tremor, and seizure. **Recommendation:** Since propranolol (Inderal®) and other nonselective beta blockers (e.g., Blocadren®, Cartrol®, Corgard®, and Visken®) tend to cause narrowing of the bronchi, they should generally be avoided by persons with asthma. |
| Theophylline (**Primatene® Tablets, Slo-bid®, Theo-Dur®, Theo-24®, Uniphyl®**, and others)  | Radioactive iodine ($I^{131}$) [used to treat an overactive thyroid] | Could result in theophylline toxicity, signs of which include nausea, vomiting, diarrhea, headache, irritability, nervousness, rapid heartbeat, insomnia, tremor, and seizure. |
| Theophylline (**Primatene® Tablets, Slo-bid®, Theo-Dur®, Theo-24®, Uniphyl®**, and others)  | Rifampin (**Rifadin®, Rifamate®, Rimactane®**) [used in combination with at least one other drug, rifampin is used to treat tuberculosis; also used in the treatment of individuals who are carriers of meningitis] | Decreased amount of theophylline in the blood, possibly leading to a decreased effect (i.e., inadequate control of asthma). **Recommendation:** Your doctor may need to adjust your theophylline dose if rifampin is started or stopped. |

| ASTHMA DRUG | INTERACTING DRUG | RESULT |
|---|---|---|

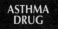

**Theophylline (Primatene® Tablets, Slo-bid®, Theo-Dur®, Theo-24®, Uniphyl®, and others)**

Cigarette smoking

Smoking leads to a decrease in the amount of theophylline in the blood, possibly leading to a reduced effect (i.e., inadequate control of asthma).

**Recommendation:** If you are a smoker, your doctor may prescribe a larger dose of theophylline for you (compared with a nonsmoker) to achieve the same effect. (Do *not* change the dosage of theophylline yourself; only your doctor should do this.)

**Theophylline (Primatene® Tablets, Slo-bid®, Theo-Dur®, Theo-24®, Uniphyl®, and others)**

**Thiabendazole (Mintezol®)**

[for treatment of parasitic worms, such as threadworms and trichinosis]

Can lead to a substantial increase in the amount of theophylline in the blood. Theophylline toxicity may result; symptoms include nausea, vomiting, diarrhea, headache, irritability, rapid heartbeat, insomnia, tremor, and seizure.

**Recommendation:** Your doctor may need to adjust your theophylline dose if thiabendazole is started or stopped.

**Theophylline (Primatene® Tablets, Slo-bid®, Theo-Dur®, Theo-24®, Uniphyl®, and others)**

Troleandomycin **(TAO®)**

[for treatment of upper and lower respiratory tract infections]

Increased amount of theophylline in the blood, possibly leading to theophylline toxicity. Symptoms include nausea, vomiting, diarrhea, headache, irritability, nervousness, rapid heartbeat, insomnia, tremor, and seizure.

**Recommendation:** Your doctor may need to adjust your theophylline dose if troleandomycin is started or stopped.

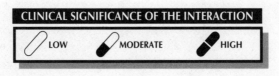

CLINICAL SIGNIFICANCE OF THE INTERACTION

LOW    MODERATE    HIGH

Theophylline (**Primatene® Tablets, Slo-bid®, Theo-Dur®, Theo-24®, Uniphyl®,** and others)

Verapamil (**Calan®, Isoptin®, Verelan®**)

[for treatment of high blood pressure and angina]

Verapamil may increase the amount of theophylline in the blood, possibly leading to theophylline toxicity (symptoms include nausea, vomiting, diarrhea, headache, irritability, nervousness, rapid heartbeat, insomnia, tremor, and seizure).

Other antihypertensive drugs in this class—diltiazem (Cardizem®) and nifedipine (Adalat®, Procardia®)—are less likely to increase theophylline concentrations, and may do so in only a small percentage of persons.

**Recommendation:** It may be necessary for your doctor to adjust the dose of theophylline if verapamil is started or stopped, or if its dosage is changed. (Of course, only your doctor should change medication dosage, when appropriate.)

## CHAPTER 5

# DRUGS FOR STOMACH AND INTESTINAL PROBLEMS

Although the gastrointestinal tract includes organs such as the mouth, esophagus ("food pipe" carrying food from the mouth to the stomach), stomach, small and large intestines, liver, pancreas, and gallbladder, this chapter will focus primarily on the stomach and intestines. The stomach secretes digestive juices that help turn solid food into a thick souplike paste. The contents of the stomach are then emptied into the small intestine, where most of the nutrients from the food are absorbed into the bloodstream. Most of the water in food is absorbed in the large intestine.

The main food-digesting juices secreted by the lining of the stomach are hydrochloric acid and a chemical known as pepsinogen. Hydrochloric acid converts pepsinogen into the active form called pepsin. Pepsin is an enzyme—a protein that speeds up a chemical reaction in the body—that aids in the digestion of proteins from food. Acid without pepsin has little digestive power.[1,2] The stomach is protected from its own corrosive acid by a layer of mucus.

Although the digestive system is amazingly efficient, malfunctions do arise. One of the possible problems faced by more than 25 million Americans[3] is an *ulcer,* an open sore or crater in the lining of the stomach or the duodenum, the first part of the small intestine. Researchers speculate that when the stomach secretes an excessive amount of acid (and it's not entirely clear why this happens), the protective mucous layer is eaten away at one spot. This area is now vulnerable to the stomach's lining. Not everyone with ulcers, however, has excess acid, so other factors appear to be involved as well.

A *gastric* ulcer develops in the stomach; as its name implies, a *duodenal* ulcer develops in the duodenum, which is a more common site for ulcers than the stomach.[4] *Peptic* ulcer is a general term, referring to an ulcer in the stomach, duodenum, or esophagus.

## The Development of an Ulcer

Excessive production of stomach acid is thought to increase the risk of developing a duodenal ulcer. Gastric ulcer, however, is *not* thought to be related to excessive acid secretion. Rather, many clinicians theorize that gastric ulcers are linked to a weakening in the resistance of the stomach's lining to its own digestive juices (what causes this decline is unknown).

Several reports indicate that the consumption of alcohol or caffeine may increase the flow of stomach acid. Use of certain analgesic drugs, known as non-steroidal anti-inflammatory drugs (such as aspirin, ibuprofen, indomethacin, and naproxen, to name a few), has been linked to ulcers. Prolonged use of these medications taken in high doses can damage the lining of the stomach.

Another factor that many reports associate with ulcer is the presence of a bacterium, *Helicobacter pylori* (formerly named Campylobacter), in the stomach or small intestine. Researchers have found that when they kill this bacterium with antibiotics, they may be able to cure a chronic, protracted ulcer.[5] Whether the bacterium is actually the cause of the ulcer or simply must be present, along with other factors, for the ulcer to develop, continues to be debated. The link between this bacterium and ulcer is still unclear; many individuals carry these bacteria in their stomach, yet do not develop any symptoms. It's possible that only certain strains of this bacterium can produce illness.

In the beginning stage, an ulcer often causes discomfort similar to indigestion. As the ulcer progresses, pain may follow. Food often relieves the pain of a duodenal ulcer by buffering, or neutralizing, the excess acid. With gastric ulcers, however, food aggravates the pain in approximately 50 percent of cases.[6] (In fact, many gastric-ulcer sufferers lose weight, even becoming anorectic, because of the abdominal pain that often follows eating.) If the ulcer progresses, it can cause bleeding—if the hole is deep enough and strikes a blood vessel—which can become life-threatening.

Not all ulcers, however, are painful. Some of them are "silent" and do not cause any symptoms, such as pain. The number of people with silent ulcer is not clear, but one study indicated that approximately one third of persons with acute gastrointestinal bleeding suffer from silent ulcer.[7] Silent ulcers are particularly dangerous because early warning signs are absent; as a result, a life-threatening bleeding episode may be the first sign that something is wrong.

## Medications Used to Treat or Prevent Ulcers

Several medications are available to treat ulcers. Most of these medications work by counteracting the effect of the stomach's acid. One group of drugs—known as histamine receptor inhibitors (also called $H_2$-receptor antagonists)—work by inhibiting the stomach's ability to produce acid. Commonly used drugs in this class include cimetidine (Tagamet®), ranitidine (Zantac®), and famotidine (Pepcid®). Another drug, sucralfate (Carafate®), works in a different way—by forming a protecting coating in the stomach and duodenum. This coating creates a barrier between a duodenal ulcer and further acid attack so that healing of the ulcer is promoted (similar to the way a bandage protects a wound from further damage). Antacids work by neutralizing hydrochloric acid. When an antacid is used for ulcers, it should be only under a doctor's supervision.

A medication that dramatically suppresses the secretion of stomach acid is omeprazole (Prilosec®). Omeprazole works by deactivating the enzyme that pumps acid (hydrogen ions) into the stomach. Omeprazole is used in the short-term treatment of duodenal ulcers. It is particularly useful in treating ulcers that do not respond to standard therapy with a histamine-receptor inhibitor. This medication has been used to treat symptoms of *gastrinoma*, a condition in which a tumor produces a hormone causing the stomach to secrete acid. Other conditions that respond to this drug are *erosive esophagitis* and *gastroesophageal reflux* disease—both disorders involve acid seeping from the stomach into the esophagus. The acid eats through the lining of the esophagus, resulting in severe pain and heartburn.

The role of diet in the management of ulcer therapy remains controversial, although most experts claim that ulcer patients need not be on a restricted diet. As mentioned earlier, because some reports indicate that caffeine and alcohol may increase the stomach's secretion of acid, consumption of these should be limited. If you smoke, you should stop. A substantial amount of evidence indicates that ulcers heal more slowly—and recur more frequently—in cigarette smokers than in nonsmokers.

# Inflammatory Bowel Disease

A group of chronic inflammatory disorders involving the gastrointestinal tract is known as *inflammatory bowel disease* (IBD). IBD is often divided into two groups of diseases: ulcerative colitis and Crohn's disease. Individuals with ulcerative colitis typically suffer from bloody diarrhea, abdominal pain, and cramps. Sufferers of Crohn's disease have similar symptoms, but the diarrhea is often without blood and these individuals may complain of general fatigue. Crohn's disease may involve different portions of the intestine, and symptoms typically vary depending on which portion is affected. The bowel often develops a thickened wall and narrowed lumen (i.e., the hollow space through which the digested food passes) in Crohn's disease, sometimes to the extent that the flow of intestinal contents is obstructed. Drug treatment for ulcerative colitis and Crohn's disease consists mainly of sulfasalazine (Azulfidine®) and corticosteroids (see Chapter 8 for more information on corticosteroids).

Another gastrointestinal illness sounds like IBD, but is far more common. The abbreviation—IBS—almost begs confusion with the more serious IBD. But these letters stand for *irritable bowel syndrome,* a disorder that sends millions of patients to a physician each year. Symptoms of IBS may include abdominal cramping, diarrhea or constipation (sometimes the two alternate in the same individual), excessive gas, and passage of mucus.

Irritable bowel syndrome tends to be difficult to treat, and several different classes of drugs have been used to relieve it. These include antispasmotic medications, which contain atropinelike drugs (e.g., bellafoline combined with phenobarbital [Belladenal®] and chlordiazepoxide combined with clidinium [Librax®]), as well as antidiarrheal agents such as loperamide (Imodium®), diphenoxylate (Lomotil®), and difenoxin (Motofen®), which inhibit contraction of the intestines. Antidepressants (see Chapter 9) may be useful in the treatment of IBS. Short-term use of opiates (see Chapter 1) in low doses has been helpful for some individuals with severe diarrhea resulting from IBS.

| GASTROINTESTINAL DRUG | INTERACTING DRUG | RESULT |
|---|---|---|

Cimetidine **(Tagamet®)**

Alcohol

Cimetidine may produce a small increase in blood alcohol concentrations (resulting in a greater degree of intoxication) under certain circumstances. Other antiulcer $H_2$-antagonist drugs include famotidine (Pepcid®), nizatidine (Axid®), and ranitidine (Zantac®). Although some evidence suggests that ranitidine slightly increases blood alcohol levels, most studies suggest that ranitidine has little or no effect on alcohol. Little information is available on nizatidine, but it may have less effect than cimetidine. Famotidine does not appear to affect blood alcohol levels.

**Recommendation:** Persons taking any of the antiulcer $H_2$-antagonist drugs would do well to avoid alcohol because alcohol may worsen most of the diseases for which these drugs are used (e.g., peptic ulcers, esophagitis, etc.). If alcohol is used with these drugs, be alert for the possibility that you may get a little more effect from the alcohol than you expect. This effect of enhanced intoxication occurs only in certain persons taking this combination.

---

Cimetidine **(Tagamet®)**

Alprazolam **(Xanax®)** [for treatment of anxiety]

Cimetidine may increase the plasma concentration of alprazolam, which could lead to an increased effect as evidenced by decreased alertness, an impaired ability to concentrate, dizziness, incoordination, forgetfulness, and drowsiness.

**Recommendation:** If you must take a benzodiazepine (i.e., a type of drug such as alprazolam) for the treatment of anxiety while you are taking cimetidine, your doctor may need to monitor your response to the antianxiety medication more carefully than usual. Two antianxiety benzodiazepines that do not appear to be affected by cimetidine are lorazepam (Ativan®) and oxazepam (Serax®).

Another way to reduce the risk of this interaction is to use ranitidine (Zantac®)

| GASTROINTESTINAL DRUG | INTERACTING DRUG | RESULT |
|---|---|---|

*(cont.)*
Cimetidine

Alprazolam

or famotidine (Pepcid®) rather than cimetidine; they are probably less likely to interact with benzodiazepines than cimetidine.

---

Cimetidine **(Tagamet®)**

Amiodarone **(Cordarone®)**

[for life-threatening arrhythmias—irregularities of the heartbeat and heart rhythm—of the ventricles (lower heart chambers)]

May result in an increased concentration of amiodarone. If the amount of amiodarone in the blood reaches a high enough level, amiodarone toxicity could result, as shown by symptoms such as nausea, slowed heart rate, lightheadedness, sensitivity to light, fatigue, tremor, lack of coordination, and fainting.

This effect may not appear until several weeks after these two drugs are being taken concomitantly.

---

Cimetidine **(Tagamet®)**

Amitriptyline **(Elavil®, Endep®)**

[for treatment of depression]

Can result in an increased blood concentration of amitriptyline, possibly to a toxic level. Symptoms of amitriptyline toxicity include severe dry mouth, blurred vision, fast heartbeat, difficulty or inability to urinate, and constipation.

Amitriptyline is in a class of drug known as a tricyclic antidepressant. Other tricyclic antidepressants may be similarly affected by cimetidine. They include amoxapine (Asendin®), desipramine (Pertofrane®, Norpramin®), doxepin (Adapin®, Sinequan®), imipramine (Janimine®, Tofranil®), nortriptyline (Aventyl®, Pamelor®), protriptyline (Vivactil®), and trimipramine (Surmontil®).

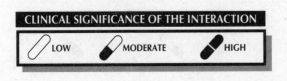

CLINICAL SIGNIFICANCE OF THE INTERACTION

LOW    MODERATE    HIGH

143

| GASTROINTESTINAL DRUG | INTERACTING DRUG | RESULT |
|---|---|---|

*(cont.)*

**Cimetidine** / **Amitriptyline**

**Recommendation:** It may be necessary for your doctor to adjust the dose of amitriptyline if cimetidine is started or stopped, or if its dosage is changed. (Of course, only your doctor should change medication dosages, when appropriate.)

Your doctor may choose to use ranitidine (Zantac®), famotidine (Pepcid®), or nizatidine (Axid®) instead of cimetidine, because they are less likely to interact.

---

**Cimetidine (Tagamet®)**

Anticoagulants (oral), such as dicumarol and wafarin **(Coumadin®, Panwarfin®)**

[for the prevention of blood clots]

May result in increased anticoagulant effect; some persons may develop bleeding, such as blood in urine, coughing up of blood, black stools (or red blood in stools), vomiting blood or substance resembling coffee grounds, bruising, or other bleeding.

This interaction is dose-related, which means larger doses of cimetidine (e.g., 800 mg or more daily) are more likely to interact with warfarin than smaller doses.

**Recommendation:** Avoid this combination. If you are taking warfarin and must use an antiulcer drug, discuss with your doctor whether you can take ranitidine (Zantac®), famotidine (Pepcid®), or nizatidine (Axid®); all of these antiulcer drugs are less likely to interact with warfarin than cimetidine (Tagamet®).

Your level of anticoagulation should be monitored by your doctor if you are taking both cimetidine and an anticoagulant.

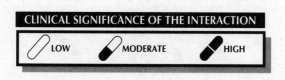

CLINICAL SIGNIFICANCE OF THE INTERACTION

LOW    MODERATE    HIGH

Cimetidine
**(Tagamet®)**

Carbamazepine
**(Tegretol®)**

[for epilepsy, trigeminal neuralgia (spasms of pain in the face), and other disorders]

Persons receiving carbamazepine who then begin taking cimetidine may experience higher concentrations of carbamazepine for about one week, which could lead to an increased effect during this time period.

High concentrations of carbamazepine can lead to symptoms such as dizziness, drowsiness, nausea, vomiting, twitching, and blurred vision. These symptoms may occur after the first few days of taking cimetidine if you are already taking carbamazepine.

**Recommendation:** If you must take cimetidine and are already receiving carbamazepine, be alert for the presence of the symptoms mentioned above and discuss them with your doctor. Ranitidine (Zantac®), and probably famotidine (Pepcid®) and nizatidine (Axid®), probably do not cause this problem.

If cimetidine is used, your doctor may monitor carbamazepine blood levels for several days after initiating cimetidine therapy.

Cimetidine
**(Tagamet®)**

Carmustine **(BiCNU®)**

[for cancer therapy]

Carmustine is a powerful drug; one of its adverse effects is the suppression of bone marrow. Since bone marrow is one of the places where leukocytes—a type of white blood cell needed to ward off infection—are produced, suppression of bone marrow can lead to infection. Cells in the bone marrow also manufacture platelets, substances required for blood clotting.

Cimetidine may enhance carmustine's ability to suppress the activity of bone marrow cells, and thus, can increase the risk of developing an infection or bleeding.

**Recommendation:** Your doctor may need to check for excessive effects of carmustine if cimetidine is used concurrently.

| GASTROINTESTINAL DRUG | INTERACTING DRUG | RESULT |
|---|---|---|

Cimetidine
**(Tagamet®)**

Chlordiazepoxide
**(Librium®)**

[for treatment of anxiety]

Cimetidine may increase the plasma concentraton of chlordiazepoxide, which could lead to an increased effect as evidenced by decreased alertness, an impaired ability to concentrate, dizziness, incoordination, forgetfulness, and drowsiness.

This interaction may be more severe in elderly persons or in iidividuals with liver disease, who are more sensitive to the action of chlordiazepoxide.

**Recommendation:** If you must take a benzodiazepine (i.e., a type of drug such as chlordiazepoxide) for the treatment of anxiety while you are taking cimetidine, your doctor may need to monitor your response to the antianxiety medication more carefully than usual. Two antianxiety benzodiazepines that do not appear to be affected by cimetidine are lorazepam (Ativan®) and oxazepam (Serax®).

Another way to reduce the risk of this interaction is to use ranitidine (Zantac®) or famotidine (Pepcid®) rather than cimetidine; they are probably less likely to interact with benzodiazepines than cimetidine.

Cimetidine
**(Tagamet®)**

Chloroquine **(Aralen®)**

[used in the treatment of malaria]

Cimetidine may increase blood chloroquine concentrations, which may increase the risk of chloroquine toxicity. Symptoms of chloroquine toxicity can include blurred vision, lightheadedness, fainting, hearing loss, and muscle weakness. If any of these occur, see your doctor.

**Recommendation:** Your doctor may wish to substitute famotidine (Pepcid®), ranitidine (Zantac®), or nizatidine (Axid®) for cimetidine, since they may be less likely to interact with chloroquine.

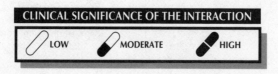

CLINICAL SIGNIFICANCE OF THE INTERACTION

LOW        MODERATE        HIGH

| GASTROINTESTINAL DRUG | INTERACTING DRUG | RESULT |
| --- | --- | --- |

Cimetidine **(Tagamet®)**

Clorazepate **(Tranxene®)**

[for treatment of anxiety]

Cimetidine may increase the plasma concentration of clorazepate, which could lead to an increased effect, such as decreased alertness, an impaired ability to concentrate, dizziness, incoordination, forgetfulness, and drowsiness.

This interaction may be more severe in elderly persons, who are more sensitive to the action of clorazepate.

**Recommendation:** If you must take a benzodiazepine (i.e., a type of drug such as clorazepate) for the treatment of anxiety while you are taking cimetidine, your doctor may need to monitor your response to the antianxiety medication more carefully than usual. Two antianxiety benzodiazepines that do not appear to be affected by cimetidine are lorazepam (Ativan®) and oxazepam (Serax®).

Another way to reduce the risk of this interaction is to use ranitidine (Zantac®) or famotidine (Pepcid®) rather than cimetidine; they are probably less likely to interact with benzodiazepines than cimetidine.

Cimetidine **(Tagemet®)**

Desipramine **(Pertofrane®, Norpramin®)**

[for treatment of depression]

Can result in an increased blood concentration of desipramine, possibly to a toxic level. Symptoms of desipramine toxicity include severe dry mouth, blurred vision, fast heartbeat, difficulty or inability to urinate, and constipation.

Desipramine is in a class of drug known as a tricyclic antidepressant. Other tricyclic antidepressants may be similarly affected by cimetidine. They include amitriptyline (Elavil®, Endep®), amoxapine (Asendin®), doxepin (Adapin®, Sinequan®), imipramine (Janimine®, Tofranil®), nortriptyline (Aventyl®, Pamelor®), protriptyline (Vivactil®), and trimipramine (Surmontil®).

**Recommendation:** It may be necessary for your doctor to adjust the

147

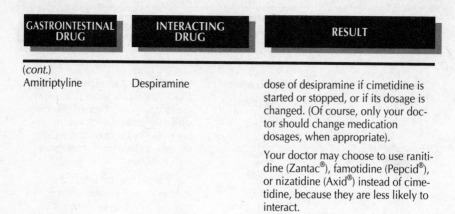

*(cont.)*
Amitriptyline          Despiramine

dose of desipramine if cimetidine is started or stopped, or if its dosage is changed. (Of course, only your doctor should change medication dosages, when appropriate).

Your doctor may choose to use ranitidine (Zantac®), famotidine (Pepcid®), or nizatidine (Axid®) instead of cimetidine, because they are less likely to interact.

Cimetidine (**Tagamet**®)

Diazepam (**Valium**®)

[for treatment of anxiety]

Cimetidine may increase the plasma concentration of diazepam, which could lead to an increased effect as evidenced by decreased alertness, an impaired ability to concentrate, dizziness, incoordination, forgetfulness, and drowsiness.

This interaction may be more severe in elderly persons or in individuals with liver disease, who are more sensitive to the action of diazepam.

**Recommendation:** If you must take a benzodiazepine (a type of drug such as diazepam) for the treatment of anxiety while you are taking cimetidine, your doctor may need to monitor your response to the antianxiety medication more carefully than usual. Two antianxiety benzodiazepines that do not appear to be affected by cimetidine are lorazepam (Ativan®) and oxazepam (Serax®).

Another way to reduce the risk of this interaction is to use ranitidine (Zantac®) or famotidine (Pepcid®) rather than cimetidine; they are probably less likely to interact with benzodiazepines than cimetidine.

**CLINICAL SIGNIFICANCE OF THE INTERACTION**

LOW        MODERATE        HIGH

Cimetidine (**Tagamet**®)

Diltiazem (**Cardizem**®, **Cardizem SR**®, **Cardizem CD**®)

[for treatment of angina or hypertension]

Cimetidine may cause increased diltiazem blood levels, possibly leading to diltiazem toxicity (symptoms include low blood pressure, dizziness, and flushing).

**Recommendation:** It may be necessary for your doctor to adjust the dose of diltiazem if cimetidine is started, stopped, or changed in dosage. (Of course, only your doctor should change medication dosage, when appropriate.)

Cimetidine (**Tagamet**®)

**Doxepin** (Adapin®, Sinequan®)

[for treatment of depression]

Can result in an increased blood concentration of doxepin, possibly to a toxic level. Symptoms of doxepin toxicity include severe dry mouth, blurred vision, fast heartbeat, difficulty or inability to urinate, and constipation.

Doxepin is in a class of drug known as a tricyclic antidepressant. Other tricyclic antidepressants may be similarly affected by cimetidine. They include amitriptyline (Elavil®, Endep®), amoxapine (Asendin®), despiramine (Pertofrane®, Norpramin®), imipramine (Janimine®, Tofranil®), nortriptyline (Aventyl®, Pamelor®), protriptyline (Vivactil®), and trimipramine (Surmontil®).

**Recommendation:** It may be necessary for your doctor to adjust the dose of doxepin if cimetidine is started or stopped, or if its dosage is changed. (Of course, only your doctor should change medication dosages, when appropriate).

Your doctor may choose to use ranitidine (Zantac®), famotidine (Pepcid®), or nizatidine (Axid®) instead of cimetidine, because they are less likely to interact.

| GASTROINTESTINAL DRUG | INTERACTING DRUG | RESULT |
|---|---|---|

Cimetidine **(Tagamet®)**

Flecainide **(Tambocor®)**

[for life-threatening arrhythmias—irregularities of the heartbeat and heart rhythm—of the ventricles (lower heart chambers)]

Cimetidine may increase the amount of flecainide in the blood. Flecainide toxicity may cause blurred vision, heart failure, or abnormal heart rhythms. Adverse effects of this interaction are more likely to occur in persons with impaired kidney function.

---

Cimetidine **(Tagamet®)**

Flurazepam **(Dalmane®)**

[for treatment of insomnia]

Cimetidine may cause an increase in the blood level of flurazepam, possibly leading to increased sedation, decreased alertness, an impaired ability to concentrate, forgetfulness, and drowsiness.

This interaction may be more severe in elderly persons.

**Recommendation:** If you must take cimetidine and a sleeping pill, temazepam (Restoril®), does not appear to be affected by cimetidine. Another alternative is to use the antiulcer drug ranitidine (Zantac®) or famotidine (Pepcid®) rather than cimetidine; they appear to be less likely to interact with flurazepam than cimetidine.

---

Cimetidine **(Tagamet®)**

Glipizide **(Glucotrol®)**

[for treatment of diabetes mellitus, a condition that results in abnormally high blood sugar levels]

Cimetidine may increase the blood level of glipizide, which may cause an excessively low blood sugar level (an excessive drop in blood sugar levels is undesirable). This may produce symptoms including cold sweats, trembling, and an increased heart rate.

This interaction may be caused by reducing the amount of acid in the stomach, so the same problem may be seen with other antiulcer drugs that decrease stomach acid, such as famotidine (Pepcid®), nizatidine (Axid®), ranitidine (Zantac®), omeprazole (Prilosec®), and antacids.

**Recommendation:** Diabetics taking glipizide should watch for any change in their sugar levels when cimetidine is started or discontinued.

| GASTROINTESTINAL DRUG | INTERACTING DRUG | RESULT |
|---|---|---|

*(cont.)*
Cimetidine      Glipizide

Sucralfate (Carafate®) may be a good alternative for diabetics with ulcers because preliminary reports suggest that this medication appears less likely to significantly change blood sugar levels. (Glipizide and sucralfate should be taken at different times to reduce the possibility of sucralfate binding with glipizide in the stomach. Separate doses of these two medication by several hours if possible.)

---

Cimetidine **(Tagamet®)**

Glyburide **(DiaBeta®, Micronase®)**

[for treatment of diabetes mellitus, a condition that results in abnormally high blood sugar levels]

Cimetidine may increase the blood level of glyburide, which may cause an excessively low blood sugar level (an excessive drop in blood sugar levels is undesirable). This may produce symptoms including cold sweats, trembling, and an increased heart rate.

This interaction may be caused by reducing the amount of acid in the stomach, so the same problem may be seen with other antiulcer drugs that decrease stomach acid, such as famotidine (Pepcid®), nizatidine (Axid®), ranitidine (Zantac®), omeprazole (Prilosec®), and antacids.

**Recommendation**: Diabetics taking glyburide should watch for any change in their sugar levels when cimetidine is started or discontinued. Sucralfate (Carafate®) may be a good alternative for diabetics with ulcers because preliminary reports suggest that this medication appears less likely to significantly change blood sugar levels. (Glyburide and sucralfate should be taken at different times to reduce the possibility of sucralfate binding with glyburide in the stomach. Separate doses of these two medications by several hours if possible.)

---

**CLINICAL SIGNIFICANCE OF THE INTERACTION**

LOW     MODERATE     HIGH

Cimetidine **(Tagamet®)**

Imipramine **(Janimine®, Tofranil®)**

[for treatment of depression]

Can result in an increased blood concentration of imipramine, possibly to a toxic level. Symptoms of imipramine toxicity include severe dry mouth, blurred vision, fast heartbeat, difficulty or inability to urinate, and constipation.

Imipramine is in a class of drug known as a tricyclic antidepressant. Other tricyclic antidepressants may be similarly affected by cimetidine. They include amitriptyline (Elavil®, Endep®), amoxapine (Asendin®), desipramine (Pertofrane®, Norpramin®), doxepin (Adapin®, Sinequan®), nortriptyline (Aventyl®, Pamelor®), protriptyline (Vivactil®), and trimipramine (Surmontil®).

**Recommendation:** It may be necessary for your doctor to adjust the dose of imipramine if cimetidine is started or stopped, or if its dosage is changed. (Of course, only your doctor should change medication dosages, when appropriate).

Your doctor may choose to use ranitidine (Zantac®), famotidine ), or nizatidine (Axid®) instead of cimetidine, because they are less likely to interact.

Cimetidine **(Tagamet®)**

Ketoconazole **(Nizoral®)**

[for treatment of various fungus infections]

Stomach acid is needed for the proper absorption (and thus effectiveness) of oral ketoconazole. Since cimetidine reduces the secretion of stomach acid, cimetidine tends to reduce the absorption of ketoconazole.

**Recommendation:** Your doctor may need to adjust the dosing times of these drugs so that the ketoconazole is given when the effect of cimetidine is low. Alternatively, the manufacturer of ketoconazole describes a method of dissolving the ketoconazole in a very mild acid before administration. Your doctor or pharmacist may help you with this.

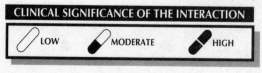

CLINICAL SIGNIFICANCE OF THE INTERACTION

LOW    MODERATE    HIGH

| GASTROINTESTINAL DRUG | INTERACTING DRUG | RESULT |
| --- | --- | --- |
| Cimetidine (Tagamet®)  | Labetalol (Normodyne®, Trandate®)<br><br>[for treatment of high blood pressure] | Increased levels of labetalol in the blood may result when cimetidine is also taken, possibly leading to an excessive reduction in blood pressure, slowed heart rate, and difficulty breathing. |
| Cimetidine (Tagamet®)  | Lidocaine (Xylocaine®)<br><br>[used to treat abnormal heart rhythms; for topical anesthesia during minor surgery; also available as an over-the-counter medication for topical use on skin to relieve pain, itching, and inflammation, but such topical use is unlikely to interact with cimetidine] | When lidocaine is used to treat heart arrhythmias, cimetidine can increase the concentration of lidocaine, possibly leading to lidocaine toxicity, symptoms of which include drowsiness, dizziness, confusion, numbness or tingling, nausea, visual disturbances, ringing in the ears, muscle twitching, tremor, and seizures.<br><br>**Recommendation:** Persons receiving lidocaine with cimetidine should have their blood level of lidocaine monitored by their doctor.<br><br>Ranitidine (Zantac®) may be a good alternative to cimetidine in persons who are receiving lidocaine because ranitidine has a minimal effect on lidocaine. |
| Cimetidine (Tagamet®) | Meperidine (Demerol®, Mepergan®)<br><br>[for relief of moderate to severe pain] | Cimetidine may increase the effect of meperidine, possibly leading to increased sedation and impaired breathing.<br><br>**Recommendation:** Since ranitidine (Zantac®) and probably famotidine (Pepcid®) and nizatidine (Axid®) appear less likely to interact with narcotic analgesics, such as meperidine, they may be preferable to cimetidine. |
| Cimetidine (Tagamet®)  | Metoprolol (Lopressor®)<br><br>[for treatment of high blood pressure, angina, and to reduce the rate of death in persons with suspected or definite heart attack] | Increased levels of metoprolol in the blood may result when cimetidine is also taken, possibly leading to an excessive reduction in blood pressure, slowed heart rate, and difficulty breathing. |

| GASTROINTESTINAL DRUG | INTERACTING DRUG | RESULT |
|---|---|---|

Cimetidine **(Tagamet®)**

Metronidazole **(Flagyl®, Metric 21®, Protostat®)**

[for treatment of certain bacterial infections]

Especially when the metronidazole is given orally or intravenously, could lead to increased serum levels of metronidazole, which could cause dizziness, vertigo (a sensation in which you feel as if you are revolving in space or your surroundings are revolving around you), nausea, numbness, and tingling.

---

Cimetidine **(Tagamet®)**

Moricizine **(Ethmozine®)**

[for the treatment of certain types of arrhythmias, i.e., irregularities of the heartbeat and heart rhythm]

May increase the amount of moricizine in the body, possibly leading to dizziness, nausea, vomiting, lethargy, palpitations, fainting, and excessively low blood pressure.

**Recommendation:** It may be necessary for your doctor to adjust the dose of moricizine if cimetidine is started or stopped, or if its dosage is changed. (Of course, only your doctor should change medication dosages, when appropriate.)

---

Cimetidine **(Tagamet®)**

Nifedipine **(Adalat®, Procardia®)**

[for treatment of angina and high blood pressure]

May increase the amount of nifedipine in the blood. Possible nifedipine toxicity—evidenced by symptoms such as dizziness, flushing, and headache—may occur.

---

Cimetidine **(Tagamet®)**

Nortriptyline **(Aventyl®, Pamelor®)**

[for treatment of depression]

Can result in an increased blood concentration of nortriptyline, possibly to a toxic level. Symptoms of nortriptyline toxicity include severe dry mouth, blurred vision, fast heartbeat, difficulty or inability to urinate, and constipation.

Nortriptyline is in a class of drug known as a tricyclic antidepressant. Other tricyclic antidepressants may be similarly affected by cimetidine. They include amitriptyline (Elavil®,

| GASTROINTESTINAL DRUG | INTERACTING DRUG | RESULT |
|---|---|---|

(*cont.*)
Cimetidine

Nortriptyline

Endep®), amoxapine (Asendin®), desipramine (Pertofrane®, Norpramin®), doxepin (Adapin®, Sinequan®), imipramine (Janimine®, Tofranil®), protriptyline (Vivactil®), and trimipramine (Surmontil®).

**Recommendation:** It may be necessary for your doctor to adjust the dose of nortriptyline if cimetidine is started or stopped, or if its dosage is changed. (Of course, only your doctor should change medication dosages, when appropriate).

Your doctor may choose to use ranitidine (Zantac®), famotidine (Pepcid®), or nizatidine (Axid®) instead of cimetidine, because they are less likely to interact.

Cimetidine **(Tagamet®)**

Phenytoin **(Dilantin®)**

[for the prevention of seizures]

Cimetidine increases the amount of phenytoin in the blood, possibly leading to phenytoin toxicity. Symptoms of phenytoin toxicity include rapid, involuntary eye movements, muscular incoordination, slurred speech, and confusion.

**Recommendation:** Be alert for symptoms of phenytoin toxicity when phenytoin is taken with cimetidine. Your doctor should monitor phenytoin blood levels when cimetidine therapy is initiated.

In persons who are stabilized on phenytoin and cimetidine, discontinuation of cimetidine may cause levels of phenytoin to drop, resulting in a decreased effect. Ranitidine (Zantac®) and famotidine (Pepsid®) appear less likely to interact with phenytoin in this way and would be preferable to cimetidine in most persons receiving phenytoin.

**CLINICAL SIGNIFICANCE OF THE INTERACTION**

LOW    MODERATE    HIGH

Cimetidine **(Tagamet®)**

Prazepam **(Centrax®)**

[for treatment of anxiety]

Cimetidine may increase the amount of prazepam in the blood, which could lead to an increased effect as evidenced by decreased alertness, an impaired ability to concentrate, dizziness, incoordination, forgetfulness, and drowsiness.

This interaction may be more severe in elderly persons, who are more sensitive to the action of prazepam.

**Recommendation:** If you must take a benzodiazepine (i.e., a type of drug such as prazepam) for the treatment of anxiety while you are taking cimetidine, your doctor may need to monitor your response to the antianxiety medication more carefully than usual. Two antianxiety benzodiazepines that do not appear to be affected by cimetidine are lorazepam (Ativan®) and oxazepam (Serax®).

Another way to reduce the risk of this interaction is to use ranitidine (Zantac®) or famotidine (Pepcid®) rather than cimetidine; they are probably less likely to interact with benzodiazepines than cimetidine.

---

Cimetidine **(Tagamet®)**

Procainamide **(Procan SR®, Pronestyl®)**

[for the treatment of ventricular arrhythmias (irregularities of the heartbeat and heart rhythm of the lower chambers of the heart)]

Cimetidine may increase the amount of procainamide in the blood, possibly leading to symptoms such as nausea, vomiting, malaise, weakness, lightheadedness, and palpitations.

**Recommendation:** Persons with kidney impairment probably should not take these two drugs together because cimetidine increases the amount of procainamide in the body by interfering with the kidney's ability to get rid of procainamide. Another antiulcer drug, ranitidine (Zantac®), causes a small increase in procainamide levels (smaller than that caused by the cimetidine-procainamide interaction). Famotidine (Pepsid®) does not appear to increase procainamide levels.

| GASTROINTESTINAL DRUG | INTERACTING DRUG | RESULT |
|---|---|---|

Cimetidine **(Tagamet®)**

Propranolol **(Inderal®)**

[for treatment of high blood pressure and angina; also used to prevent migraine headaches]

May increase the amount of propranolol in the blood when cimetidine is also taken, possibly leading to an excessive reduction in blood pressure, slowed heart rate, difficulty breathing, and cold hands and cold feet.

**Recommendation:** Be aware of this interaction when taking both cimetidine and propranolol. Another antiulcer drug, such as ranitidine (Zantac®), may be preferable when propranolol must be taken.

---

Cimetidine **(Tagamet®)**

Quinidine **(Cardioquin®, Duraquin®, Quinaglute®, Quinidex®, Quinora®)**

[for arrhythmias, or irregularities of the heartbeat and heart rhythm]

Cimetidine taken with quinidine can lead to an elevated concentration of quinidine in the blood. Notify your doctor if you observe signs such as ringing in your ears, vertigo (a sensation in which you feel as if you are revolving in space or your surroundings are revolving around you), dizziness, confusion, blurred vision, nausea, lightheadedness, fainting, and tremor.

**Recommendation:** It may be necessary for your doctor to adjust the dose of quinidine if cimetidine is started or stopped, or if its dosage is changed. (Of course, only your doctor should change medication dosages, when appropriate).

Another alternative is to use either the antiulcer drug ranitidine (Zantac®) or famotidine (Pepcid®) rather than cimetidine; they appear to be less likely to interact with quinidine than cimetidine.

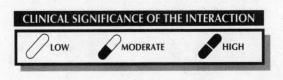

CLINICAL SIGNIFICANCE OF THE INTERACTION

LOW   MODERATE   HIGH

| GASTROINTESTINAL DRUG | INTERACTING DRUG | RESULT |
| --- | --- | --- |

Cimetidine
(**Tagamet**®)

Theophylline **(Theo-Dur**®, **Theo-24**®, **Slobid**®, **Slo-Phyllin**®, **Uniphyl**®, and others)

[for relief of asthma]

Increased levels of theophylline in the blood may result when cimetidine is also taken, causing symptoms of theophylline toxicity in some patients. These symptoms include nausea, vomiting, diarrhea, headache, irritability, restlessness, nervousness, rapid heartbeat, insomnia, tremor, and seizure.

Your doctor may need to adjust the amount of theophylline in your blood if you begin or discontinue taking cimetidine or if the dose of cimetidine changes. (Do *not* change the dosage of either drug yourself; only your doctor should do this.)

**Recommendation:** Your doctor should monitor the amount of theophylline in your blood after you have begun cimetidine therapy. You may wish to ask your doctor about other antiulcer drugs, such as ranitidine (Zantac®) or famotidine (Pepcid®), which are less likely to interact with theophylline.

Cimetidine
(**Tagamet**®)

Tolbutamide (**Orinase**®)

[for treatment of diabetes mellitus, a condition that results in abnormally high blood sugar levels]

Cimetidine can increase the amount of tolbutamide in the blood. It is not known whether this enhances the blood sugar–lowering effect of tolbutamide.

**Recommendation:** Diabetics taking tolbutamide should watch for any change in their sugar levels when cimetidine is started or discontinued. Sucralfate (Carafate®) may be a good alternative medication for diabetics with ulcers because preliminary reports suggest that this medication appears less likely to significantly change tolbutamide blood levels.

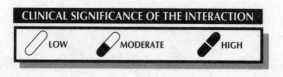

CLINICAL SIGNIFICANCE OF THE INTERACTION

LOW    MODERATE    HIGH

| GASTROINTESTINAL DRUG | INTERACTING DRUG | RESULT |
|---|---|---|

Cimetidine **(Tagamet®)**

Triazolam **(Halcion®)**

[for treatment of insomnia]

Cimetidine may cause an increased amount of triazolam in the blood, possibly leading to increased sedation, decreased alertness, an impaired ability to concentrate, forgetfulness, and drowsiness.

This interaction may be more severe in elderly persons who are more sensitive to the action of triazolam.

**Recommendation:** If you must take cimetidine and a sleeping pill, temazepam (Restoril®) does not appear to be affected by cimetidine. Another alternative is to use the antiulcer drug ranitidine (Zantac®) or famotidine (Pepcid®) rather than cimetidine; they appear to be less likely to interact with triazolam than cimetidine.

Cimetidine **(Tagamet®)**

Verapamil **(Calan®, Isoptin®)**

[for treatment of angina and high blood pressure]

May increase verapamil levels, possibly leading to toxicity. Symptoms of toxicity include excessive slowing of the heart rate, decreased blood pressure, headache, flushing, and edema (fluid accumulation).

Famotidine **(Pepcid®)**

Ketoconazole **(Nizoral®)**

[for the treatment of fungal infections]

Stomach acid is needed for the proper absorption (and thus effectiveness) of oral ketoconazole. Since famotidine reduces the secretion of stomach acid, famotidine is likely to reduce the absorption of ketoconazole.

**Recommendation:** Your doctor may need to adjust the dosing times of these drugs so that the ketoconazole is given when the effect of famotidine is low. Alternatively, the manufacturer of ketoconazole describes a method of dissolving the ketoconazole in a very mild acid before administration. Your doctor or pharmacist may help you with this.

| GASTROINTESTINAL DRUG | INTERACTING DRUG | RESULT |
|---|---|---|

Nizatidine (**Axid**®)

Ketoconazole (**Nizoral**®)

[for the treatment of fungal infections]

Stomach acid is needed for the proper absorption (and thus effectiveness) of oral ketoconazole. Since nizatidine reduces the secretion of stomach acid, nizatidine is likely to reduce the absorption of ketoconazole.

**Recommendation:** Your doctor may need to adjust the dosing times of these drugs so that the ketoconazole is given when the effect of nizatidine is low. Alternatively, the manufacturer of ketoconazole describes a method of dissolving the ketoconazole in a very mild acid before administration. Your doctor or pharmacist may help you with this.

Omeprazole (**Prilosec**®)

Ketoconazole (**Nizoral**®)

[for the treatment of fungal infections]

Stomach acid is needed for the proper absorption (and thus effectiveness) of oral ketoconazole. Since omeprazole reduces the secretion of stomach acid, omeprazole is likely to reduce the absorption of ketoconazole.

**Recommendation:** The manufacturer of ketoconazole describes a method of dissolving the ketoconazole in a very mild acid before administration. Your doctor or pharmacist may help you with this.

Omeprazole (**Prilosec**®)

Phenytoin (**Dilantin**®)

[for the prevention of seizures]

Omeprazole taken with phenytoin may lead to increased plasma levels of phenytoin; some persons receiving these two drugs simultaneously may be at risk of phenytoin toxicity, signs of which include rapid, involuntary eye movement, muscular incoordination, slurred speech, and confusion. This interaction is more likely in people taking more than 20 mg a day of omeprazole.

**CLINICAL SIGNIFICANCE OF THE INTERACTION**

LOW　　MODERATE　　HIGH

| GASTROINTESTINAL DRUG | INTERACTING DRUG | RESULT |
|---|---|---|
| Omeprazole (**Prilosec**®) | Warfarin (**Coumadin**®, **Panwarfin**®)<br><br>[for the prevention of blood clots] | Omeprazole may increase the anticoagulant effect of warfarin; the effect is usually small, but some persons may have a slightly increased risk of bleeding, such as blood in urine, coughing up of blood, black stools (or red blood in stools), vomiting of blood or substance resembling coffee grounds, bruising, or other bleeding. |
| Ranitidine (**Zantac**®) | Cefpodoxime proxetil (**Vantin**®)<br><br>[used to treat various bacterial infections] | Ranitidine reduces the absorption of cefpodoxime proxetil. Other antiulcer drugs—cimetidine (Tagamet®), famotidine (Pepcid®), and nizatidine (Axid®)—probably have the same effect.<br><br>The effect of these antiulcer drugs on other cephalosporins (the class of antibiotic to which cefpodoxime proxetil belongs) is not known.<br><br>**Recommendation:** Separation of the doses may not prevent this interaction, so be on the lookout for signs that the antibiotic is not working. |
| Ranitidine (**Zantac**®) | Cefuroxime axetil (**Ceftin**®)<br><br>[used to treat various bacterial infections, such as infections of the throat, ear, urinary tract, and others] | Ranitidine reduces the absorption of cefuroxime. Other antiulcer drugs—cimetidine (Tagamet®), famotidine (Pepcid®), and nizatidine (Axid®)—probably have the same effect.<br><br>The effect of these antiulcer drugs on other cephalosporins (the class of antibiotic to which cefuroxime belongs) is not known.<br><br>**Recommendation:** Separation of the doses may not prevent this interaction, so be on the lookout for signs that the antibiotic is not working. |

| GASTROINTESTINAL DRUG | INTERACTING DRUG | RESULT |
|---|---|---|

Ranitidine (**Zantac**®)

Glipizide (**Glucotrol**®)

[for treatment of diabetes mellitus, a condition that results in abnormally high blood sugar levels]

Ranitidine has been reported to increase the amount of glipizide in the blood, which enhances the effect of lowering the amount of sugar in the blood. (Symptoms of an excessive drop in blood sugar levels include cold sweats, trembling, and an increased heart rate.)

When ranitidine is started or discontinued, diabetics taking glipizide should watch for any change in their sugar levels.

This interaction may be caused by reducing the amount of acid in the stomach, so the same problem may be seen with other antiulcer drugs that decrease stomach acid, such as cimetidine (Tagamet®), famotidine (Pepcid®), nizatidine (Axid®), omeprazole (Prilosec®), and antacids.

**Recommendation:** Diabetics should carefully check their sugar levels after beginning or ending therapy with ranitidine. Sucralfate (Carafate®) may be a good alternative for diabetics with ulcers because preliminary reports suggest that this medication is less likely to significantly change blood sugar levels. (Glipizide and sucralfate should be taken several hours apart to reduce the possibility of sucralfate binding with glipizide in the stomach. Separate doses of these two medications as much as possible.)

Ranitidine (**Zantac**®)

Ketoconazole (**Nizoral**®)

[for the treatment of fungal infections]

Stomach acid is needed for the proper absorption (and thus effectiveness) or oral ketoconazole. Since ranitidine reduces the secretion of stomach acid, ranitidine is likely to reduce the absorption of ketoconazole.

**Recommendation:** Your doctor may need to adjust the dosing times of

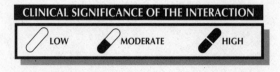

CLINICAL SIGNIFICANCE OF THE INTERACTION

LOW      MODERATE      HIGH

| GASTROINTESTINAL DRUG | INTERACTING DRUG | RESULT |
|---|---|---|
| (cont.)<br>Ranitidine | Ketoconazole | these drugs so that the ketoconazole is given when the effect of ranitidine is low. Alternatively, the manufacturer of ketoconazole describes a method of dissolving the ketonazole in a very mild acid before administration. Your doctor or pharmacist may help you with this. |
| Ranitidine **(Zantac®)** | Nifedipine **(Adalat®, Procardia®)**<br><br>[for treatment of angina and high blood pressure] | May mildly increase the amount of nifedipine in the blood, but not as much as cimetidine (see cimetidine-nifedipine interaction , p. 154). |
| Ranitidine **(Zantac®)** | Triamterene **(Dyazide®, Dyrenium®, Maxzide®)**<br><br>[for the treatment of high blood pressure in persons who are at risk of developing low levels of potassium] | Ranitidine may cause a slight decrease in triamterene blood levels, possibly leading to a reduced ability of triamterene to promote fluid loss and reduce blood pressure. |
| Sucralfate **(Carafate®)** | Ciprofloxacin **(Cipro®)**<br><br>[for the treatment of various infections, including urinary tract and lower respiratory tract infections] | When taken together, sucralfate may reduce the absorption of ciprofloxacin. As a result, this antibiotic may not work as effectively when taken with sucralfate.<br><br>**Recommendation:** Do not take ciprofloxacin and sucralfate simultaneously. Ciprofloxacin should be taken at least two hours before or at least six hours after taking sucralfate. |
| Sucralfate **(Carafate®)** | Norfloxacin **(Noroxin®)**<br><br>[for the treatment of urinary tract infections] | When taken together, sucralfate is highly likely to markedly reduce the absorption and effectiveness of norfloxacin.<br><br>**Recommendation:** Do not take norfloxacin and sucralfate simultaneously. Norfloxacin should be taken at least two hours before or at least six hours after taking sucralfate. |

Sulfasalazine (**Azulfidine**®)

Digoxin (**Lanoxin**®)

[for heart failure and heart abnormalities, such as atrial fibrillation and atrial flutter]

Sulfasalazine taken together with digoxin may decrease the absorption and effectiveness of digoxin.

Your doctor should monitor the amount of digoxin in your blood when adding sulfasalazine therapy.

**Recommendation:** Do not take digoxin and sulfasalazine simultaneously. Digoxin should be taken at least two hours before or at least six hours after taking sulfasalazine.

**CLINICAL SIGNIFICANCE OF THE INTERACTION**

LOW    MODERATE    HIGH

# HEART DRUGS: DRUGS FOR ANGINA, IRREGULAR HEARTBEAT, AND CONGESTIVE HEART FAILURE

To work properly, the heart needs a constant flow of oxygen-rich blood. When this supply is oxygen-deficient, a condition called *angina pectoris* results. When the heart is deprived of oxygen for a long enough time to result in death of heart tissue (a few minutes), a heart attack follows; however, if oxygen deprivation is only temporary, heart muscle is not permanently damaged, and the condition is labeled angina.

The causes of an inadequate supply of oxygen to the heart are varied. One of the most frequent culprits is the coronary arteries, the very vessels that normally supply the heart with oxygen-rich blood. These arteries may be narrowed or blocked because of fatty deposits clinging to their walls. Or, the muscles in the coronary arteries may go into spasm, causing brief periods of narrowing, which also deprives the heart of needed oxygen.

Chest pain is the most common symptom of angina; the pain typically lasts from fifteen to thirty seconds, and is generally a tightness or squeezing sensation that may extend from the left chest to the left arm or shoulder, neck, or jaw. Although discomforting, the pain may serve as a useful warning sign so that the sufferer sees his or her doctor, who can take action to improve the condition. Angina is more elusive in the thousands of persons who suffer from "silent angina," a condition in which symptoms do not appear even though the coronary arteries may be narrowed. Certain diagnostic procedures—such as a stress test and continuous electrocardiographic monitoring—may help to identify which persons have silent angina.

## What Precipitates an Anginal Attack?

Physical exertion is one of the classic triggers of anginal pain. Exertion brings on the most common type of angina, known as classic angina. The heart's demand for oxygen increases when you exercise or strenuously exert yourself (such as climbing up many flights of stairs or lifting heavy objects). If this demand for oxygen cannot be met, chest pain results. Extreme cold and emotional stress have also been implicated as triggers of anginal pain.

Another condition, known as aortic stenosis, can cause angina. In this disorder the valve between the heart and the major artery that carries blood to the rest of the body—the aorta—becomes narrowed. Only a well-trained physician can determine whether angina is caused by narrowed coronary arteries or aortic stenosis. Certain medical tests, such as an echocardiogram and cardiac catheterization, may be needed to help make this determination.

## Medications Used to Treat or Prevent Angina

Three "families" of drugs are primarily used to treat or prevent angina: beta blockers, calcium-channel blockers, and nitrates. Beta blockers reduce the force of the heart's contraction and slow the heart rate; as a result, the heart's workload is reduced. Beta blockers used to treat angina include acebutolol (Sectral®), atenolol (Tenormin®), metoprolol (Lopressor®), nadolol (Corgard®), and propranolol (Inderal®).

Calcium-channel blockers are useful in the prevention of an anginal attack. Muscles in the heart and walls of blood vessels need calcium to contract. Calcium-channel blockers prevent calcium from entering these muscles; as a result, blood vessels in the heart and throughout the body relax. Relaxation of coronary arteries in the heart allows more oxygen to reach the heart tissue, which helps to prevent an attack of angina. By relaxing blood vessels throughout the body, calcium-channel blockers ease the workload of the heart, and help to reduce high blood pressure (see Chapter 7). Calcium-channel blockers used to treat angina include diltiazem (Cardizem®), nicardipine (Cardene®), nifedipine (Adalat®, Procardia®), and verapamil (Calan®, Isoptin®).

Bepridil (Vascor®) is a drug used to treat angina pectoris in persons who do not respond well to or cannot take other antianginal drugs; its use can lead to potentially severe adverse effects (such as an abnormal heartbeat, called ventricular arrhythmia).[1]

Nitrates also dilate blood vessels by relaxing muscle tissue that surrounds the vessels. These drugs reduce oxygen demand and increase its availability by dilating coronary arteries. Nitrates for angina include isosorbide dinitrate (Dilatrate-SR®, Isordil®, Sorbitrate®) and nitroglycerin (Deponit®, Minitran®, Nitro-Bid®, Nitrodisc®, Nitro-Dur®, Nitrogard®, Nitrong®, Nitrostat®). Unlike the beta blockers and calcium-channel blockers, the nitrates can be used to bring relief of pain once an anginal attack begins.

## Arrhythmia: Defects in the Heart's Electrical System

Heart arrhythmia is an abnormal heartbeat or heart rhythm. The heartbeat of a person with an arrhythmia may be irregular, or the beat may be regular but inappropriate—either too slow or too fast. When the heart beats too slowly, the condition is called bradycardia; a rapid heartbeat is known as tachycardia.

The heart is not just a simple pump; it is a complex electro-mechanical organ. The heart is able to generate tiny electrical impulses and conduct these signals to various parts of the heart to begin performing a particular function. Flaws, however, may develop in this electrical system; when they do, an arrhythmia results.

In the heart's right atrium (one of the heart's two upper chambers) is found a group of specialized cells known as the pacemaker. In healthy individuals these trigger an electrical impulse about once a second. This signal is conducted through the atria, triggering them to squeeze blood into the ventricles (the two large, bottom-most chambers of the heart that pump blood to the rest of the body). The ventricles are stimulated to contract after another group of specialized cells, the atrio-ventricular (A-V) node, transmits an electrical signal to a branch of conducting fibers called the "His bundle." All of these electrical activities are measured on an electrocardiogram, or ECG.

Arrhythmias may result when the initiation or conduction of electrical impulses goes awry. An arrhythmia may be related to a disorder of the pacemaker, the A-V node, the His bundle, or other sites in the heart. Or, an inadequate supply of oxygen-rich blood to the heart itself may cause an arrhythmia. Depending on the type of arrhythmia, the result may be symptoms such as lightheadedness, dizziness, chest pain, fainting, or even death.

One of the most common types of arrhythmia is known as a premature ventricular contraction (PVC). This abnormality occurs when a ventricle contracts sooner than it should. This may feel like a skipped beat or a "thump" in the chest. Normally, the pacemaker sends out an electrical signal that is transmitted throughout the atria before the ventricles contract. In PVC, however, an abnormal electrical impulse originates in one of the ventricles, causing the ventricle to contract *before* the pacemaker sends out its electrical signal. PVCs are usually harmless unless heart disease is also present.

Another type of arrhythmia is ventricular tachycardia, which means the ventricles contract faster than normal. At this quickened pace, the heart cannot pump efficiently and several symptoms may develop, such as dizziness, shortness of breath, chest pain, fainting, and shock. Although three out of every four persons who suffer from ventricular tachycardia report some symptoms, this disorder is particularly dangerous for the remaining 25 percent of persons who do not experience any symptoms; the first sign that anything is amiss in the symptomless sufferer is sudden death (which is why ventricular tachycardia is often referred to as "sudden death" arrhythmia). Therefore, many doctors recommend that anyone with a family history of heart disease, especially sudden death, should be evaluated by a cardiologist.

Ventricular tachycardia is common in persons with ischemic heart disease, a condition in which the heart tissue is supplied with an inadequate supply of oxygen-rich blood.[2] Excessively low levels of potassium, high levels of calcium, and inflammation or infection of the heart have been associated with ventricular tachycardia.[3] Left unchecked, ventricular tachycardia may progress to a more severe arrhythmia—ventricular fibrillation—a life-threatening disorder in which the heart cannot pump at all to the rest of the body.

## Drug Treatment of Arrhythmias

Various drugs are used to treat arrhythmias. The type of arrhythmia often affects the physician's selection of a particular antiarrhythmic agent. Some of the medications used to treat arrhythmias include adenosine (Adenocard®), amiodarone (Cordarone®), bretylium (Bretylol®), digoxin (Lanoxin®), disopyramide (Norpace®), flecainide (Tambocor®), lidocaine (Xylocaine®), mexiletine (Mexitil®), moricizine (Ethmozine®), procainamide (Pronestyl®, Procan SR®), propafenone (Rythmol®), quinidine (Cardioquin®, Duraquin®, Quinaglute®, Quinidex®, Quinora®), tocainide (Tonocard®), and others. Certain beta blockers and calcium-channel blockers are also used to treat arrhythmia.

## Congestive Heart Failure

Another serious condition of the heart is *congestive heart failure* (CHF). This disorder, which affects more than two million Americans—over one quarter of whom will require hospitalization each year—results when the heart can no longer pump effectively.

Several factors may lead to heart failure, such as weakened heart muscle (often this leads to an inability of the ventricles to eject a suitable fraction of the blood they contain). The result is typically an accumulation of fluid in the lungs, feet, ankles, and hands. Other symptoms of CHF include shortness of breath or wheezing, signifying a buildup of fluid in the lungs; weakness; frequent urination; and swollen, distended neck veins. As fluid accumulates, the person with CHF typically gains weight.

The heart itself often aggravates the problem in an attempt to compensate for its inability to pump normally. For example, the heart may become enlarged or beat more rapidly; this may help in the short run, but, over an extended period of time, such responses may lead to a further weakening of heart muscle.

## Medications Used to Treat Congestive Heart Failure

Drug treatment of CHF generally involves three medications: digitalis, diuretics, and vasodilators. Digitalis is a derivative of the foxglove plant; the purified form of this drug—digoxin (Lanoxin®)—is widely used today to strengthen the heart's pumping force. Diuretics help to relieve fluid accumulation (see Chapter 7 for a more detailed description of diuretic drugs).

Vasodilators help to reduce the heart's workload by causing the muscles surrounding the arteries to relax, which leads to a decrease in blood pressure. With relaxation of the coronary arteries (those in the heart itself), the amount of oxygen-rich blood delivered to the heart is increased. Vasodilators include several different types of drugs; one type useful in treating the symptoms of CHF is the angiotensin-converting enzyme—ACE for short—inhibitors. The ACE inhibitors approved for treating congestive heart failure include captopril (Capoten®) and enalapril (Vasotec®). Other vasodilators include hydralazine (Apresoline®), minoxidil (Loniten®), nitroglycerin, nitroprusside (Nipride®), and prazosin (Minipress®).

| HEART DRUG | INTERACTING DRUG | RESULT |
| --- | --- | --- |
| Acebutolol **(Sectral®)**  | Antidiabetic drugs: <br><br> • acetohexamide **(Dymelor®)** <br> • chlorpropamide **(Diabinese®)** <br> • glipizide **(Glucotrol®)** <br> • glyburide **(DiaBeta®, Micronase®)** <br> • insulin **(Humulin®, Lente®, Novolin®,** • and others <br> • tolazamide **(Tolinase®)** <br> • tolbutamide **(Orinase®),** and others <br><br> [for treatment of diabetes mellitus, a condition that results in excessively high amounts of sugar in the blood and urine] | Although the heart typically beats faster (tachycardia) when blood sugar levels are low, this symptom may be absent when acebutolol is taken. This effect may occur when antidiabetic agents are combined with other drugs that are in the same class as acebutolol, such as atenolol (Tenormin®), betaxolol (Kerlone®), carteolol (Cartrol®), esmolol (Brevibloc®), labetalol (Normodyne®, Trandate®), metoprolol (Lopressor®), nadolol (Corgard®), pindolol (Visken®), propranolol (Inderal®), and timolol (Blocadren®). |
| Acebutolol **(Sectral®)**  | Guanadrel **(Hylorel®),** guanethidine **(Ismelin®),** and reserpine **(Serpasil®, Regroton®)** <br><br> [for treatment of high blood pressure] | May lead to low blood pressure, which could lead to slowed heartbeat and fainting. |
| Acebutolol **(Sectral®)**  | Indomethacin **(Indocin®)** <br><br> [for reduction of inflammation; used to reduce the pain and swelling associated with arthritis, tendinitis, and bursitis] | Reduction in the antihypertensive or antianginal effect of acebutolol. Indomethacin belongs to a class of drugs known as nonsteroidal anti-inflammatory drugs (NSAIDs); this effect may occur with other NSAIDs, such as piroxicam (Feldene®) and naproxen (Anaprox®, Naprosyn®). Sulindac (Clinoril®) appears less likely to interfere with the antihypertensive effect of acebutolol. <br><br> **Recommendation:** Your doctor may want to check your blood pressure if you start, stop, or change the dosage of an NSAID. |

ACE inhibitors:

- benazepril (**Lotensin**®)
- captopril (**Capoten**®)
- enalapril (**Vasotec**®)
- fosinopril (**Monopril**®)
- lisinopril (**Prinivil**®, **Zestril**®)
- quinapril (**Accupril**®)
- ramipril (**Altace**®)

Amiloride (**Midamor**®)

[used in combination with other medications to treat high blood pressure; also used to treat disorders that involve excess fluid accumulation]

Both ACE inhibitors and amiloride tend to increase serum potassium levels. Their effects may be additive, resulting in excessively high potassium levels in some people.

**Recommendation:** Discuss this interaction with your doctor.

---

ACE inhibitors:

- benazepril (**Lotensin**®)
- captopril (**Capoten**®)
- enalapril (**Vasotec**®)
- fosinopril (**Monopril**®)
- lisinopril (**Prinivil**®, **Zestril**®)
- quinapril (**Accupril**®)
- ramipril (**Altace**®)

Loop diuretics:

- bumetanide (**Bumex**®)
- ethacrynic acid (**Edecrin**®)
- furosemide (**Lasix**®)

[to reduce high blood pressure and fluid accumulation]

Some persons may require the combined use of an ACE inhibitor and loop diuretic to control their medical condition. However, if ACE inhibitor therapy is started in the presence of loop diuretic therapy (which has been sufficient to reduce the blood volume), some patients may experience a precipitous fall in blood pressure. Symptoms of excessively low blood pressure levels include lightheadness and fainting.

If your doctor suspects that you may be sensitive to ACE inhibitors due to diuretic-induced reduction in blood volume, he or she may reduce the diuretic dose or stop the diuretic temporarily before starting ACE inhibitor therapy. Your doctor may also start with a low dose of the ACE inhibitor and increase the dose gradually.

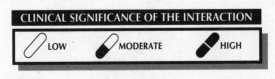

CLINICAL SIGNIFICANCE OF THE INTERACTION

LOW      MODERATE      HIGH

| | | |
| --- | --- | --- |
| ACE inhibitors:<br><br>• benazepril **(Lotensin®)**<br>• captopril **(Capoten®)**<br>• enalapril **(Vasotec®)**<br>• fosinopril **(Monopril®)**<br>• lisinopril **(Prinivil®, Zestril®)**<br>• quinapril **(Accupril®)**<br>• ramipril **(Altace®)** | Potassium **(K-Tab®, Kaon-CL Tabs®, Micro-K®, Ten-K®**, and others)<br><br>[used to supplement potassium levels or to prevent potassium depletion] | ACE inhibitors tend to increase serum potassium levels. Concurrent use of potassium supplements may result in excessively high potassium levels in the body. Salt substitutes containing potassium should be used with caution. |

| | | |
| --- | --- | --- |
| ACE inhibitors:<br><br>• benazepril **(Lotensin®)**<br>• captopril **(Capoten®)**<br>• enalapril **(Vasotec®)**<br>• fosinopril **(Monopril®)**<br>• lisinopril **(Prinivil®, Zestril®)**<br>• quinapril **(Accupril®)**<br>• ramipril **(Altace®)** | Spironolactone **(Aldactone®)**<br><br>[used in combination with other medications to treat high blood pressure; also used to treat disorders that involve excess fluid accumulation] | Both ACE inhibitors and spironolactone tend to increase serum potassium levels. Their effects may be additive, resulting in excessively high potassium levels in some people.<br><br>**Recommendation:** Discuss this interaction with your doctor. |

| HEART DRUG | INTERACTING DRUG | RESULT |
|---|---|---|
| ACE inhibitors:<br><br>• benazepril **(Lotensin®)**<br>• captopril **(Capoten®)** enalapril **(Vasotec®)**<br>• fosinopril **(Monopril®)**<br>• lisinopril **(Prinivil®, Zestril®)**<br>• quinapril **(Accupril®)**<br>• ramipril **(Altace®)** | Thiazide and thiazide-like diuretics:<br><br>• chlorothiazide **(Diuril®)**<br>• chlorthalidone **(Hygroton®)**<br>• hydrochlorothiazide **(Esidrix®, HydroDIURIL®, Oretic®, and others)**<br>• metolazone **(Diulo®, Zaroxolyn®)**<br><br>[to reduce high blood pressure]<br><br> | In most persons, combined use of an ACE inhibitor with a thiazide diuretic works well to help control hypertension or congestive heart failure. However, if ACE inhibitor therapy is started in the presence of diuretic therapy (which has been sufficient to reduce the blood volume), some patients may experience a precipitous (fall in blood pressure. Symptoms of excessively low blood pressure levels include lightheadedness and fainting.<br><br>If your doctor suspects that you may be sensitive to ACE inhibitors due to diuretic-induced reduction in blood volume, he or she may reduce the diuretic dose or stop the diuretic temporarily before starting ACE inhibitor therapy. Your doctor may also start with a low dose of the ACE inhibitor and increase the dose gradually. |
| ACE inhibitors:<br><br>• benazepril **(Lotensin®)**<br>• captopril **(Capoten®)**<br>• enalapril **(Vasotec®)**<br>• fosinopril **(Monopril®)**<br>• lisinopril **(Prinivil®, Zestril®)**<br>• quinapril **(Accupril®)**<br>• ramipril **(Altace®)**<br><br> | Triamterene **(Dyrenium®)**<br><br>[used to treat disorders that involve excess fluid accumulation] | Both ACE inhibitors and triamterene tend to increase serum potassium levels. Their effects may be additive, resulting in excessively high potassium levels in some people.<br><br>**Recommendation:** Discuss this interaction with your doctor. |

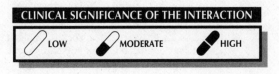

CLINICAL SIGNIFICANCE OF THE INTERACTION

LOW    MODERATE    HIGH

| HEART DRUG | INTERACTING DRUG | RESULT |
|---|---|---|
| Adenosine (**Adenocard**®) 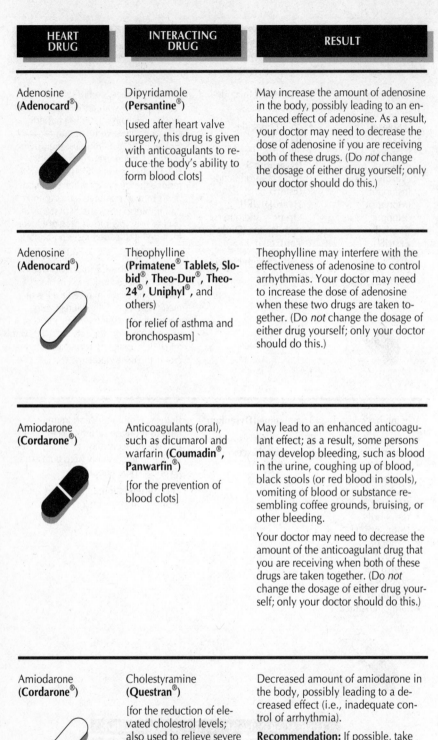 | Dipyridamole (**Persantine**®) [used after heart valve surgery, this drug is given with anticoagulants to reduce the body's ability to form blood clots] | May increase the amount of adenosine in the body, possibly leading to an enhanced effect of adenosine. As a result, your doctor may need to decrease the dose of adenosine if you are receiving both of these drugs. (Do *not* change the dosage of either drug yourself; only your doctor should do this.) |
| Adenosine (**Adenocard**®) | Theophylline (**Primatene**® **Tablets, Slobid**®, **Theo-Dur**®, **Theo-24**®, **Uniphyl**®, and others) [for relief of asthma and bronchospasm] | Theophylline may interfere with the effectiveness of adenosine to control arrhythmias. Your doctor may need to increase the dose of adenosine when these two drugs are taken together. (Do *not* change the dosage of either drug yourself; only your doctor should do this.) |
| Amiodarone (**Cordarone**®) | Anticoagulants (oral), such as dicumarol and warfarin (**Coumadin**®, **Panwarfin**®) [for the prevention of blood clots] | May lead to an enhanced anticoagulant effect; as a result, some persons may develop bleeding, such as blood in the urine, coughing up of blood, black stools (or red blood in stools), vomiting of blood or substance resembling coffee grounds, bruising, or other bleeding. Your doctor may need to decrease the amount of the anticoagulant drug that you are receiving when both of these drugs are taken together. (Do *not* change the dosage of either drug yourself; only your doctor should do this.) |
| Amiodarone (**Cordarone**®) | Cholestyramine (**Questran**®) [for the reduction of elevated cholestrol levels; also used to relieve severe itching associated with partial biliary obstruction] | Decreased amount of amiodarone in the body, possibly leading to a decreased effect (i.e., inadequate control of arrhythmia). **Recommendation:** If possible, take amiodarone at least two hours before or four hours after the cholestyramine. |

| HEART DRUG | INTERACTING DRUG | RESULT |
|---|---|---|

Amiodarone **(Cordarone®)**

Cimetidine **(Tagamet®)**

[for relief of stomach and intestinal ulcers]

May result in an increased concentration of amiodarone. If the amount of amiodarone in the blood reaches a high enough level, amiodarone toxicity could result, with symptoms such as nausea, slowed heart rate, light-headedness, sensitivity to light, fatigue, tremor, lack of coordination, and fainting.

This effect may not be seen for several weeks after these two drugs are being taken concomitantly.

---

Amiodarone **(Cordarone®)**

Digoxin **(Lanoxin®)**

[for heart failure and heart abnormalities, such as atrial fibrillation and atrial flutter]

Increased amount of digoxin in the body, possibly leading to digoxin toxicity. Symptoms of digoxin toxicity include nausea, vomiting, poor appetite, weakness, lethargy, visual abnormalities, and irregular heartbeat.

Your doctor may need to decrease the amount of digoxin you are receiving when both of these drugs are taken together. (Do *not* change the dosage of either drug yourself; only your doctor should do this.)

---

Amiodarone **(Cordarone®)**

Flecainide **(Tambocor®)**

[used to treat heart arrhythmias]

Enhanced effect of flecainide. Symptoms of increased effect of flecainide include dizziness, faintness, headache, blurred vision, and rapid or irregular heartbeat.

Your doctor may need to decrease the amount of flecainide you are receiving when both of these drugs are taken together. (Do *not* change the dosage of either drug yourself; only your doctor should do this.)

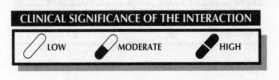

CLINICAL SIGNIFICANCE OF THE INTERACTION

LOW     MODERATE     HIGH

Amiodarone **(Cordarone®)**

Metoprolol **(Lopressor®)**

[for treatment of high blood pressure and angina]

In a few cases, combined use of amiodarone with either metoprolol or propranolol (drugs in a class known as beta blockers) has been followed by slowed or irregular heartbeat and even cardiac arrest (i.e., stopping of the heart).

It is not known whether other antihypertensive drugs in the beta-blocker class would produce a similar effect, but if they do the most likely would be those that are degraded primarily in the liver, such as acebutolol (Sectral®), betaxolol (Kerlone®), penbutolol (Levatol®), and pindolol (Visken®). In one case, atenolol (Tenormin®), another antihypertensive in the beta-blocker class, did not seem to interact with amiodarone. It is possible that other beta blockers eliminated mainly by the kidneys—such as nadolol (Corgard®)—would also fail to interact.

Amiodarone **(Cordarone®)**

Phenytoin **(Dilantin®)**

[for the prevention of seizures]

When these drugs are given together, the amount of phenytoin in the body is substantially increased, possibly leading to rapid involuntary movement of the eye, muscular incoordination, and confusion.

In addition, the amount of amiodarone in the body may decrease, leading to inadequate control of arrhythmia.

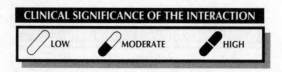

**CLINICAL SIGNIFICANCE OF THE INTERACTION**

LOW    MODERATE    HIGH

| HEART DRUG | INTERACTING DRUG | RESULT |
|---|---|---|
| Amiodarone (**Cordarone**®)  | Procainamide (**Procan**®**SR, Pronestyl**®) [for treatment of irregular heartbeat and heart rhythm] | This combination increases the amount of procainamide in the body, possibly leading to toxicity; symptoms of procainamide toxicity include nausea, vomiting, malaise, weakness, lightheadedness, arrhythmia, and excessively low blood pressure levels. Your doctor may need to decrease the dosage of procainamide when these drugs are given together. (Do *not* change the dosage of either drug yourself; only your doctor should do this.) |
| Amiodarone (**Cordarone**®)  | Propranolol (**Inderal**®) [for treatment of high blood pressure, angina pectoris, and irregular heartbeats; also used to prevent migraine headaches] | May lead to slowed or irregular heartbeat, and possibly stopping of the heart (i.e., cardiac arrest). **Recommendation:** Persons taking these drugs together should be monitored carefully. |
| Amiodarone (**Cordarone**®) | Quinidine (**Cardioquin**®, **Duraquin**®, **Quinaglute**®, **Quinidex**®, **Quinora**®) [for arrhythmias, or irregularities of the heartbeat and heart rhythm] | May result in an increased amount of quinidine in the body, possibly leading to abnormal heart function. (Nerve impulses travel through the heart at a particular speed. When amiodarone and quinidine are combined, certain nerve impulses may travel more slowly.) |

Captopril
(**Capoten**®)

Allopurinol (**Zyloprim**®, **Lopurin**®)

[for treatment of gout]

Hypersensitivity reactions—such as skin eruptions, fever, and pain in joints—may result from the combination of captopril and allopurinol.

---

Captopril
(**Capoten**®)

Aspirin (**Alka-Seltzer**® **Antacid and Pain Reliever, Anacin**®, **Ascriptin**®, **Bayer**®, **Bufferin**®, **Ecotrin**®, and many others)

[for relief of pain and fever; pain often relieved due to reduced inflammation]

Repeated doses of aspirin decrease the antihypertensive effect of captopril in some persons.

Not much is known about the effect of aspirin on ACE inhibitors other than captopril, but it is possible that other ACE inhibitors also interact.

**Recommendation:** Occasional doses of aspirin probably do not affect captopril. If aspirin is used often, however, blood pressure should be monitored frequently to ensure the aspirin is not interfering with the antihypertensive effect.

---

Captopril
(**Capoten**®)

Azathioprine (**Imuran**®)

[for immune suppression, which is needed after organ transplantation to prevent rejection of the transplanted organ]

The likelihood of neutropenia (a decrease in the number of a specific type of white blood cell) occurring may be greater than when using either drug alone.

Captropril
(**Capoten**®)

Nonsteroidal anti-inflammatory drugs:

- diclofenac (**Voltaren**®)
- diflunisal (**Dolobid**®)
- etodolac (**Lodine**®)
- fenoprofen (**Nalfon**®)
- flurbiprofen (**Ansaid**®)
- ibuprofen (**Advil**®, **Motrin**®, **Nuprin**®, **Rufen**®)
- indomethacin (**Indocin**®)
- ketoprofen (**Orudis**®)
- ketorolac (**Toradol**®)
- meclofenamate (**Meclomen**®)
- nabumetone (**Relafen**®)
- naproxen (**Naprosyn**®)
- naproxen sodium (**Anaprox**®)
- phenylbutazone (**Butazolidin**®)
- piroxicam (**Feldene**®)
- sulindac (**Clinoril**®)
- tolmetin (**Tolectin**®)

[for reducing inflammation of joints and muscles and pain caused by inflammation]

Indomethacin may inhibit the antihypertensive effect of captopril and probably other ACE inhibitors. Other nonsteroidal anti-inflammatory drugs (NSAIDS)—with the possible exception of sulindac (Clinoril®)—probably have a similar effect.

**Recommendation:** Your doctor may want to check your blood pressure if you start, stop, or change the dosage of an NSAID.

Digitoxin
(**Crystodigin**®)

Aminoglutethimide
(**Cytadren**®)

[used to treat certain patients with Cushing's syndrome, a hormonal disorder]

Aminoglutethimide may reduce the amount of digitoxin in the body.

**Recommendation:** Your doctor may use digoxin (another form of digitalis) rather than digitoxin to minimize this interaction.

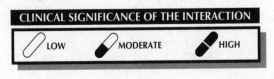

CLINICAL SIGNIFICANCE OF THE INTERACTION

LOW   MODERATE   HIGH

| HEART DRUG | INTERACTING DRUG | RESULT |
|---|---|---|
| Digitoxin (**Crystodigin**®) | Amphotericin B (**Fungizone**®) [used to treat certain fungal infections] | The potassium loss resulting from amphotericin B may increase the risk of digitoxin toxicity. Symptoms of digitoxin toxicity include nausea, vomiting, poor appetite, weakness, lethargy, visual abnormalities, and irregular heartbeat. |
| Digitoxin (**Crystodigin**®) | Barbiturates: <br>• amobarbital (**Amytal**®) <br>• butabarbital (**Butisol**®) <br>• butalbital <br>• pentobarbital (**Nembutal**®) <br>• phenobarbital (**Luminal**®, **Solfoton**®) <br>• primidone (**Mysoline**®) <br>• secobarbital (**Seconal**®), and others <br>[used to treat insomnia and anxiety; certain barbiturates are used to prevent seizures] | Phenobarbital may reduce the amount of digitoxin in the blood, thereby reducing the effect of the digitoxin. (Other barbiturates are expected to act similarly.) <br><br>It may be necessary for your doctor to adjust the dose of digitoxin if a barbiturate is started or stopped, or if its dosage is changed. (Do *not* change the dosage of either drug yourself; only your doctor should do this.) |
| Digitoxin (**Crystodigin**®) | Diuretics (potassium-losing): <br>• bumetanide (**Bumex**®) <br>• chlorothiazide (**Diuril**®) <br>• chlorthalidone (**Hygroton**®) <br>• ethacrynic acid (**Edecrin**®) <br>• furosemide (**Lasix**®) <br>• hydrochlorothiazide (**Esidrix**®, **HydroDIURIL**®, **Oretic**®, and others) <br>• indapamide (**Lozol**®) <br>• methyclothiazide (**Enduron**®) <br>• metolazone (**Diulo**®, **Zaroxolyn**®) <br>• polythiazide (**Renese**®) | Certain diuretics can cause a loss of potassium in the body. As the amount of potassium in the body decreases, the likelihood of digitoxin toxicity increases. Symptoms of digitoxin toxicity include nausea, poor appetite, weakness, lethargy, and visual abnormalities. <br><br>**Recommendation:** Your doctor may wish to check your potassium level periodically, especially if you are taking large doses of diuretics and/or if your dietary intake of potassium is low. |

| HEART DRUG | INTERACTING DRUG | RESULT |
|---|---|---|

Digitoxin (**Crystodigin**®)

Rifampin (**Rifadin**®, **Rimactane**®)

[used in combination with at least one other drug, rifampin is used to treat tuberculosis; also used in the treatment of individuals who are carriers of meningitis]

Rifampin may substantially reduce the amount of digitoxin in the blood, diminishing the effect of the digitoxin.

Digoxin (**Lanoxin**®)

Charcoal

[used to treat flatulence, or excess gas]

Charcoal significantly reduces the amount of digoxin absorbed in the body; as a result the effect of the digoxin is reduced.

**Recommendation:** Take digoxin two hours before or six hours after taking charcoal.

Digoxin (**Lanoxin**®)

Cyclosporine (**Sandimmune**®)

[for immune suppression, which is needed after organ transplantation to prevent rejection of the transplanted organ]

Cyclosporine may result in an increased amount of digoxin in the body, possibly leading to digoxin toxicity (symptoms of which include nausea, poor appetite, weakness, lethargy, and visual abnormalities).

Your doctor may need to decrease the amount of digoxin you are receiving if cyclosporine is added to your drug therapy. (Do *not* change the dosage of either drug yourself; only your doctor should do this.)

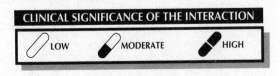

CLINICAL SIGNIFICANCE OF THE INTERACTION

LOW    MODERATE    HIGH

---

Digoxin (**Lanoxin**®)

Diuretics (potassium-losing):

- bumetanide (**Bumex**®)
- chlorothiazide (**Diuril**®)
- chlorthalidone (**Hygroton**®)
- ethacrynic acid (**Edecrin**®)
- furosemide (**Lasix**®)
- hydrochlorothiazide (**Esidrix**®, **HydroDIURIL**®, **Oretic**®, and others)
- indapamide (**Lozol**®)
- methyclothiazide (**Enduron**®)
- metolazone (**Diulo**®, **Zaroxolyn**®)
- polythiazide (**Renese**®)

Certain diuretics can cause a loss of potassium in the body. As the amount of potassium in the body decreases, the likelihood of digoxin toxicity increases. Symptoms of digoxin toxicity include nausea, poor appetite, weakness, lethargy, and visual abnormalities.

**Recommendation:** Your doctor may wish to check your potassium level periodically, especially if you are taking large doses of diuretics and/or if your dietary intake of potassium is low.

---

Digoxin (**Lanoxin**®)

Erythromycin (**E-Mycin**®, **Ilosone**®, **Robimycin**®, **Wyamycin**® S, and others)

[for treatment of various bacterial infections, such as pneumonia and infections of the ear and throat]

In about 10 percent of the population, erythromycin may increase blood digoxin concentrations, possibly increasing the risk of digoxin toxicity. Symptoms of digoxin toxicity include nausea, vomiting, poor appetite, weakness, lethargy, visual abnormalities, and irregular heartbeat.

It is possible that some other antibiotics (e.g., tetracyclines) may produce a similar effect.

---

Digoxin (**Lanoxin**®)

Hydroxychloroquine (**Plaquenil**®)

[used in the treatment of malaria, systemic lupus erythmatosus, and rheumatoid arthritis]

Hydroxychloroquine may increase blood digoxin levels, possibly increasing the risk of digoxin toxicity. Symptoms of digoxin toxicity include nausea, vomiting, poor appetite, weakness, lethargy, visual abnormalities, and irregular heartbeat.

| HEART DRUG | INTERACTING DRUG | RESULT |
|---|---|---|

Digoxin **(Lanoxin®)**

Rifampin **(Rifadin®, Rimactane®)**

[used in combination with at least one other drug, rifampin is used to treat tuberculosis; also used in the treatment of individuals who are carriers of meningitis]

Rifampin may reduce the amount of digoxin in the blood; in some persons, this effect may be large enough to diminish the effect of the digoxin.

Digoxin **(Lanoxin®)**

Spironolactone **(Aldactone®)**

[for treatment of high blood pressure; also used to treat disorders that involve excess fluid accumulation]

Spironolactone may cause an increase in the amount of digoxin in the body, possibly to toxic levels. Symptoms of digoxin toxicity include nausea, poor appetite, weakness, lethargy, and visual abnormalities.

Spironolactone may also interfere with the ability of certain laboratory tests used to determine the amount of digoxin in the body.

**Recommendation:** Although many people take this combination without difficulty, you should be alert for alterations in digoxin effect if spironolactone is started or stopped.

Digoxin **(Lanoxin®)**

Sulfasalazine **(Azulfidine®)**

[for treatment of various bacterial infections; also used to reduce intestinal inflammation associated with ulcerative colitis]

Sulfasalazine taken together with digoxin may decrease the absorption and effectiveness of digoxin.

**Recommendation:** Your doctor should monitor the amount of digoxin in your blood when adding sulfasalazine therapy.

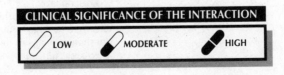

CLINICAL SIGNIFICANCE OF THE INTERACTION

LOW　　MODERATE　　HIGH

| HEART DRUG | INTERACTING DRUG | RESULT |
| --- | --- | --- |

Diltiazem
(**Cardizem**®)

Calcium

[a mineral needed for the heart, muscles, and nerves to function properly; also needed for strong bones and teeth]

When large doses of calcium are taken there is a possible reduced effect of diltiazem.

This interaction is not usually significant unless the calcium is given intravenously.

Diltiazem
(**Cardizem**®)

Carbamazepine
(**Tegretol**®)

[for epilepsy, trigeminal neuralgia (spasms of pain in the face), and other disorders]

May increase carbamazepine concentration in the body, possibly leading to double vision, headaches, abnormal muscle coordination, or dizziness.

Possible damage to nervous system could result from this interaction. Reduced effect of the diltiazem may also occur.

**Recommendation:** It may be necessary for your doctor to adjust the dose of carbamazepine if diltiazem is started or stopped, or if its dosage is changed. (Of course, only your doctor should change medication dosage, when appropriate.)

Nifedipine, which does not affect the amount of carbamazepine in the body, may be an alternative to diltiazem if a calcium-channel blocker must be given with carbamazepine.

Diltiazem
(**Cardizem**®)

Cimetidine (**Tagamet**®)

[for relief of stomach and intestinal ulcers]

Cimetidine may increase diltiazem levels, possibly leading to toxicity (symptoms of which include low blood pressure, dizziness, and flushing).

**Recommendation:** It may be necessary for your doctor to adjust the dose of diltiazem if cimetidine is started or stopped, or if its dosage is changed. (Of course, only your doctor should change medication dosages, when appropriate.)

| HEART DRUG | INTERACTING DRUG | RESULT |
|---|---|---|

Diltiazem
(Cardizem®)

Cyclosporine
(Sandimmune®)

[for immune suppression, which is needed after organ transplantation to prevent rejection of the transplanted organ]

Increased concentration of cyclosporine in the body. Increased blood levels of cyclosporine have been associated with nephrotoxicity (kidney damage).

**Recommendation:** It may be necessary for your doctor to adjust the dose of cyclosporine if diltiazem is started or stopped, or if its dosage is changed. (Of course, only your doctor should change medication dosages, when appropriate.)

---

Diltiazem
(Cardizem®)

Digitalis drugs:

• digitoxin
  (Crystodigin®)
• digoxin (Lanoxin®)

[for heart failure and other heart abnormalities]

Diltiazem may increase digitoxin effect somewhat, possibly increasing the likelihood of side effects occurring. Symptoms of digitoxin toxicity include nausea, poor appetite, weakness, lethargy, and visual disturbances.

Diltiazem may also slightly increase digoxin effect, but in most cases, this increased effect is so small that problems rarely result.

Nifedipine (Adalat®, Procardia®), another drug in the same class as diltiazem, does not appear to increase the amount of digitoxin or digoxin in the body.

---

Diltiazem
(Cardizem®)

Lithium (Cibalith-S®, Eskalith®, Lithane®, Lithobid®, and others)

[for manic-depressive disorder]

Could lead to neurotoxicity (problems involving the nervous system). Possible symptoms include nausea, vomiting, muscular incoordination, and ringing in the ears.

---

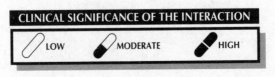

CLINICAL SIGNIFICANCE OF THE INTERACTION

LOW    MODERATE    HIGH

Diltiazem **(Cardizem®)**

Propranolol **(Inderal®)**

[for treatment of high blood pressure, angina pectoris, and irregular heartbeats; also used to prevent migraine headaches]

Diltiazem can increase the amount of propranolol in the blood, and may also lead to reductions in the blood pressure and slowing of the heart rate. This is usually a favorable interaction that may be used intentionally by your doctor, but occasionally the blood pressure or heart rate may become excessively low.

**Recommendation:** When diltiazem is added to propranolol (or conversely, when propranolol is added to diltiazem), watch for any symptoms of excessive lowering of blood pressure or heart rate (e.g., dizziness, faintness). Diltiazem probably has a similar effect with other beta blockers (antihypertensive medications that are in the same class as propranolol) although the magnitude of the additive effect may be different. Beta blockers include acebutolol (Sectral®), atenolol (Tenormin®), betaxolol (Kerlone®), carteolol (Cartrol®), esmolol (Brevibloc®), labetalol (Normodyne®, Trandate®), metoprolol (Lopressor®), nadolol (Corgard®), pindolol (Visken®), and timolol (Blocardren®).

Disopyramide **(Norpace®)**

Barbiturates:

- amobarbital **(Amytal®)**
- butabarbital **(Butisol®)**
- butalbital
- pentobarbital **(Nembutal®)**
- phenobarbital **(Luminal®, Solfoton®)**
- primidone **(Mysoline®)**
- secobarbital **(Seconal®),** and others

[used to treat insomnia and anxiety; certain barbiturates are used to prevent seizures]

Phenobarbital may decrease the effectiveness of disopyramide, even to the point of increasing the likelihood of arrhythmias occurring.

**Recommendation:** Your doctor should monitor the concentration of disopyramide (he or she does this with a blood test) when phenobarbital—or another barbiturate—is prescribed for you (or when you are told to stop taking a barbiturate).

Disopyramide
**(Norpace®)**

Lidocaine **(Xylocaine®)**

[used to treat abnormal heart rhythms; for topical anesthesia during minor surgery; also available as an over-the-counter medication for relief of pain, itching, and inflammation, but such topical use is unlikely to interact with disopyramide]

May lead to arrhythmia or heart failure. Persons taking these drugs concurrently should be monitored carefully.

**Disopyramide**
(Norpace®)

Phenytoin **(Dilantin®)**

[for the prevention of seizures]

Causes a decreased amount of disopyramide in the body, possibly leading to inadequate control of arrhythmia. Interestingly, in the body, disopyramide is changed to another chemical, which accumulates in the body and may cause "anticholinergic" effects, such as dry mouth, blurred vision, fast heartbeat, difficulty or inability to urinate, and constipation.

Disopyramide
**(Norpace®)**

Rifampin **(Rifadin®, Rifamate®, Rimactane®)**

[used in combination with at least one other drug, rifampin is used to treat tuberculosis; also used in the treatment of individuals who are carriers of meningitis]

May cause a reduced amount of disopyramide in the body, possibly leading to decreased antiarrhythmia control.

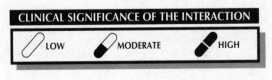

CLINICAL SIGNIFICANCE OF THE INTERACTION

LOW    MODERATE    HIGH

| HEART DRUG | INTERACTING DRUG | RESULT |
| --- | --- | --- |
| Encainide **(Enkaid®)** 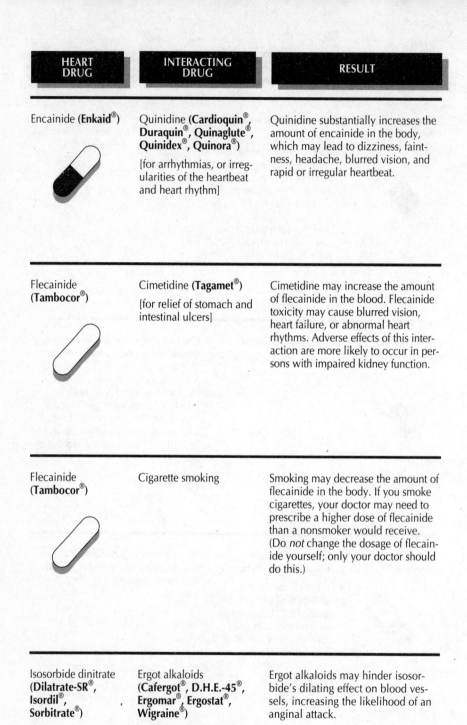 | Quinidine **(Cardioquin®, Duraquin®, Quinaglute®, Quinidex®, Quinora®)** [for arrhythmias, or irregularities of the heartbeat and heart rhythm] | Quinidine substantially increases the amount of encainide in the body, which may lead to dizziness, faintness, headache, blurred vision, and rapid or irregular heartbeat. |
| Flecainide **(Tambocor®)** | Cimetidine **(Tagamet®)** [for relief of stomach and intestinal ulcers] | Cimetidine may increase the amount of flecainide in the blood. Flecainide toxicity may cause blurred vision, heart failure, or abnormal heart rhythms. Adverse effects of this interaction are more likely to occur in persons with impaired kidney function. |
| Flecainide **(Tambocor®)** | Cigarette smoking | Smoking may decrease the amount of flecainide in the body. If you smoke cigarettes, your doctor may need to prescribe a higher dose of flecainide than a nonsmoker would receive. (Do *not* change the dosage of flecainide yourself; only your doctor should do this.) |
| Isosorbide dinitrate **(Dilatrate-SR®, Isordil®, Sorbitrate®)** | Ergot alkaloids **(Cafergot®, D.H.E.-45®, Ergomar®, Ergostat®, Wigraine®)** [for treatment of migraine] | Ergot alkaloids may hinder isosorbide's dilating effect on blood vessels, increasing the likelihood of an anginal attack. |

| HEART DRUG | INTERACTING DRUG | RESULT |
|---|---|---|

Lidocaine **(Xylocaine®, Anestacon®**, and others)

Cimetidine **(Tagamet®)**

[for relief of stomach and intestinal ulcers]

When lidocaine is used to treat heart arrhythmias, cimetidine can increase the concentration of lidocaine, possibly leading to lidocaine toxicity. Symptoms of lidocaine toxicity include drowsiness, dizziness, confusion, numbness or tingling, nausea, visual disturbances, ringing in the ears, muscle twitching, tremor, and seizures.

**Recommendation:** Persons receiving lidocaine with cimetidine should have their blood level of lidocaine monitored by their doctor.

Ranitidine (Zantac®), a drug in the same class as cimetidine, may be a good alternative to cimetidine in persons who are receiving lidocaine because ranitidine has a minimal effect on lidocaine.

Lidocaine **(Xylocaine®, Anestacon®**, and others)

Phenobarbital **(Luminal®, Solfoton®)**

[used to treat insomnia and anxiety; also used to prevent seizures]

Phenobarbital may reduce the effectiveness of lidocaine; your doctor may need to use a slightly larger dose of lidocaine in the presence of phenobarbital. (Of course, only your doctor should alter the dosage of any medication.)

Other barbiturates may have a similar effect on lidocaine.

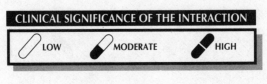

CLINICAL SIGNIFICANCE OF THE INTERACTION

LOW    MODERATE    HIGH

Metoprolol **(Lopressor®)**

Antidiabetic drugs:

- acetohexamide **(Dymelor®)**
- chlorpropamide **(Diabinese®)**
- glipizide **(Glucotrol®)**
- glyburide **(DiaBeta®, Micronase®)**
- insulin **(Humulin®, Lente®, Novolin®,** and others)
- tolazamide **(Tolinase®)**
- tolbutamide **(Orinase®),** and others

[for treatment of diabetes mellitus, a condition that results in excessively high amounts of sugar in the blood and urine]

Although the heart typically beats faster (tachycardia) when blood sugar levels are low, this symptom may be absent when metoprolol is taken. This effect may occur when antidiabetic agents are combined with other drugs that are in the same class as metoprolol, such as acebutolol (Sectral®), atenolol (Tenormin®), betaxolol (Kerlone®), carteolol (Cartrol®), esmolol (Brevibloc®), labetalol (Normodyne®, Trandate®), nadolol (Corgard®), pindolol (Visken®), propranolol (Inderal®), and timolol (Blocadren®).

Metoprolol **(Lopressor®)**

Barbiturates:

- amobarbital **(Amytal®)**
- butabarbital **(Butisol®)**
- butalbital
- pentobarbital **(Nembutal®)**
- phenobarbital **(Luminal®, Solfoton®)**
- primidone **(Mysoline®)**
- secobarbital **(Seconal®),** and others

[used to treat insomnia and anxiety; certain barbiturates are used to prevent seizures]

Barbiturates may reduce the concentration of metoprolol, possibly leading to inadequate control of high blood pressure or a worsening of other disorders for which metoprolol is used.

It may be necessary for your doctor to adjust the dose of metoprolol if a barbiturate is started or stopped, or if its dosage is changed. (Of course, only your doctor should change medication dosages, when appropriate.)

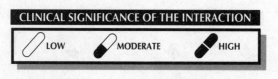

CLINICAL SIGNIFICANCE OF THE INTERACTION

LOW    MODERATE    HIGH

Metoprolol
(**Lopressor**®)

Cimetidine (**Tagamet**®)

[for relief of stomach and intestinal ulcers]

Increased levels of metoprolol in the blood when cimetidine is also taken, possibly leading to an excessive reduction in blood pressure, slowed heart rate, and difficulty breathing.

---

Metoprolol
(**Lopressor**®)

Lidocaine (**Xylocaine**®)

[used to treat abnormal heart rhythms; for topical anesthesia during minor surgery; also available as an over-the-counter medication for relief of pain, itching, and inflammation, but such topical use is unlikely to interact with metoprolol]

Increased lidocaine effect, perhaps to the point of lidocaine toxicity (symptoms of which include dizziness, lethargy, nausea, confusion, agitation, ringing in ears).

This interaction is more likely to occur when lidocaine is given intravenously.

---

Metoprolol
(**Lopressor**®)

Oral contraceptives, such as **Brevicon**®, **Demulen**®, **Enovid**®, **Lo/Ovral**®, **Norinyl**®, **Ortho Novum**®, **Ovcon**®, **Ovral**®, **Tri-Norinyl**®, **Triphasil**®, and many others

[for prevention of pregnancy]

Oral contraceptives may increase the concentration of metoprolol in the blood. While it is not known whether this will result in an increased antihypertensive effect, you should have your blood pressure checked regularly to ensure that it is not too low. (This is an unusual interaction because many other antihypertensive drugs may interact with oral contraceptives in a way that results in an *increase* in blood pressure levels. When metoprolol was combined with an oral contraceptive, however, the opposite effect—reduced blood pressure—was observed.)

Metoprolol is part of a family of drugs known as beta blockers. It is not known whether oral contraceptives produce a similar interaction with other beta-blocker drugs—such as propranolol (Inderal®)—but such an interaction is likely.

**Recommendation:** Your doctor may want to monitor your blood pressure for any changes if an oral contraceptive is started or stopped in the presence of metoprolol therapy.

191

| HEART DRUG | INTERACTING DRUG | RESULT |
|---|---|---|

**Metoprolol (Lopressor®)**

Propafenone (**Rhythmol®**)

[for treatment of life-threatening ventricular arrhythmias (i.e., irregular heartbeat)]

Receiving these drugs together may result in a substantially increased amount of metoprolol in the body, possibly leading to excessive reduction in blood pressure, lethargy, slowed heart rate, difficulty breathing, and cold hands and feet.

---

**Metoprolol (Lopressor®)**

Propoxyphene (**Darvocet-N®, Darvon®, Darvon® with A.S.A.®, Dolene®, and Wygesic®**)

[for relief of mild to moderate pain]

Propoxyphene can increase the concentration of metoprolol, possibly leading to excessive reduction in blood pressure, lethargy, slowed heart rate, difficulty breathing, and cold hands and feet.

**Recommendation:** In most cases, the way to avoid this interaction is to use a pain reliever other than propoxyphene.

---

**Metoprolol (Lopressor®)**

Quinidine (**Cardioquin®, Duraquin®, Quinaglute®, Quinidex®, Quinora®**)

[for arrhythmias, or irregularities of the heartbeat and heart rhythm]

Quinidine can increase the amount of metoprolol in the body, possibly leading to an excessive reduction in blood pressure, lethargy, slowed heart rate, difficulty breathing, and cold hands and feet.

---

**Metoprolol (Lopressor®)**

Rifampin (**Rifadin®, Rifamate®, Rimactane®**)

[used in combination with at least one other drug, rifampin is used to treat tuberculosis; also used in the treatment of individuals who are carriers of meningitis]

Rifampin may reduce the concentration of metoprolol, possibly leading to decreased effect (i.e., less control of high blood pressure levels or angina).

**Recommendation:** Your doctor may want to check your blood pressure if you start, stop, or change the dosage of rifampin.

**CLINICAL SIGNIFICANCE OF THE INTERACTION**

LOW   MODERATE   HIGH

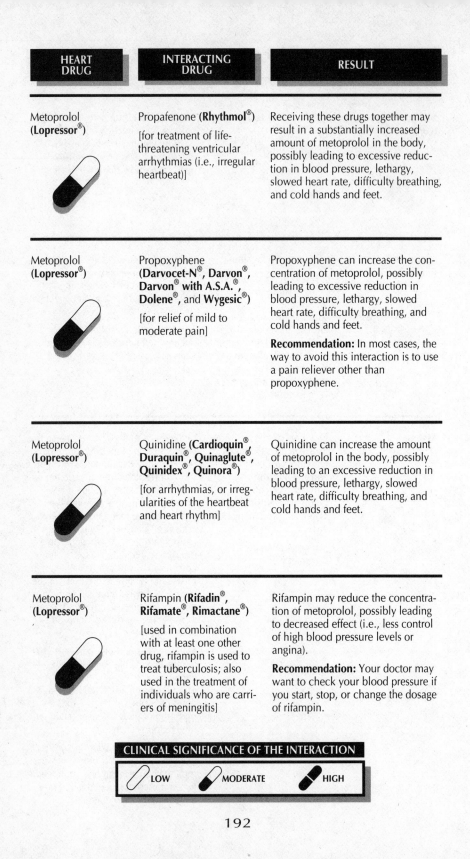

| HEART DRUG | INTERACTING DRUG | RESULT |
| --- | --- | --- |
| Mexiletine (**Mexitil**®) | Acetazolamide (**Diamox**®) [used in glaucoma therapy and for certain types of seizures] | Medications, such as acetazolamide, that cause the urine to become much more alkaline (i.e., less acidic) than it normally is may result in an increased amount of mexiletine in the body. This may lead to toxicity, signs of which include dizziness, lightheadedness, nausea, vomiting, and tremor. This interaction may also occur with other drugs similar to acetazolamide, such as dichlorphenamide (Daranide®) and methazolamide (Neptazane®), which are also used to treat glaucoma. |
| Mexiletine (**Mexitil**®) | Phenytoin (**Dilantin**®) [for the prevention of seizures] | Phenytoin substantially reduces the amount of mexiletine in the body, possibly reducing the effectiveness of mexiletine. Your doctor may need to increase the dose of mexiletine to achieve the same level of antiarrhythmic control when phenytoin is taken concomitantly. (Do *not* change the dosage of either drug yourself; only your doctor should do this.) |
| Mexiletine (**Mexitil**®) | Rifampin (**Rifadin**®, **Rifamate**®, **Rimactane**®) [used in combination with at least one other drug, rifampin is used to treat tuberculosis; also used in the treatment of individuals who are carriers of meningitis] | Rifampin substantially reduces the amount of mexiletine in the body, possibly reducing the effectiveness of mexiletine. Your doctor may need to increase the dose of mexiletine to achieve the same level of antiarrhythmic control when rifampin is taken concomitantly. (Do *not* change the dosage of either drug yourself; only your doctor should do this.) |
| Mexiletine (**Mexitil**®) | Sodium bicarbonate (**Alka-Seltzer**®, **Arm & Hammer**®) [antacid used to relieve heartburn and acid indigestion; some Alka-Seltzer® products are used to relieve pain and symptoms of the common cold] | Chemicals, such as sodium bicarbonate, that cause the urine to become much more alkaline (i.e., less acidic) than it normally is, may result in an increased amount of mexiletine in the body. This may lead to toxicity, signs of which include dizziness, lightheadedness, nausea, vomiting, and tremor. |

Mexiletine **(Mexitil®)**

Theophylline **(Primatene® Tablets, Slo-bid®, Theo-Dur®, Theo-24®, and others)**

[for relief of asthma and bronchospasm]

Elevated amount of theophylline in the blood, possibly leading to theophylline toxicity. Signs of toxicity include nausea, vomiting, diarrhea, headache, irritability, rapid heart rate, and insomnia.

**Recommendation:** It may be necessary for your doctor to adjust the dose of theophylline if mexiletine is started or stopped, or if its dosage is changed. (Of course, only your doctor should change medication dosages, when appropriate.)

Moricizine **(Ethmozine®)**

Cimetidine **(Tagamet®)**

[for relief of stomach and intestinal ulcers]

May increase the amount of moricizine in the body, possibly leading to dizziness, nausea, vomiting, lethargy, palpitations, fainting, and excessively low blood pressure.

**Recommendation:** It may be necessary for your doctor to adjust the dose of moricizine if cimetidine is started or stopped, or if its dosage is changed. (Of course, only your doctor should change medication dosages, when appropriate.

Nadolol **(Corgard®)**

Antidiabetic drugs:

acetohexamide **(Dymelor®)**
• chlorpropamide **(Diabinese®)**
• glipizide **(Glucotrol®)**
• glyburide **(DiaBeta®, Micronase®)**
• insulin **(Humulin®, Lente®, Novolin®, and others)**
• tolazamide **(Tolinase®)**
• tolbutamide **(Orinase®), and others**

[for treatment of diabetes mellitus, a condition that results in excessively

Several results have been reported:

1. Secretion of insulin may be inhibited by nadolol, thereby leading to higher blood sugar levels than normal.

2. High blood pressure and markedly slowed heartbeat may result when blood sugar levels are low.

3. Reduced circulation to the hands and feet.

4. Although the heart typically beats faster (tachycardia) when blood sugar levels are low, this symptom may be absent when nadolol is taken.

**Recommendation:** If possible, diabetics should avoid nonselective beta blockers (which act on the heart,

| HEART DRUG | INTERACTING DRUG | RESULT |
|---|---|---|

*(cont.)*
Nadolol

high amounts of sugar in the blood and urine]

lungs, and blood vessels) such as nadolol. If a beta blocker is necessary, cardioselective beta blockers—such as acebutolol (Sectral®), atenolol (Tenormin®), betaxolol (Kerlone®), or metoprolol (Lopressor®)—are usually recommended. These act primarily on the heart.

---

Nadolol **(Corgard®)**

Epinephrine—contained in products such as **Ana-Kit®, AsthmaHaler®, AsthmaNefrin®, Bronkaid® Mist, Epifrin®, EpiPen®, Epitrate®, Eppy/N®, Glaucon®, Medihaler-Epi®, Primatene® Mist, Sus-Phrine®**, and others

[for temporary relief of shortness of breath and wheezing caused by bronchial asthma; Ana-Kit® and EpiPen® are used for the emergency treatment of allergic reactions to insect stings or bites, food, and other substances that trigger a serious allergic reaction]

The outcome depends on the condition for which the person is being treated, and on how the epinephrine is given.

**Persons with anaphylactic shock:** Some people develop a severe, possibly life-threatening, allergic reaction (called anaphylactic shock) to insect stings or bites and certain medications or foods. Symptoms of anaphylactic shock include hives, wheezing, difficulty breathing, abdominal pain, incontinence, fever, and loss of consciousness; death may also occur. Epinephrine injections help reverse anaphylactic shock, but in persons taking a specific type of antihypertensive drug (i.e., nonselective beta blocker, such as nadolol), the epinephrine may not work very well and other measures often must be taken.

**Persons *not* in anaphylactic shock:** People taking nadolol who receive epinephrine for something other than anaphylactic shock are at risk of developing excessively high blood pressure levels. If the epinephrine is injected with the intention of systemic effects (i.e., reaching most of the tissues and organs in the body), the blood pressure may increase dramatically. If, however, the epinephrine is inhaled into the lungs, put in

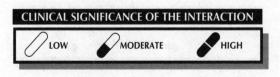

CLINICAL SIGNIFICANCE OF THE INTERACTION

LOW   MODERATE   HIGH

| HEART DRUG | INTERACTING DRUG | RESULT |
|---|---|---|

(*cont.*)
Nadolol

Epinephrine

the eye, or injected for only local effects (e.g., by a dentist or dermatologist), the risk of a hypertensive reaction appears to be much less (unless a much larger than usual amount of epinephrine is used).

**Recommendation:** It is best for people who are at risk of anaphylactic shock (e.g., those allergic to beestings) to avoid taking nadolol or other beta blockers.

---

Nadolol (**Corgard**®)

Lidocaine (**Xylocaine**®)

[used to treat abnormal heart rhythms; for topical anesthesia during minor surgery; also available as an over-the-counter medication for relief of pain, itching, and inflammation, but such topical use is unlikely to interact with nadolol]

May increase the lidocaine effect, perhaps to the point of lidocaine toxicity (symptoms of which include dizziness, lethargy, nausea, confusion, agitation, ringing in ears).

This interaction is more likely to occur when lidocaine is given intravenously.

---

Nicardipine (**Cardene**®)

Cyclosporine (**Sandimmune**®)

[for immune suppression, which is needed after organ transplantation to prevent rejection of the transplanted organ]

Increased concentration of cyclosporine in the body. Increased blood levels of cyclosporine have been associated with kidney damage.

**Recommendation:** It may be necessary for your doctor to adjust the dose of cyclosporine if nicardipine is started or stopped, or if its dosage is changed. (Of course, only your doctor should change medication dosages, when appropriate.)

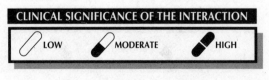

CLINICAL SIGNIFICANCE OF THE INTERACTION

LOW      MODERATE      HIGH

196

Nicardipine **(Cardene®)**

Propranolol **(Inderal®)**

[for treatment of high blood pressure, angina pectoris, and irregular heartbeats; also used to prevent migraine headaches]

Nicardipine and propranolol may have additive effects in lowering the blood pressure. This is usually a positive effect, and may be used intentionally by your doctor to treat angina or high blood pressure. Occasionally, however, the blood pressure may become excessively low.

**Recommendation:** When nicardipine is added to propranolol (or conversely, when propranolol is added to nicardipine), watch for any symptoms of excessive lowering of blood pressure (e.g., dizziness, faintness). Nicardipine probably has a similar effect with other beta blockers (antihypertensive medications that are in the same class as propranolol) although the magnitude of the additive effect may be different. Beta blockers include acebutolol (Sectral®), atenolol (Tenormin®), betaxolol (Kerlone®), carteolol (Cartrol®), esmolol (Brevibloc®), labetalol (Normodyne®, Trandate®), metoprolol (Lopressor®), nadolol (Corgard®), pindolol (Visken®), and timolol (Blocadren®)

Nifedipine **(Adalat®, Procardia®)**

Barbiturates:

- amobarbital **(Amytal®)**
- butabarbital **(Butisol®)**
- butalbital
- pentobarbital **(Nembutal®)**
- phenobarbital **(Luminal®, Solfoton®)**
- primidone **(Mysoline®)**
- secobarbital **(Seconal®),** and others

[used to treat insomnia and anxiety; certain barbiturates are used to prevent seizures]

Significant decrease in the amount of nifedipine available in the body, possibly leading to a decreased effect of the nifedipine. This effect is particularly likely when nifedipine is taken orally.

Much of the evidence for this interaction comes from studies of phenobarbital, but other barbiturates are expected to interact similarly.

Persons receiving a barbiturate may require higher than usual doses of nifedipine. (Of course, *never* alter the dosage of any medication without your doctor's consent and supervision.)

| HEART DRUG | INTERACTING DRUG | RESULT |
|---|---|---|
| Nifedipine (**Adalat**®, **Procardia**®) | Cimetidine (**Tagamet**®) [for relief of stomach and intestinal ulcers] | Cimetidine may increase the amount of nifedipine in the body. Possible nifedipine toxicity—such as dizziness, flushing, and headache—may occur. |
| Nifedipine (**Adalat**®, **Procardia**®) | Diltiazem (**Cardizem**®) [for the treatment of angina pectoris] | When taken together, diltiazem significantly increases the amount of nifedipine in the body. This may lead to dizziness, flushing, and headache. |
| Nifedipine (**Adalat**®, **Procardia**®) | Quinidine (**Cardioquin**®, **Duraquin**®, **Quinaglute**®, **Quinidex**®, **Quinora**®) [for arrhythmias, or irregularities of the heartbeat and heart rhythm] | Increased amount of nifedipine in the body, possibly leading to nifedipine toxicity such as dizziness, flushing, and headache. |
| Nifedipine (**Adalat**®, **Procardia**®) | Ranitidine (**Zantac**®) [for relief of stomach and intestinal ulcers] | Ranitidine may increase nifedipine levels in the body, but not as much as cimetidine (see nifedipine-cimetidine interaction, above). |
| Nifedipine (**Adalat**®, **Procardia**®) | Vincristine (**Oncovin**®) [for treatment of certain types of cancer] | Significantly increased amount of vincristine in the body, possibly resulting in numbness, tingling, weakness, and constipation. |

| HEART DRUG | INTERACTING DRUG | RESULT |
|---|---|---|
| Nitroglycerin (**Deponit**®, **Minitran**®, **Nitro-Bid**®, **Nitrodisc**®, **Nitro-Dur**®, **Nitrogard**®, **Nitrong**®, **Nitrostat**®) | Alcohol | Could result in excessively low blood pressure with lightheadedness, rapid heart rate, and fainting.<br><br>**Recommendation:** Reduce or eliminate your alcohol intake if you think you may be experiencing this interaction. |
| Nitroglycerin (**Deponit**®, **Minitran**®, **Nitro-Bid**®, **Nitrodisc**®, **Nitro-Dur**®, **Nitrogard**®, **Nitrong**®, **Nitrostat**®) | Aspirin | When nitroglycerin is taken by sublingual route (i.e., under the tongue), aspirin may interact with it to increase the amount of nitroglycerin in the body, possibly leading to low blood pressure levels, headache, and dizziness.<br><br>It is not known whether this interaction also occurs with nitroglycerin in the oral form. |
| Nitroglycerin (**Deponit**®, **MInitran**®, **Nitro-Bid**®, **Nitrodisc**®, **Nitro-Dur**®, **Nitrogard**®, **Nitrong**®, **Nitrostat**®) | Ergot alkaloids (**Cafergot**®, **D.H.E.-45**®, **Ergomar**®, **Ergostat**® E. **Wigraine**®)<br><br>[for treatment of migraine] | Ergot alkaloids may hinder nitroglycerin's dilating effect on blood vessels, increasing the likelihood of an anginal attack. |

**CLINICAL SIGNIFICANCE OF THE INTERACTION**

LOW    MODERATE    HIGH

Pindolol (**Visken**®)

Epinephrine—contained in products such as **Ana-Kit**®, **AsthmaHaler**®, **AsthmaNefrin**®, **Bronkaid**® **Mist, Epifrin**®, **EpiPen**®, **Epitrate**®, **Eppy-N**®, **Glaucon**®, **Medihaler-Epi**®, **Primatene**® **Mist, Sus-Phrine**®, and others

[for temporary relief of shortness of breath and wheezing caused by bronchial asthma; Ana-Kit® and EpiPen® are used for the emergency treatment of allergic reactions to insect stings or bites, food, and other substances that trigger a serious allergic reaction]

The outcome depends on the condition for which the person is being treated, and on how the epinephrine is given.

**Persons with anaphylactic shock:** Some people develop a severe, possibly life-threatening, allergic reaction (called anaphylactic shock) to insect stings or bites and certain medications or foods. Symptoms of anaphylactic shock include hives, wheezing, difficulty breathing, abdominal pain, incontinence, fever, and loss of consciousness; death may also occur. Epinephrine injections help reverse anaphylactic shock, but in persons taking a specific type of antihypertensive drug (i.e., nonselective beta blocker, such as pindolol), the epinephrine may not work very well and other measures often must be taken.

**Persons *not* in anaphylactic shock:** People taking pindolol who receive epinephrine for something other than anaphylactic shock are at risk of developing excessively high blood pressure levels. If the epinephrine is injected with the intention of "systemic" effects (i.e., reaching most of the tissues and organs in the body), the blood pressure may increase dramatically. If, however, the epinephrine is inhaled into the lungs, put in the eye, or injected for only local effects (e.g., by a dentist of dermatologist), the risk of a hypertensive reaction appears to be much less (unless a much larger than usual amount of epinephrine is used).

**Recommendation:** It is best for people who are at risk of anaphylactic shock (e.g., those allergic to beestings) to avoid taking pindolol or other beta blockers.

**CLINICAL SIGNIFICANCE OF THE INTERACTION**

LOW    MODERATE    HIGH

| HEART DRUG | INTERACTING DRUG | RESULT |
|---|---|---|

Procainamide **(Procan SR®, Pronestyl®)**

Ambenonium **(Mytelase®)**

[used to treat myasthenia gravis, an autoimmune disorder involving muscular weakness; also used to treat other conditions, such as urinary retention (difficulty or inability to urinate)]

Cholinergic therapy improves nerve functioning in people with myasthenia gravis (a neuromuscular disorder). Those receiving cholinergic therapy (such as ambenonium) may not respond as well to therapy when procainamide is also given. This interaction may result in a worsening of symptoms of myasthenia gravis, such as muscle weakness, double vision, and difficulty swallowing or breathing.

---

Procainamide **(Procan SR®, Pronestyl®)**

Cimetidine **(Tagamet®)**

[for relief of stomach and intestinal ulcers]

Cimetidine may increase the concentration of procainamide in the body, possibly leading to symptoms such as nausea, vomiting, malaise, weakness, lightheadedness, and palpitations.

**Recommendation:** Persons with kidney impairment probably should not take these two drugs together because cimetidine increases the amount of procainamide in the body by interfering with the kidney's ability to get rid of procainamide. Ranitidine (Zantac®) causes a small increase in procainamide levels (smaller than that caused by the cimetidine-procainamide interaction). Famotidine (Pepsid®) does not appear to increase procainamide levels.

---

Procainamide **(Procan SR®, Pronestyl®)**

Neostigmine **(Prostigmin®)**

[used to treat myasthenia gravis, an autoimmune disorder involving muscular weakness; also used to treat other conditions, such as urinary retention (difficulty or inability to urinate)]

Cholinergic therapy improves nerve functioning in people with myasthenia gravis (a neuromuscular disorder). Those receiving cholinergic therapy (such as neostigmine) may not respond as well to therapy when procainamide is also given. This interaction may result in a worsening of symptoms of myasthenia gravis, such as muscle weakness, double vision, and difficulty swallowing or breathing.

| HEART DRUG | INTERACTING DRUG | RESULT |
|---|---|---|

Procainamide **(Procan SR®, Pronestyl®)**

Pyridostigmine **(Mestinon®)**

[used to treat myasthenia gravis, an autoimmune disorder involving muscular weakness; also used to treat other conditions, such as urinary retention (difficulty or inability to urinate)]

Cholinergic therapy improves nerve functioning in people with myasthenia gravis (a neuromuscular disorder). Those receiving cholinergic therapy (such as pyridostigmine) may not respond as well to therapy when procainamide is also given. This interaction may result in a worsening of symptoms of myasthenia gravis, such as muscle weakness, double vision, and difficulty swallowing or breathing.

---

Procainamide **(Procan SR®, Pronestyl®)**

Trimethoprim **(Proloprim®; Bactrim®** and **Septra®** also contain trimethoprim)

[for the treatment of urinary tract infections]

May lead to a substantial increase in the amount of procainamide in the body, possibly leading to toxicity. Signs of this toxicity include nausea, vomiting, malaise, weakness, and lightheadedness.

---

Propafenone **(Rhythmol®)**

Anticoagulants (oral), such as warfarin **(Coumadin®, Panwarfin®)**

[for the prevention of blood clots]

Propafenone increases the amount of warfarin in the body, possibly leading to an increased anticoagulant effect. Some persons may develop bleeding, such as blood in the urine, coughing up of blood, black stools (or red blood in stools), vomiting of blood or substance resembling coffee grounds, bruising, or other bleeding.

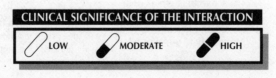

CLINICAL SIGNIFICANCE OF THE INTERACTION

LOW    MODERATE    HIGH

| HEART DRUG | INTERACTING DRUG | RESULT |
| --- | --- | --- |

Propafenone **(Rhythmol®)**

Digoxin **(Lanoxin®)**

[for heart failure and heart abnormalities, such as atrial fibrillation and atrial flutter]

Propafenone may increase the amount of digoxin in the body, possibly leading to digoxin toxicity (symptoms of which include nausea, poor appetite, weakness, lethargy, and visual abnormalities).

---

Propafenone **(Rhythmol®)**

Food

Food may substantially increase the amount of propafenone in the body. Increased levels of propafenone may lead to dizziness, nausea, weakness, lethargy, and blurred vision.

**Recommendation:** Take propafenone in a consistent manner with regard to meals. If your doctor tells you to take propafenone with food, do so consistently every time you take this medication.

---

Propafenone **(Rhythmol®)**

Rifampin **(Rifadin®, Rifamate®, Rimactane®)**

[used in combination with at least one other drug, rifampin is used to treat tuberculosis; also used in the treatment of individuals who are carriers of meningitis]

Rifampin reduces the amount of propafenone in the body, possibly reducing the antiarrhythmic effectiveness.

---

Propranolol **(Inderal®)**

Antacids that contain aluminum or magnesium, such as **Gaviscon®, Gelusil®, Maalox®, Mylanta®, Phillips' Milk of Magnesia®,** and others

[for relief of acid indigestion, heartburn, and abdominal pain caused by too much acid in the stomach]

The absorption of propranolol may be reduced when taken simultaneously with aluminum- or magnesium-containing antacids.

**Recommendation:** Take the antacid at least four hours before or two hours after taking propranolol.

| HEART DRUG | INTERACTING DRUG | RESULT |
|---|---|---|

Propranolol
(**Inderal**®)

Antidiabetic drugs:

- acetohexamide (**Dymelor**®)
- chlorpropamide (**Diabinese**®)
- glipizide (**Glucotrol**®)
- glyburide (**DiaBeta**®, **Micronase**®)
- insulin (**Humulin**®, **Lente**®, **Novolin**®, and others)
- tolazamide (**Tolinase**®)
- tolbutamide (**Orinase**®), and others

[for treatment of diabetes mellitus, a condition that results in excessively high amounts of sugar in the blood and urine]

Several results have been reported:

1. Secretion of insulin may be inhibited by propranolol, thereby leading to higher blood sugar levels than normal.

2. High blood pressure and markedly slowed heartbeat may result when blood sugar levels are low.

3. Reduced circulation to the hands and feet.

4. Although the heart typically beats faster (tachycardia) when blood sugar levels are low, this symptom may be absent when propranolol is given.

**Recommendation:** If possible, diabetics should avoid nonselective beta blockers (which act on the heart, lungs, and blood vessels) such as propranolol. If a beta blocker is necessary, cardioselective beta blockers—such as acebutolol (Sectral®), atenolol (Tenormin®), betaxolol (Kerlone®), or metoprolol (Lopressor®)—are usually recommended. These act primarily on the heart.

---

Propranolol
(**Inderal**®)

Barbiturates:

- amobarbital (**Amytal**®)
- butabarbital (**Butisol**®)
- butalbital
- pentobarbital (**Nembutal**®)
- phenobarbital (**Luminal**®, **Solfoton**®)
- primidone (**Mysoline**®)
- secobarbital (**Seconal**®), and others

[used to treat insomnia and anxiety; certain barbiturates are used to prevent seizures]

Barbiturates may reduce the amount of propranolol in the blood, possibly leading to reduced propranolol effect (i.e., inadequate control of blood pressure or worsening of other conditions for which propranolol is used).

Although this interaction has occurred with the barbiturate phenobarbital, other barbiturates are expected to have a similar effect on propranolol.

It may be necessary for your doctor to adjust the dose of propranolol if a barbiturate is started or stopped, or if its dosage is changed. (Of course, only your doctor should change medication dosages, when appropriate.)

| HEART DRUG | INTERACTING DRUG | RESULT |
|---|---|---|

Propranolol
**(Inderal®)**

Chlorpromazine
**(Thorazine®)**

[for the treatment of various psychotic disorders; also used to relieve nausea]

These drugs enhance the effect of each other. As a result, an increased amount of propranolol in the body may lead to an excessive reduction in blood pressure, lethargy, slowed heart rate, difficulty breathing, and cold hands and feet.

An increased amount of chlorpromazine in the body may lead to drowsiness, dry mouth, dizziness, blurred vision, constipation, difficulty urinating, fainting, and involuntary body movements (e.g., tremor, restless movement, facial grimacing).

Propranolol
**(Inderal®)**

Cimetidine **(Tagamet®)**

[for relief of stomach and intestinal ulcers]

When cimetidine is taken with propranolol, the amount of propranolol in the blood may increase, possibly leading to an excessive reduction in blood pressure, slowed heart rate, difficulty breathing, and cold hands and feet.

**Recommendation:** Be aware of this interaction when taking both cimetidine and propranolol. Use of another antiulcer drug, such as ranitidine (Zantac®), may be preferable when propranolol must be taken.

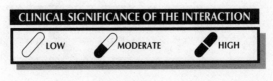

CLINICAL SIGNIFICANCE OF THE INTERACTION

LOW    MODERATE    HIGH

Propranolol
(**Inderal**®)

Epinephrine—contained in products such as **Ana-Kit**®, **AsthmaHaler**®, **AsthmaNefrin**®, **Bronkaid**® **Mist, Epifrin**®, **EpiPen**®, **Epitrate**®, **Eppy/N**®, **Glaucon**®, **Medihaler-Epi**®, **Primatene**® **Mist, Sus-Phrine**®, and others

[for temporary relief of shortness of breath and wheezing caused by bronchial asthma; Ana-Kit® and EpiPen® are used for the emergency treatment of allergic reactions to insect stings or bites, food, and other substances that trigger a serious allergic reaction]

The outcome depends on the condition for which the person is being treated, and on how the epinephrine is given.

**Persons with anaphylactic shock:** Some people develop a severe, possibly life-threatening, allergic reaction (called anaphylactic shock) to insect stings or bites and certain medications or foods. Symptoms of anaphylactic shock include hives, wheezing, difficulty breathing, abdominal pain, incontinence, fever, and loss of consciousness; death may also occur. Epinephrine injections help reverse anaphylactic shock, but in persons taking a specific type of antihypertensive drug (i.e., nonselective beta blocker, such as propranolol), the epinephrine may not work very well and other measures often must be taken.

**Persons *not* in anaphylactic shock:** People taking propranolol who receive epinephrine for something other than anaphylactic shock are at risk of developing excessively high blood pressure levels. If the epinephrine is injected with the intention of systemic effects (i.e., reaching most of the tissues and organs in the body), the blood pressure may increase dramatically. If, however, the epinephrine is inhaled into the lungs, put in the eye, or injected for only local effects (e.g., by a dentist or dermatologist), the risk of a hypertensive reaction appears to be much less (unless a much larger than usual amount of epinephrine is used).

**Recommendation:** It is best for people who are at risk of anaphylactic shock (e.g., those allergic to beestings) to avoid taking propranolol or other beta blockers.

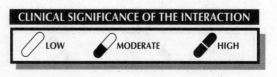

CLINICAL SIGNIFICANCE OF THE INTERACTION

LOW    MODERATE    HIGH

| Propranolol (**Inderal**®) | Ergot alkaloids (**Cafergot**®, **D.H.E.-45**®, **Ergomar**®, **Ergostate**® **Wigraine**®)<br><br>[for treatment of migraine] | Possibly enhances the vasoconstrictive (i.e., narrowing of the blood vessels) effect of ergot alkaloids. This may lead to coldness, numbness or tingling of extremities, pain in legs with exertion, and cramps. |

| Propranolol (**Inderal**®) | Felodipine (**Plendil**®)<br><br>[for treatment of high blood pressure] | Felodipine and propranolol may have an additive effect in lowering the blood pressure. This is usually a positive effect, and may be used intentionally by your doctor to treat angina or high blood pressure. Occasionally, however, the blood pressure may become excessively low. |

**Recommendation:** When felodipine is added to propranolol (or conversely, when propranolol is added to felodipine), watch for any symptoms of excessive lowering of blood pressure (e.g., dizziness, faintness). Felodipine probably has a similar effect with other beta blockers (antihypertensive medications that are in the same class as propranolol) although the magnitude of the additive effect may be different. Other beta blockers include acebutolol (Sectral®), atenolol (Tenormin®), betaxolol (Kerlone®), carteolol (Cartrol®), esmolol (Brevibloc®), labetalol (Normodyne, Trandate®), metoprolol (Lopressor®), nadolol (Corgard®), pindolol (Visken®), and timolol (Blocadren®).

| HEART DRUG | INTERACTING DRUG | RESULT |
|---|---|---|

Propranolol
(Inderal®)

Isoproterenol (Isuprel®, Duo-Medihaler®, and others)

[used as a bronchodilator to relieve bronchospasms associated with asthma, bronchitis, and emphysema]

Propranolol, as well as other beta blockers (the class of drug of propranolol), may reduce the bronchodilating effect of isoproterenol in asthmatic persons. Other beta blockers include acebutolol (Sectral®), atenolol (Tenormin®), betaxolol (Kerlone®), carteolol (Cartrol®), esmolol (Brevibloc®), labetalol (Normodyne®, Trandate®), metoprolol (Lopressor®), nadolol (Corgard®), pindolol (Visken®), and timolol (Blocadren®).

---

Propranolol
(Inderal®)

Isradipine (DynaCirc®)

[for treatment of high blood pressure]

Isradipine and propranolol may have an additive effect in lowering the blood pressure. This is usually a positive effect, and may be used intentionally by your doctor to treat angina or high blood pressure. Occasionally, however, the blood pressure may become excessively low.

**Recommendation:** When isradipine is added to propranolol (or conversely, when propranolol is added to isradipine), watch for any symptoms of excessive lowering of blood pressure (e.g., dizziness, faintness). Isradipine probably has a similar effect with other beta blockers (antihypertensive medications that are in the same class as propranolol) although the magnitude of the additive effect may be different. Other beta blockers include acebutolol (Sectral®), atenolol (Tenormin®), betaxolol (Kerlone®), carteolol (Cartrol®), esmolol (Brevibloc®), labetalol (Normodyne®, Trandate®), metoprolol (Lopressor®), nadolol (Corgard®), pindolol (Visken®), and timolol (Blocadren®).

---

**CLINICAL SIGNIFICANCE OF THE INTERACTION**

LOW    MODERATE    HIGH

| HEART DRUG | INTERACTING DRUG | RESULT |
|---|---|---|

Propranolol
**(Inderal®)**

Lidocaine **(Xylocaine®)**

[used to treat abnormal heart rhythms; for topical anesthesia during minor surgery; also available as an over-the counter medication for relief of pain, itching, and inflammation, but such topical use is unlikely to interact with propranolol]

Increases the lidocaine effect, perhaps to the point of lidocaine toxicity (symptoms of which include dizziness, lethargy, nausea, confusion, agitation, ringing in ears).

This interaction is more likely to occur when lidocaine is given intravenously.

Propranolol
**(Inderal®)**

Nifedipine **(Adalat®, Procardia®, Procardia XL®)**

[for treatment of high blood pressure and angina pectoris]

Nifedipine and propranolol may have an additive effect in lowering the blood pressure. This is usually a positive effect, and may be used intentionally by your doctor to treat angina or high blood pressure. Occasionally, however, the blood pressure may become excessively low.

**Recommendation:** When nifedipine is added to propranolol (or conversely, when propranolol is added to nifedipine), watch for any symptoms of excessive lowering of blood pressure (e.g., dizziness, faintness). Nifedipine probably has a similar effect with other beta blockers (antihypertensive medications that are in the same class as propranolol) although the magnitude of the additive effect may be different. Other beta blockers include acebutolol (Sectral®), atenolol (Tenormin®), betaxolol (Kerlone®), carteolol (Cartrol®), esmolol (Brevibloc®), labetalol (Normodyne®, Trandate®), metoprolol (Lopressor®), nadolol (Corgard®), pindolol (Visken®), and timolol (Blocadren®).

209

| HEART DRUG | INTERACTING DRUG | RESULT |
| --- | --- | --- |
| Propranolol **(Inderal®)**  | Propafenone **(Rhythmol®)** [for treatment of life-threatening ventricular arrhythmias (i.e., irregular heartbeat)] | Receiving these drugs together may result in a substantially increased amount of propranolol in the body, possibly leading to an excessive reduction in blood pressure, slowed heart rate, difficulty breathing, and cold hands and feet. |
| Propranolol **(Inderal®)**  | Propoxyphene **(Darvocet-N®, Darvon®, Darvon® with A.S.A.®, Dolene®, and Wygesic®)** [for relief of mild to moderate pain] | Can increase the concentration of propranolol, possibly leading to an excessive reduction in blood pressure, slowed heart rate, difficulty breathing, and cold hands and feet. |
| Propranolol **(Inderal®)**  | Rifampin **(Rifadin®, Rifamate®, Rimactane®)** [used in combination with at least one other drug, rifampin is used to treat tuberculosis; also used in the treatment of individuals who are carriers of meningitis] | Reduced propranolol effect. A larger dose of propranolol may be needed in the presence of rifampin therapy. (Do *not* change the dosage of either drug yourself; only your doctor should do this.) |

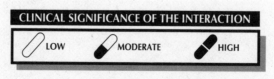

**CLINICAL SIGNIFICANCE OF THE INTERACTION**
LOW   MODERATE   HIGH

| HEART DRUG | INTERACTING DRUG | RESULT |
|---|---|---|

Propranolol **(Inderal®)**

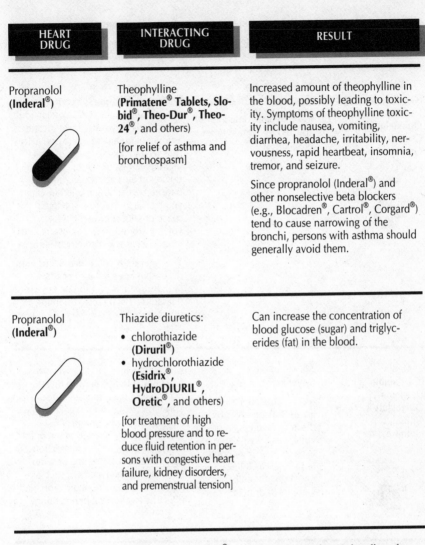

Theophylline **(Primatene® Tablets, Slo-bid®, Theo-Dur®, Theo-24®, and others)**

[for relief of asthma and bronchospasm]

Increased amount of theophylline in the blood, possibly leading to toxicity. Symptoms of theophylline toxicity include nausea, vomiting, diarrhea, headache, irritability, nervousness, rapid heartbeat, insomnia, tremor, and seizure.

Since propranolol (Inderal®) and other nonselective beta blockers (e.g., Blocadren®, Cartrol®, Corgard®) tend to cause narrowing of the bronchi, persons with asthma should generally avoid them.

---

Propranolol **(Inderal®)**

Thiazide diuretics:

- chlorothiazide **(Diruril®)**
- hydrochlorothiazide **(Esidrix®, HydroDIURIL®, Oretic®, and others)**

[for treatment of high blood pressure and to reduce fluid retention in persons with congestive heart failure, kidney disorders, and premenstrual tension]

Can increase the concentration of blood glucose (sugar) and triglycerides (fat) in the blood.

---

Propranolol **(Inderal®)**

Thioridazine **(Mellaril®)**

[for the treatment of various psychotic disorders]

These drugs enhance the effect of one another. As a result, an increased amount of propranolol in the body may lead to an excessive reduction in blood pressure, slowed heart rate, difficulty breathing, and cold hands and feet.

An increased amount of thioridazine in the body may lead to drowsiness, dry mouth, blurred vision, constipation, and difficulty urinating.

| HEART DRUG | INTERACTING DRUG | RESULT |
|---|---|---|

Quinidine
**(Cardioquin®,
Duraquin®,
Quinaglute®,
Quinidex®,
Quinora®)**

Acetazolamide
**(Diamox®)**

[used in glaucoma ther-
apy and for certain types
of seizures]

Medications, such as acetazolamide,
that cause the urine to become much
more alkaline (i.e., less acidic) than it
normally is may result in an increased
amount of quinidine in the body. This
may lead to toxicity, signs of which
include nausea, vomiting, headache,
ringing in the ears, visual disturbances, vertigo (a sensation in which
you feel as if you are revolving in
space or your surroundings are revolving around you), confusion, and
in severe cases, psychiatric disorders.

This interaction may also occur with
drugs that are similar to acetazolamide, such as dichlorphenamide
(Daranide®) and methazolamide
(Neptazane®).

Quinidine
**(Cardioquin®,
Duraquin®,
Quinaglute®,
Quinidex®,
Quinora®)**

Ambenonium
**(Mytelase®)**

[used to treat myasthenia
gravis, an autoimmune
disorder involving mus-
cular weakness; also
used to treat other conditions, such as urinary
retention (difficulty or
inability to urinate)]

Cholinergic therapy improves nerve
functioning in people with myasthenia gravis (a neuromuscular disorder).
Those receiving cholinergic therapy
(such as ambenonium) may not respond as well to therapy when quinidine is also given. This interaction
may result in a worsening of symptoms of myasthenia gravis, such as
muscle weakness, double vision, and
difficulty swallowing or breathing.

Quinidine
**(Cardioquin®,
Duraquin®,
Quinaglute®,
Quinidex®,
Quinora®)**

Antacids (oral) that con-
tain aluminum and mag-
nesium, such as
**Gaviscon®, Gelusil®,
Maalox®, Mylanta®,
Phillips' Milk of
Magnesia®**, and others

[for relief of acid indigestion, heartburn, and
abdominal pain caused
by too much acid in
the stomach]

Antacids containing the combination
of aluminum and magnesium are able
to make the urine more alkaline (i.e.,
less acidic), causing an increased
amount of quinidine in the body. The
amount of quinidine may increase
enough to reach toxicity. Symptoms
of quinidine toxicity include nausea,
vomiting, headache, ringing in the
ears, visual disturbances, vertigo (a
sensation in which you feel as if you
are revolving in space or your surroundings are revolving around you),
confusion, and, in severe cases, psychiatric disorders.

| HEART DRUG | INTERACTING DRUG | RESULT |
|---|---|---|

Quinidine **(Cardioquin®, Duraquin®, Quinaglute®, Quinidex®, Quinora®)**

Barbiturates:

- amobarbital **(Amytal®)**
- butabarbital **(Butisol®)**
- butalbital
- pentobarbital **(Nembutal®)**
- phenobarbital **(Luminal®, Solfoton®)**
- primidone **(Mysoline®)**
- secobarbital **(Seconal®),** and others

[used to treat insomnia and anxiety; certain barbiturates are used to prevent seizures]

Barbiturates may reduce the amount of quinidine in the body, possibly leading to decreased effectiveness of quinidine.

Your doctor may need to change the dose of quinidine if he or she prescribes a barbiturate for you or you discontinue barbiturate therapy. (Do *not* change the dosage of either drug yourself; only your doctor should do this.)

Quinidine **(Cardioquin®, Duraquin®, Quinaglute®, Quinidex®, Quinora®)**

Cimetidine **(Tagamet®)**

[for relief of stomach and intestinal ulcers]

Cimetidine taken with quinidine can lead to an elevated concentration of quinidine in the blood. Notify your doctor if you observe signs such as ringing in your ears, vertigo (a sensation in which you feel as if you are revolving in space or your surroundings are revolving around you), dizziness, confusion, blurred vision, nausea, lightheadedness, fainting, and tremor.

**Recommendation:** It may be necessary for your doctor to adjust the dose of quinidine if cimetidine is started or stopped, or if its dosage is changed. (Of course, only your doctor should change medication dosages, when appropriate.)

Another alternative is to use the antiulcer drug ranitidine (Zantac®) or famotidine (Pepcid®) rather than cimetidine: they appear to be less likely to interact with quinidine than cimetidine.

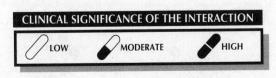

CLINICAL SIGNIFICANCE OF THE INTERACTION

LOW    MODERATE    HIGH

| HEART DRUG | INTERACTING DRUG | RESULT |
| --- | --- | --- |

Quinidine **(Cardioquin®, Duraquin®, Quinaglute®, Quinidex®, Quinora®)**

Codeine **(Empirin® with codeine, Novahistine® DH, Nucofed®, Phenergan® VC, Robitussin®-DAC, Tylenol® with codeine)**

[used to relieve pain and to suppress cough]

Quinidine may decrease the ability of codeine to relieve pain.

**Recommendation:** Codeine may not be the best choice for persons who need pain relief and are also receiving quinidine because the analgesic effectiveness of codeine may be reduced.

---

Quinidine **(Cardioquin®, Duraquin®, Quinaglute®, Quinidex®, Quinora®)**

Desipramine **(Pertofrane®, Norpramin®)**

[for the treatment of depression]

Quinidine causes an increased amount of desipramine in the blood, possibly leading to side effects such as severe dry mouth, blurred vision, fast heartbeat, difficulty or inability to urinate, and constipation.

It may be necessary for your doctor to adjust the dose of desipramine if quinidine is started or stopped, or if its dosage is changed. (Of course, only your doctor should change medication dosages, when appropriate.)

---

Quinidine **(Cardioquin®, Duraquin®, Quinaglute®, Quinidex®, Quinora®)**

Digitoxin **(Crystodigin®)**

[for heart failure and other heart abnormalities]

Quinidine increases the effect of digitoxin; in certain persons, this may lead to toxicity. Symptoms of digitoxin toxicity include nausea, poor appetite, weakness, lethargy, and visual abnormalities.

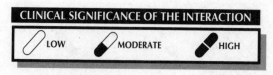

CLINICAL SIGNIFICANCE OF THE INTERACTION

LOW    MODERATE    HIGH

Quinidine **(Cardioquin®, Duraquin®, Quinaglute®, Quinidex®, Quinora®)**

Digoxin **(Lanoxin®)**

[for heart failure and heart abnormalities, such as atrial fibrillation and atrial flutter]

Quinidine increases the effect of digoxin; in certain persons, this may lead to toxicity. Symptoms of digoxin toxicity include nausea, poor appetite, weakness, lethargy, and visual abnormalities.

**Recommendation:** It may be necessary for your doctor to adjust the dose of digoxin if quinidine is started or stopped, or if its dosage is changed. (Of course, only your doctor should change medication dosages, when appropriate.)

Quinidine **(Cardioquin®, Duraquin®, Quinaglute®, Quinidex®, Quinora®)**

Imipramine **(Janimine®, Tofranil®)**

[for the treatment of depression]

Quinidine may cause an increased amount of imipramine in the body, possibly leading to side effects such as severe dry mouth, blurred vision, fast heartbeat, difficulty or inability to urinate, and constipation.

Quinidine **(Cardioquin®, Duraquin®, Quinaglute®, Quinidex®, Quinora®)**

Kaolin-Pectin **(Donnagel®)**

[used to relieve diarrhea]

Kaolin-pectin reduces the amount of quinidine in the body, possibly leading to decreased antiarrhythmic effectiveness.

**Recommendation:** Take quinidine two hours before or four hours after taking kaolin-pectin.

| HEART DRUG | INTERACTING DRUG | RESULT |
|---|---|---|

Quinidine **(Cardioquin®, Duraquin®, Quinaglute®, Quinidex®, Quinora®)**

Neostigmine **(Prostigmin®)**

[used to treat myasthenia gravis, an autoimmune disorder involving muscular weakness; also used to treat other conditions, such as urinary retention (difficulty or inability to urinate)]

Cholinergic therapy improves nerve functioning in people with myasthenia gravis (a neuromuscular disorder). Those receiving cholinergic therapy (such as neostigmine) may not respond as well to therapy when quinidine is also given. This interaction may result in a worsening of symptoms of myasthenia gravis, such as muscle weakness, double vision, and difficulty swallowing or breathing.

Quinidine **(Cardioquin®, Duraquin®, Quinaglute®, Quinidex®, Quinora®)**

Phenytoin **(Dilantin®)**

[for the prevention of seizures]

Phenytoin substantially reduces the amount of quinidine in the body, possibly reducing the antiarrhytmic effectiveness of quinidine. Your doctor may need to increase the dose of quinidine to achieve the same level of antiarrhythmic control when phenytoin is taken concomitantly. (Do *not* change the dosage of either drug yourself; only your doctor should do this.)

Quinidine **(Cardioquin®, Duraquin®, Quinaglute®, Quinidex®, Quinora®)**

Pyridostigmine **(Mestinon®)**

[used to treat myasthenia gravis, an autoimmune disorder involving muscular weakness; also used to treat other conditions, such as urinary retention (difficulty or inability to urinate)]

Cholinergic therapy improves nerve functioning in people with myasthenia gravis (a neuromuscular disorder). Those receiving cholinergic therapy (such as pyridostigmine) may not respond as well to therapy when quinidine is also given. This interaction may result in a worsening of symptoms of myasthenia gravis, such as muscle weakness, double vision, and difficulty swallowing or breathing.

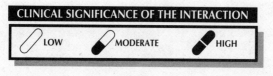

CLINICAL SIGNIFICANCE OF THE INTERACTION

LOW    MODERATE    HIGH

| HEART DRUG | INTERACTING DRUG | RESULT |
|---|---|---|

Quinidine **(Cardioquin®, Duraquin®, Quinaglute®, Quinidex®, Quinora®)**

Rifampin **(Rifadin®, Rifamate®, Rimactane®)**

[used in combination with at least one other drug, rifampin is used to treat tuberculosis; also used in the treatment of individuals who are carriers of meningitis]

Rifampin reduces the amount of quinidine in the body, possibly reducing the antiarrhythmic effectiveness of quinidine. Your doctor may need to increase the dose of quinidine to achieve the same level of antiarrhythmic control when phenytoin is taken concomitantly. (Do *not* change the dosage of either drug yourself; only your doctor should do this.)

---

Quinidine **(Cardioquin®, Duraquin®, Quinaglute®, Quinidex®, Quinora®)**

Sodium bicarbonate **(Alka-Seltzer®, Arm & Hammer®)**

[antacid used to relieve heartburn and acid indigestion; some Alka-Seltzer® products are used to relieve pain and symptoms of the common cold]

Chemicals such as sodium bicarbonate, that cause the urine to become much more alkaline (i.e, less acidic) than it normally is, may result in an increased amount of quinidine in the body. This may lead to quinidine toxicity, symptoms of which include nausea, vomiting, headache, ringing in the ears, visual disturbances, vertigo (a sensation in which you feel as if you are revolving in space or your surroundings are revolving around you), confusion, and, in severe cases, psychiatric disorders.

---

Verapamil **(Calan®, Isoptin®)**

Alcohol

Verapamil may increase the effect of alcohol. Intoxication may result to a greater degree and may last longer when verapamil is taken with alcohol.

**Recommendation:** Reduce or avoid alcohol altogether while taking verapamil. Check with your doctor.

Verapamil **(Calan®, Isoptin®)**

Barbiturates:

- amobarbital **(Amytal®)**
- butabarbital **(Butisol®)**
- butalbital
- pentobarbital **(Nembutal®)**
- phenobarbital **(Luminal®, Solfoton®)**
- primidone **(Mysoline®)**
- secobarbital **(Seconal®),** and others

[used to treat insomnia and anxiety; certain barbiturates are used to prevent seizures]

Phenobarbital (and probably other barbiturates) substantially reduces the plasma concentration of verapamil, possibly leading to a reduced effect of this antihypertensive. This effect is particularly likely when verapamil is taken orally.

Persons receiving phenobarbital or other barbiturates may require higher than usual doses of verapamil. (Of course, *never* alter the dosage of any medication without your doctor's consent and supervision.)

---

Verapamil **(Calan®, Isoptin®)**

Calcium

[a mineral needed for the heart, muscles, and nerves to function properly; also needed for strong bones and teeth]

When large doses of calcium are taken, there is a possible reduced effect of verapamil.

This interaction is not usually significant unless the calcium is given intravenously.

---

Verapamil **(Calan®, Isoptin®)**

Carbamazepine **Tegretol®)**

[for epilepsy, trigeminal neuralgia (spasms of pain in the face), and other disorders]

May increase carbamazepine concentration in the body, possibly leading to double vision, headaches, abnormal muscle coordination, or dizziness.

Reduced effect of verapamil may also occur.

**Recommendation:** It may be necessary for your doctor to adjust the dose of carbamazepine if verapamil is started or stopped or if its dosage is changed. (Of course, only your doctor should change medication dosage, when appropriate.) Nifedipine (Adalat®, Procardia®), which does not affect the amount of carbamazepine in the body, may be an alternative to verapamil if a calcium-channel blocker must be given with carbamazepine

| | | |
|---|---|---|
| Verapamil **(Calan®, Isoptin®)**  | Cimetidine **(Tagamet®)** [for relief of stomach and intestinal ulcers] | May increase verapamil levels, possibly leading to toxicity. Symptoms of toxicity include excessive slowing of the heart rate, decreased blood pressure, headache, flushing, and edema (fluid accumulation). |
| Verapamil **(Calan®, Isoptin®)**  | Cyclosporine **(Sandimmune®)** [for immune suppression, which is needed after organ transplantation to prevent rejection of the transplanted organ] | Increased concentration of cyclosporine in the body. Increased blood levels of cyclosporine have been associated with nephrotoxicity (kidney damage). **Recommendation:** It may be necessary for your doctor to adjust the dose of cyclosporine if verapamil is started or stopped, or if its dosage is changed. (Of course, only your doctor should change medication dosages, when appropriate.) |

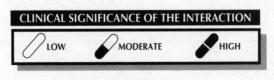

CLINICAL SIGNIFICANCE OF THE INTERACTION

LOW    MODERATE    HIGH

Verapamil (**Calan®**, **Isoptin®**)

Digoxin (**Lanoxin®**)

[for heart failure and heart abnormalities, such as atrial fibrillation and atrial flutter]

Increased digoxin effect, possibly leading to toxicity. Symptoms of toxicity include nausea, poor appetite, weakness, lethargy, and visual abnormalities.

**Recommendation:** It may be necessary for your doctor to adjust the dose of digoxin if verapamil is started or stopped, or if its dosage is changed. (Of course, only your doctor should change medication dosages, when appropriate).

Verapamil is in a drug class known as calcium-channel blockers, certain others of which—nifedipine (Adalat®, Procardia®), isradipine (DynaCirc®), and nicardipine (Cardene®)—do not appear to interact with digoxin. Reports of a diltiazem-digoxin interaction are mixed; diltiazem increased the amount of digoxin in some persons, while in others, no interaction occurred.

Verapamil (**Calan®**, **Isoptin®**)

Lithium (**Cibalith-S®**, **Eskalith®**, **Lithane®**, **Lithobid®**, and others)

[for manic-depressive disorder]

In a few isolated cases, this combination seemed to lead to neurotoxicity (problems involving the nervous system). Possible symptoms include nausea, vomiting, muscular incoordination, and ringing in the ears. This interaction may also occur with diltiazem (Cardizem®) and possibly with other calcium-channel blockers (a particular class of medication used to treat hypertension and angina).

Some persons do not seem to have any trouble with the combined use of lithium and verapamil or other calcium-channel blockers. If you are concerned about this unlikely interaction, discuss your concerns with your doctor.

| HEART DRUG | INTERACTING DRUG | RESULT |
|---|---|---|

Verapamil (**Calan®**, **Isoptin®**)

Prazosin (**Minipress®**)

[for the treatment of high blood pressure]

May lead to an excessive decrease in blood pressure in some persons. Symptoms could include dizziness, lightheadedness, and fainting.

---

Verapamil (**Calan®**, **Isoptin®**)

Propranolol (**Inderal®**)

[for treatment of high blood pressure, angina pectoris, and irregular heartbeat; also used to prevent migraine headaches]

Verapamil can increase the amount of propranolol in the blood, and may also lead to reductions in the blood pressure and slowing of the heart rate. This is usually a favorable interaction that may be used intentionally by your doctor, but occasionally the blood pressure or heart rate may become excessively low.

**Recommendation:** When verapamil is added to propranolol (or conversely, when propranolol is added to verapamil), watch for any symptoms of excessive lowering of blood pressure or heart rate (e.g., dizziness, faintness). Verapamil probably has a similiar effect with other beta blockers (antihypertensive medications that are in the same class as propranolol) although the magnitude of the additive effect may be different. Other beta blockers include acebutolol (Sectral®), atenolol (Tenormin®), betaxolol (Kerlone®), carteolol (Cartrol®), esmolol (Brevibloc®), labetalol (Normodyne®, Trandate®), metoprolol (Lopressor®), nadolol (Corgard®), pindolol (Visken®), and timolol (Blocadren®).

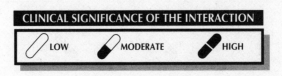

CLINICAL SIGNIFICANCE OF THE INTERACTION

LOW    MODERATE    HIGH

Verapamil **(Calan®, Isoptin®)**

Quindine **(Cardioquin®, Duraqin®, Quinaglute®, Quinidex®, Quinora®)**

[for arrhythmias, or irregularities of the heartbeat and heart rhythm]

Can cause increased levels of quinidine in the body, possibly leading to quinidine toxicity. Symptoms of quinidine toxicity include ringing in the ears, nausea, headache, blurred vision, and, in severe cases, psychiatric disorders.

**Recommendation:** If you must take quinidine with a calcium-channel blocker, diltiazem may be an option because it does not appear to interact with quinidine. Check with your doctor.

Verapamil **(Calan®, Isoptin®)**

Rifampin **(Rifadin®, Rifamate®, Rimactane®)**

[used in combination with at least one other drug, rifampin is used to treat tuberculosis; also used in the treatment of individuals who are carriers of meningitis]

A large decrease in the amount of verapamil in the body, possibly leading to a decreased effect of verapamil (i.e., worsened control of high blood pressure or angina, depending upon the reason verapamil is being taken). This effect occurs when verapamil is taken orally, but not when it is given intravenously.

**Recommendation:** It may be necessary for your doctor to adjust the dose of verapamil if rifampin is started or stopped, or if its dosage is changed. (Of course, only your doctor should change medication dosages, when appropriate.)

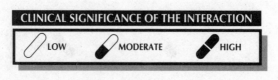

CLINICAL SIGNIFICANCE OF THE INTERACTION

LOW    MODERATE    HIGH

Verapamil **(Calan®, Isoptin®)**

Theophylline **(Primatene® Tablets, Slo-bid®, Theo-Dur®, Theo-24®, and others)**

[for treatment of asthma and bronchospasm]

Increased amount of theophylline in the blood, possibly leading to theophylline toxicity (symptoms of which include nausea, vomiting, diarrhea, headache, irritability, rapid heart rate, insomnia, and tremor).

Other antihypertensive drugs in this class—diltiazem (Cardizem®) and nifedipine (Adalat®, Procardia®)—are less likely to increase theophylline concentrations, and may do so in only a small percentage of persons.

**Recommendation:** It may be necessary for your doctor to adjust the dose of theophylline if verapamil is started or stopped, or if its dosage is changed. (Of course, only your doctor should change medication dosages, when appropriate.)

CHAPTER 7

# ANTIHYPERTENSIVE DRUGS

High blood pressure, also called hypertension, is a disorder in which there is increased resistance to the pressure of blood passing through the blood vessels. More than 60 million Americans suffer from high blood pressure. Some of the consequences of this condition include heart attack, stroke, and kidney failure.

## Medications Used to Treat Hypertension

Antihypertensive agents are used to reduce high blood pressure. More than three hundred antihypertensive drugs are available by prescription in the United States. Depending upon the particular drug, these medications act on the heart, the blood vessels, the nervous system, or the kidneys, individually or in combination. Antihypertensive medication is typically categorized into the following groups:

### Diuretics

For years, doctors' first choice of drug was—and in many cases continues to be—the diuretic. This medication is also known as the water pill because it causes the kidneys to eliminate excess water (and sodium), increasing somewhat the amount of urine you produce. Over the long term, diuretics seem to have an effect on the blood vessels, making them less likely to constrict in response to certain stimuli. A widened blood vessel has less resistance against its walls than a constricted one (known as reduced peripheral resistance in the language of physicians), which leads to decreased blood pressure levels.

Some of the most frequently used and best investigated of the antihypertensive drugs are a family of drugs known as the thiazide diuretics. These include chlorothiazide (Diuril®), hydrochlorothiazide (Esidrix®, HydroDIURIL®), bendroflumethiazide (Naturetin®), cyclothiazide (Fluidil®), hydroflumethiazide (Diucardin®), methyclothiazide (Enduron®), and others. Thiazide-like medications include chlorthalidone (Hygroton®), metolazone (Diulo®, Zaroxolyn®), and others. Some of the "loop" diuretics (so named because they work in a part of the kidney known as the loop of Henle) include: bumetanide (Bumex®), furosemide (Lasix®), ethacrynic acid (Edecrin®), and others. Another diuretic with a chemical structure different from, but related to, that of the thiazide diuretics is indapamide (Lozol®).

## Centrally acting agents

Centrally acting agents affect a group of nerves—called the vasomotor center—located in the brain. These nerves are responsible for the contraction and expansion of blood vessels. By preventing these nerves from causing the blood vessels to contract too much, centrally acting agents cause the blood vessels to remain more relaxed and open. Since blood flows more easily through a relaxed vessel than through a constricted one, the blood pressure drops. Examples of centrally acting drugs include clonidine (Catapres®), methyldopa (Aldomet®), guanabenz (Wytensin®), and others.

## Alpha blockers

Alpha receptors are found in various sites in the body including blood vessels throughout the skin. When these receptors are stimulated, blood vessels narrow. Alpha-blocking drugs prevent the stimulation of alpha receptors, which allows for the relaxation of the vessels. Alpha-blocking drugs include prazosin (Minipress®), terazosin (Hytrin®), and doxazosin (Cardura®).

## Beta blockers

Beta blockers work on receptors in the heart known as beta receptors. When stimulated by chemicals—one of the most common of which is norepinephrine—beta receptors cause the heart to beat faster and to contract more forcibly. These drugs block beta receptors, thereby leading to a decrease in the heart rate and in the forcefulness of the heart's contractions. The decrease in heart rate is more pronounced with certain beta-blocking drugs. The beta blockers lower blood pressure by reducing the amount of blood pumped through the heart with each stroke. Beta blockers include acebutolol (Sectral®), atenolol (Tenormin®), betaxolol (Kerlone®), carteolol (Cartrol®), esmolol (Brevibloc®), labetalol (Normodyne®, Trandate®), metoprolol (Lopressor®), nadolol (Corgard®), penbutolol (Levatol®), pindolol (Viskin®), propranolol (Inderal®), timolol (Blocadren®), and others.

## Calcium-channel blockers

Calcium-channel blockers prevent calcium from entering muscle—both heart muscle and muscle that surrounds blood vessels. As blood vessels widen, blood passes through them with less resistance. This decrease in resistance leads to a reduction in blood pressure. Some of the calcium-channel blockers available include verapamil (Calan®, Isoptin®, Verelan®), nifedipine (Adalat®, Procardia XL®), amlodipine (Norvasc®), diltiazem (Cardizem® CD), nicardipine (Cardene®), isradipine (DynaCirc®), felodipine (Plendil®), and others.

## Vasodilators

Vasodilators act directly on the muscles within the walls of small arteries, causing them to relax. As a result, the blood vessels expand and blood flows through them more easily. Examples of vasodilators include hydralazine (Apresoline®) and minoxidil (Loniten®).

### Adrenergic neuron blockers

Some antihypertensive drugs work on different parts of the nervous system to lower blood pressure. Reserpine (Serpasil®), for example, can interfere with nerve transmissions that contribute to high blood pressure. Guanethidine (Ismelin®) and guanadrel (Hylorel®) are other antihypertensive drugs that act at the nerve endings by blocking the release of a chemical (norepinephrine) from that area.

### Angiotensin-converting enzyme (ACE) inhibitors

An enzyme in the body converts an inactive chemical—known as angiotensin I—to angiotensin II, the pharmacologically active form. Angiotensin II causes the blood vessels to constrict, leading to increased blood pressure. The ACE inhibitors block the enzyme activity that is needed to form angiotensin II. As a result, the blood vessels do not constrict. Drugs in the ACE inhibitor class include captopril (Capoten®), enalapril (Vasotec®), and lisinopril (Prinivil®, Zestril®). More recently available ACE inhibitors are ramipril (Altace®), fosinopril (Monopril®), quinapril (Accupril®), and benazepril (Lotensin®).

# Interactions

If you are taking an antihypertensive medication, regardless of type, avoid certain over-the-counter medications for the treatment of coughs, colds, or allergies unless advised by your doctor. These medications may contain phenylephrine, phenylpropanolomine, or pseudoephedrine, chemicals which cause blood vessels to narrow or prevent their dilation. Since many antihypertensive drugs lower blood pressure by relaxing or dilating blood vessels (working either directly on the blood vessel or indirectly through the nervous system), the following over-the-counter medications—which may be available as tablets, syrup, capsules, or caplets—could interfere with the effectiveness of your antihypertensive medication:

*Phenylephrine-containing medications:* Congespirin®, Dristan®, Neo-Synephrine® Nasal Spray, Dimetane®, Novahistine® Elixir, Phenergan® VC, Robitussin® Night Relief, and others.

*Phenylpropanolamine-containing medications:* Comtrex® Multi-Symptom Cold Reliever, Naldecon® DX, Sinarest® Regular and Extra Strength, Triaminic®, Dimetapp®, Cheracol® Plus Head Cold/Cough Formula, Acutrim® Appetite Suppressant, and others.

*Pseudoephedrine-containing medications:* Actifed®, Sine-Aid®, Sine-Off®, Sinutab®, Contac® Nighttime Cold Medicine, Co-Tylenol® Cold Medicine, Sudafed®, Novahistine® DMX, Robitussin-DAC®, Tylenol® Maximum Strength Sinus Medicion, Vicks Formula 44D®, Vicks Nyquil®, and others.

The above list is not exhaustive. Furthermore, drug manufacturers occasionally reformulate their nonprescription products; as a result, to ensure that a particular product contains the drug you want (or want to avoid), always read the label of your over-the-counter medications. Check with your physician if you have any questions.

| ANTIHYPERTENSIVE DRUG | INTERACTING DRUG | RESULT |
|---|---|---|

Acebutolol (**Sectral**®)

Antidiabetic drugs

- acetohexamide (**Dymelor**®)
- chlorpropamide (**Diabinese**®)
- glipizide (**Glucotrol**®)
- glyburide (**DiaBeta**®, **Micronase**®)
- insulin (**Humulin**®, **Lente**®, **Novolin**®, and others)
- tolazamide (**Tolinase**®)
- tolbutamide (**Orinase**®), and others

[for treatment of diabetes mellitus, a condition that results in excessively high amounts of sugar in the blood and urine]

Although the heart typically beats faster (tachycardia) when blood sugar levels are low, this symptom may be absent when acebutolol is given.

---

Acebutolol (**Sectral**®)

Indomethacin (**Indocin**®)

[for reduction of inflammation; used to reduce the pain and swelling associated with arthritis, tendinitis, and bursitis]

Indomethacin, a nonsteroidal anti-inflammatory drug, may reduce the antihypertensive or antianginal effect of acebutolol. This effect may occur with other nonsteroidal anti-inflammatory agents besides indomethacin, such as piroxicam (Feldene®), naproxen (Naprosyn®), and naproxen sodium (Anaprox®). Sulindac (Clinoril®), a drug in the same class as indomethacin, appears less likely to interfere with the antihypertensive effect of acebutolol.

**Recommendation:** Your doctor may want to check your blood pressure if you start, stop, or change the dosage of an NSAID.

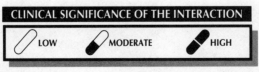

CLINICAL SIGNIFICANCE OF THE INTERACTION

LOW          MODERATE          HIGH

| ANTIHYPERTENSIVE DRUG | INTERACTING DRUG | RESULT |
|---|---|---|
| ACE inhibitors:<br><br>• benazepril (**Lotensin**®)<br>• captopril (**Capoten**®)<br>• enalapril (**Vasotec**®)<br>• fosinopril (**Monopril**®)<br>• lisinopril (**Prinivil**®, **Zestril**®)<br>• quinapril (**Accupril**®)<br>• ramipril (**Altace**®)<br><br> | Amiloride (**Midamor**®)<br><br>[used in combination with other medications to treat high blood pressure; also used to treat disorders that involve excess fluid accumulation] | Both ACE inhibitors and amiloride tend to increase serum potassium levels. Their effects may be additive, resulting in excessively high potassium levels in some people.<br><br>**Recommendation:** Discuss this interaction with your doctor. |
| ACE inhibitors:<br><br>• benazepril (**Lotensin**®)<br>• captopril (**Capoten**®)<br>• enalapril (**Vasotec**®)<br>• fosinopril (**Monopril**®)<br>• lisinopril (**Prinivil**®, **Zestril**®)<br>• quinapril (**Accupril**®)<br>• ramipril (**Altace**®)<br><br> | Loop diuretics:<br><br>• bumetanide (**Bumex**®)<br>• ethacrynic acid (**Edecrin**®)<br>• furosemide (**Lasix**®)<br><br>[for reducing high blood pressure and fluid accumulation] | Some persons may require the combined use of an ACE inhibitor and a loop diuretic to control their medical condition. If ACE inhibitor therapy, however, is started in the presence of loop diuretic therapy (which has been sufficient to reduce the blood volume), some patients may experience a precipitous fall in blood pressure. Symptoms of excessively low blood pressure levels include light-headedness and fainting.<br><br>If your doctor suspects that you may be sensitive to ACE inhibitors due to diuretic-induced reduction in blood volume, he or she may reduce the diuretic dose or stop the diuretic temporarily before starting ACE inhibitor therapy. Your doctor may also start with a low dose of ACE inhibitor and increase the dose gradually. |

| ANTIHYPERTENSIVE DRUG | INTERACTING DRUG | RESULT |
|---|---|---|
| ACE inhibitors:<br>• benazepril (**Lotensin**®)<br>• captopril (**Capoten**®)<br>• enalapril (**Vasotec**®)<br>• fosinopril (**Monopril**®)<br>• lisinopril (**Prinivil**®, **Zestril**®)<br>• quinapril (**Accupril**®)<br>• ramipril (**Altace**®)<br> | Nonsteroidal anti-inflammatory drugs:<br><br>• diclofenac (**Voltaren**®)<br>• diflunisal (**Dolobid**®)<br>• etodolac (**Lodine**®)<br>• fenoprofen (**Nalfon**®)<br>• flurbiprofen (**Ansaid**®)<br>• ibuprofen (**Advil**®, **Motrin**®, **Nuprin**®, **Rufen**®)<br>• indomethacin (**Indocin**®)<br>• ketoprofen (**Orudis**®)<br>• ketorolac (**Toradol**®)<br>• meclofenamate (**Meclomen**®)<br>• nabumetone (**Relafen**®)<br>• naproxen (**Naprosyn**®)<br>• naproxen sodium (**Anaprox**®)<br>• phenylbutazone (**Butazolidin**®)<br>• piroxicam (**Feldene**®)<br>• sulindac (**Clinoril**®)<br>• tolmetin (**Tolectin**®)<br><br>[for reducing inflammation of joints and muscles and pain caused by inflammation] | Indomethacin may inhibit the antihypertensive effect of captopril and probably other ACE inhibitors. Other nonsteroidal anti-inflammatory drugs, listed in the second column, at left—with the possible exception of sulindac (Clinoril®)—probably have a similar effect.<br><br>**Recommendation:** Your doctor may want to check your blood pressure if you start, stop, or change the dosage of an NSAID. |
| ACE inhibitors:<br>• benazepril (**Lotensin**®)<br>• captopril (**Capoten**®)<br>• enalapril (**Vasotec**®)<br>• fosinopril (**Monopril**®)<br>• lisinopril (**Prinivil**®, **Zestril**®)<br>• quinapril (**Accupril**®)<br>• ramipril (**Altace**®)<br> | Potassium (**K-Tab**®, **Kaon-CL Tabs**®, **Micro-K**®, **Ten-K**®, and others) [used to supplement potassium levels or to prevent potassium depletion] | ACE inhibitors tend to increase serum potassium levels. Concurrent use of potassium supplements may result in excessively high potassium levels in the body. Salt substitutes containing potassium should be used with caution. |

ACE inhibitors:

- benazepril (**Lotensin**®)
- captopril (**Capoten**®)
- enalapril (**Vasotec**®)
- fosinopril (**Monopril**®)
- lisinopril (**Prinivil**®, **Zestril**®)
- quinapril (**Accupril**®)
- ramipril (**Altace**®)

Spironolactone (**Aldactone**®)

[used in combination with other medications to treat high blood pressure; also used to treat disorders that involve excess fluid accumulation]

Both ACE inhibitors and spironolactone tend to increase serum potassium levels. Their effects may be additive, resulting in excessively high potassium levels in some people.

**Recommendation:** Discuss this interaction with your doctor.

---

ACE inhibitors:

- benazepril (**Lotensin**®)
- captopril (**Capoten**®)
- enalapril (**Vasotec**®)
- fosinopril (**Monopril**®)
- lisinopril (**Prinivil**®, **Zestril**®)
- quinapril (**Accupril**®)
- ramipril (**Altace**®)

Thiazide and thiazide-like diuretics:

- chlorothiazide (**Diuril**®)
- chlorthalidone (**Hygroton**®)
- hydrochlorothiazide (**Esidrix**®, **HydroDIURIL**®, **Oretic**®, and others)
- metolazone (**Diulo**®, **Zaroxolyn**®)

[to reduce high blood pressure]

In most persons, combined use of an ACE inhibitor with a thiazide diuretic works well to help control hypertension or congestive heart failure. If ACE inhibitor therapy, however, is started in the presence of diuretic therapy (which has been sufficient to reduce the blood volume), a precipitous fall in blood pressure may occur in certain persons. Symptoms of excessively low blood pressure levels include lightheadedness and fainting.

If your doctor suspects that you may be sensitive to ACE inhibitors due to diuretic-induced reduction in blood volume, he or she may reduce the diuretic dose or stop the diuretic temporarily before starting ACE inhibitor therapy. Your doctor may also start with a low dose of the ACE inhibitor and increase the dose gradually.

**CLINICAL SIGNIFICANCE OF THE INTERACTION**

| LOW | MODERATE | HIGH |

| ANTIHYPERTENSIVE DRUG | INTERACTING DRUG | RESULT |
|---|---|---|

ACE inhibitors:

- benazepril (**Lotensin**®)
- captopril (**Capoten**®)
- enalapril (**Vasotec**®)
- fosinopril (**Monopril**®)
- lisinopril (**Prinivil**®, **Zestril**®)
- quinapril (**Accupril**®)
- ramipril (**Altace**®)

Triamterene (**Dyrenium**®)

[used to treat disorders that involve excessive fluid accumulation]

Both ACE inhibitors and triamterene tend to increase serum potassium levels. Their effects may be additive, resulting in excessively high potassium levels in some people.

**Recommendation:** Discuss this interaction with your doctor.

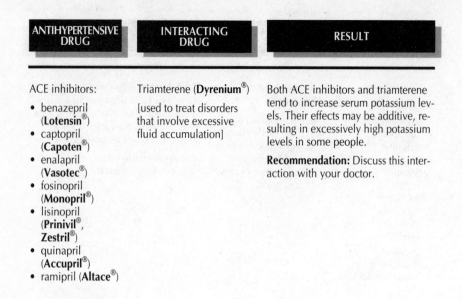

---

Atenolol (**Tenormin**®)

Ampicillin (**Omnipen**®, **Unasyn**®, and others)

[for treatment of bacterial infections]

Ampicillin may reduce the effect of the atenolol, particularly when ampicillin is used in high doses.

---

Atenolol (**Tenormin**®)

Antacids that contain aluminum, calcium, or magnesium, such as **Gaviscon**®, **Gelusil**®, **Maalox**®, **Mylanta**®, **Phillips' Milk of Magnesia**®, **Rolaids**® (sodium-free and calcium-rich), **Tums**®, and others

[for relief of acid indigestion, heartburn, and abdominal pain caused by too much acid in the stomach]

The absorption of atenolol may be reduced when taken simultaneously with aluminum-, calcium-, or magnesium-containing antacids.

**Recommendation:** Take the antacid at least four hours before or two hours after taking atenolol.

| ANTIHYPERTENSIVE DRUG | INTERACTING DRUG | RESULT |
|---|---|---|

Atenolol
(**Tenormin**®)

Antidiabetic drugs:

- acetohexamide (**Dymelor**®)
- chlorpropamide (**Diabinese**®)
- glipizide (**Glucotrol**®)
- glyburide (**DiaBeta**®, **Micronase**®)
- insulin (**Humulin**®, **Lente**®, **Novolin**®, and others)
- tolazamide (**Tolinase**®)
- tolbutamide (**Orinase**®), and others

[for treatment of diabetes mellitus, a condition that results in excessively high amounts of sugar in the blood and urine]

Although the heart typically beats faster (tachycardia) when blood sugar levels are low, this symptom may be absent when atenolol is given.

Atenolol
(**Tenormin**®)

Indomethacin (**Indocin**®)

[for reduction of inflammation; used to reduce the pain and swelling associated with arthritis, tendinitis, and bursitis]

Indomethacin may reduce the antihypertensive or antianginal effect of atenolol. This effect may occur with other nonsteroidal anti-inflammatory agents, such as diclofenac (Voltaren®), diflunisal (Dolobid®), etodolac (Lodine®), fenoprofen (Nalfon®), flurbiprofen (Ansaid®), ibuprofen (Advil®, Motrin®, Nuprin®, Rufen®), ketoprofen (Orudis®), ketorolac (Toradol®), meclofenamate (Meclomen®), nabumetone (Relafen®), naproxen (Naprosyn®), naproxen sodium (Anaprox®), piroxicam (Feldene®), sulindac (Clinoril®), and tolmetin (Tolectin®). Sulindac (Clinoril®) appears less likely to interfere with the antihypertensive effect of atenolol.

**Recommendation:** Your doctor may want to check your blood pressure if you start, stop, or change the dosage of an NSAID.

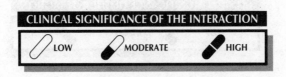

CLINICAL SIGNIFICANCE OF THE INTERACTION

LOW   MODERATE   HIGH

Bumetanide (**Bumex**®)

Aminoglycoside anti-biotics:

- amikacin (**Amikin**®)
- gentamicin (**Garamycin**®)
- kanamycin (**Kantrex**®)
- neomycin
- streptomycin
- tobramycin (**Nebcin**®), and others

[used to treat various bacterial infections]

Damage to hearing (ototoxicity) may result from the interaction of these two drugs.

---

Bumetanide (**Bumex**®)

Indomethacin (**Indocin**®) and probably other non-steroidal anti-inflamma-tory drugs

[for inflammation of joints and muscles]

Indomethacin impairs the ability of bumetanide to lower blood pressure or to rid the body of excess fluid. Other anti-inflammatory drugs—with the possible exception of sulindac (Clinoril®), a drug in the same class as indomethacin—that may interact similarly include aspirin, diclofenac (Voltaren®), diflunisal (Dolobid®), etodolac (Lodine®), fenoprofen (Nalfon®), flurbiprofen (Ansaid®), ibuprofen (Advil®, Motrin®, Nuprin®, Rufen®), ketoprofen (Orudis®), ke-torolac (Toradol®), meclofenamate (Meclomen®), nabumetone (Relafen®), naproxen (Naprosyn®), naproxen sodium (Anaprox®), piroxi-cam (Feldene®), and tolmetin (Tolectin®).

**Recommendation:** Your doctor may want to check your blood pressure if you start, stop, or change the dosage of an NSAID.

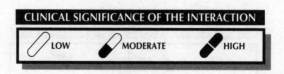

CLINICAL SIGNIFICANCE OF THE INTERACTION

LOW     MODERATE     HIGH

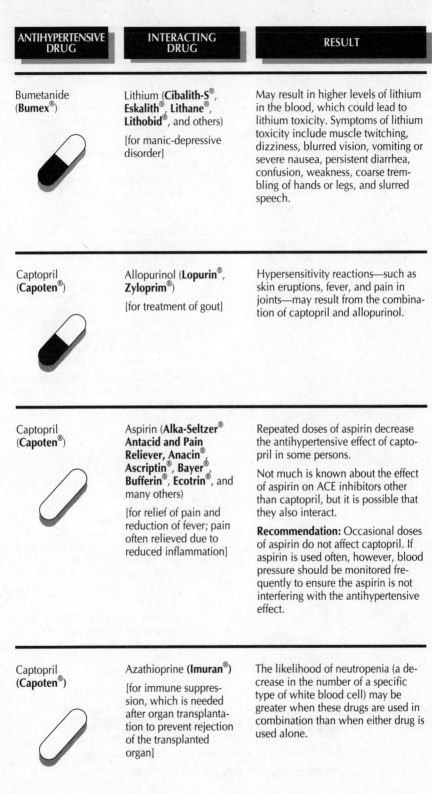

| ANTIHYPERTENSIVE DRUG | INTERACTING DRUG | RESULT |
|---|---|---|
| Bumetanide (**Bumex**®) | Lithium (**Cibalith-S**®, **Eskalith**®, **Lithane**®, **Lithobid**®, and others)<br><br>[for manic-depressive disorder] | May result in higher levels of lithium in the blood, which could lead to lithium toxicity. Symptoms of lithium toxicity include muscle twitching, dizziness, blurred vision, vomiting or severe nausea, persistent diarrhea, confusion, weakness, coarse trembling of hands or legs, and slurred speech. |
| Captopril (**Capoten**®) | Allopurinol (**Lopurin**®, **Zyloprim**®)<br><br>[for treatment of gout] | Hypersensitivity reactions—such as skin eruptions, fever, and pain in joints—may result from the combination of captopril and allopurinol. |
| Captopril (**Capoten**®) | Aspirin (**Alka-Seltzer**® **Antacid and Pain Reliever, Anacin**®, **Ascriptin**®, **Bayer**®, **Bufferin**®, **Ecotrin**®, and many others)<br><br>[for relief of pain and reduction of fever; pain often relieved due to reduced inflammation] | Repeated doses of aspirin decrease the antihypertensive effect of captopril in some persons.<br><br>Not much is known about the effect of aspirin on ACE inhibitors other than captopril, but it is possible that they also interact.<br><br>**Recommendation:** Occasional doses of aspirin do not affect captopril. If aspirin is used often, however, blood pressure should be monitored frequently to ensure the aspirin is not interfering with the antihypertensive effect. |
| Captopril (**Capoten**®) | Azathioprine (**Imuran**®)<br><br>[for immune suppression, which is needed after organ transplantation to prevent rejection of the transplanted organ] | The likelihood of neutropenia (a decrease in the number of a specific type of white blood cell) may be greater when these drugs are used in combination than when either drug is used alone. |

235

Carteolol (**Cartrol**®)

Epinephrine (**Adrenalin**®, **Ana-Kit**®, **AsthmaHaler**®, **Bronkaid**® Mist, **Epi-Pen**®, **Primatene**® Mist, **Sus-Phrine**®, and others)

[for temporary relief of shortness of breath, and wheezing caused by bronchial asthma; Ana-Kit® and EpiPen® are used for the emergency treatment of allergic reactions to insect stings or bites, food, and other substances that trigger a serious allergic reaction]

The outcome depends on the condition for which the person is being treated, and on how the epinephrine is given.

**Persons with anaphylactic shock:** Some people develop a severe, possibly life-threatening, allergic reaction (called anaphylactic shock) to insect stings or bites and certain medications or foods. Symptoms of anaphylactic shock include hives, wheezing, difficulty breathing, abdominal pain, incontinence, fever, and loss of consciousness; death may also occur. Epinephrine injections help reverse anaphylactic shock, but in persons taking a specific type of antihypertensive drug (i.e., nonselective beta blocker, such as carteolol), the epinephrine may not work very well and other measures often must be taken.

**Persons *not* in anaphylactic shock:** People taking carteolol who receive epinephrine for something other than anaphylactic shock are at risk of developing excessively high blood pressure levels. If the epinephrine is injected with the intention of systemic effects (i.e., reaching most of the tissues and organs in the body), the blood pressure may increase dramatically. If, however, the epinephrine is inhaled into the lungs, put in the eye, or injected for only local effects (e.g., by a dentist or dermatologist), the risk of a hypertensive reaction appears to be much less (unless a much larger than usual amount of epinephrine is used).

**Recommendation:** It is best for people who are at risk of anaphylactic shock (e.g., those allergic to beestings) to avoid taking carteolol or other beta blockers.

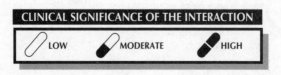

CLINICAL SIGNIFICANCE OF THE INTERACTION

LOW   MODERATE   HIGH

| ANTIHYPERTENSIVE DRUG | INTERACTING DRUG | RESULT |
|---|---|---|

Clonidine
(**Catapres**®)

Alcohol, sedatives, and barbiturates:

- butabarbital (**Butisol**®)
- mephobarbital (**Mebaral**®)
- pentobarbital (**Nembutal**®)
- phenobarbital (**Solfoton**®)
- secobarbital (**Seconal**®), and others

[barbiturates are used to treat insomina and anxiety; certain barbiturates are used to prevent seizures]

May increase the depressive effect of alcohol, sedatives, or barbiturates, possibly leading to severe drowsiness.

---

Clonidine
(**Catapres**®)

Antipsychotic medications:

- chlorpromazine (**Thorazine**®)
- haloperidol (**Haldol**®), and others

[for mental illnesses such as schizophrenia, mania, and dementia]

Severe hypotension (low blood pressure) may result, especially in individuals with heart disease.

---

Clonidine
(**Catapres**®)

Beta blockers:

- acebutolol (**Sectral**®)
- atenolol (**Tenormin**®)
- betaxolol (**Kerlone**®)
- esmolol (**Brevibloc**®)
- metoprolol (**Lopressor**®)
- nadolol (**Corgard**®)
- pindolol (**Visken**®)
- propranolol (**Inderal**®)
- timolol (**Blocadren**®), and others

[for the treatment of high blood pressure]

Increased risk of hypertensive reaction (profound increase in blood pressure) if clonidine is discontinued too rapidly while taking a beta blocker.

**Recommendation:** Do not stop taking clonidine without first consulting your doctor. Your doctor may need to gradually taper you off of the beta-blocker drug over several days before gradually discontinuing clonidine.

Clonidine (**Catapres**®)

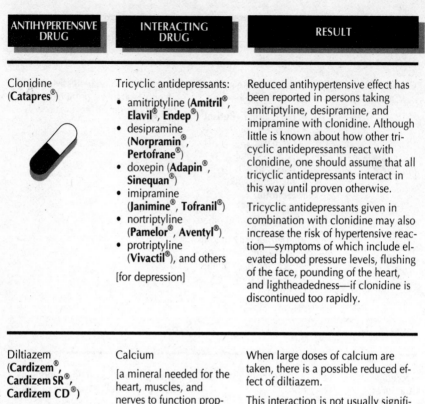

Tricyclic antidepressants:

- amitriptyline (**Amitril**®, **Elavil**®, **Endep**®)
- desipramine (**Norpramin**®, **Pertofrane**®)
- doxepin (**Adapin**®, **Sinequan**®)
- imipramine (**Janimine**®, **Tofranil**®)
- nortriptyline (**Pamelor**®, **Aventyl**®)
- protriptyline (**Vivactil**®), and others

[for depression]

Reduced antihypertensive effect has been reported in persons taking amitriptyline, desipramine, and imipramine with clonidine. Although little is known about how other tricyclic antidepressants react with clonidine, one should assume that all tricyclic antidepressants interact in this way until proven otherwise.

Tricyclic antidepressants given in combination with clonidine may also increase the risk of hypertensive reaction—symptoms of which include elevated blood pressure levels, flushing of the face, pounding of the heart, and lightheadedness—if clonidine is discontinued too rapidly.

---

Diltiazem (**Cardizem**®, **Cardizem SR**®, **Cardizem CD**®)

Calcium

[a mineral needed for the heart, muscles, and nerves to function properly; also needed for strong bones and teeth]

When large doses of calcium are taken, there is a possible reduced effect of diltiazem.

This interaction is not usually significant unless the calcium is given intravenously.

---

Diltiazem (**Cardizem**®, **Cardizem SR**®, **Cardizem CD**®)

Carbamazepine (**Tegretol**®)

[for epilepsy, trigeminal neuralgia (spasms of pain in the face), and other disorders]

May increase carbamazepine concentration in the body, possibly leading to double vision, headaches, abnormal muscle coordination, or dizziness.

Possible damage to the nervous system could result from this interaction. A reduced effect of the diltiazem may also occur.

**Recommendation:** It may be necessary for your doctor to adjust the dose of carbamazepine if diltiazem is started or stopped, or if its dosage is changed. (Of course, only your doctor should change medication dosage, when appropriate.)

Nifedipine (Adalat®, Procardia®), which does not affect the amount of

*(cont.)*
Diltiazem

carbamazepine in the body, may be an alternative to diltiazem if a calcium-channel blocker must be given with carbamazepine.

| | | |
| --- | --- | --- |
| Diltiazem (**Cardizem®, Cardizem SR®, Cardizem CD®**) | Cimetidine (**Tagamet®**) [for relief of stomach and intestinal ulcers] | May increase diltiazem levels, possibly leading to toxicity (symptoms of diltiazem toxicity include low blood pressure, dizziness, and flushing). **Recommendation:** It may be necessary for your doctor to adjust the dose of diltiazem if cimetidine is started or stopped, or if its dosage is changed. (Of course, only your doctor should change medication dosage, when appropriate.) |
| Diltiazem (**Cardizem®, Cardizem SR®, Cardizem CD®**) | Cyclosporine (**Sandimmune®**) [for immune suppression, which is needed after organ transplantation to prevent rejection of the transplanted organ] | May increase the amount of cyclosporine in the body. Increased blood levels of cyclosporine have been associated with nephrotoxicity (kidney damage). |
| Diltiazem (**Cardizem®, Cardizem SR®, Cardizem CD®**) | Digitalis drugs: • digitoxin (**Crystodigin®**) • digoxin (**Lanoxin®**) [for heart failure and other heart abnormalities] | Diltiazem may increase digitoxin effect somewhat, possibly increasing the likelihood of side effects occurring. Symptoms of digitoxin toxicity include nausea, poor appetite, weakness, lethargy, and visual disturbances. Diltiazem may also slightly increase digoxin effect, but in most cases, this increased effect is so small that problems rarely result. Nifedipine (Adalat®, Procardia®), a drug in the same class as diltiazem, does not appear to increase the amount of digitoxin or digoxin in the body. |

**CLINICAL SIGNIFICANCE OF THE INTERACTION**

LOW    MODERATE    HIGH

239

Diltiazem (**Cardizem®**, **Cardizem SR®**, **Cardizem CD®**)

Lithium (**Cibalith-S®**, **Eskalith®**, **Lithane®**, **Lithobid®**, and others)

[for manic-depressive disorder]

Could lead to neurotoxicity. Possible symptoms include nausea, vomiting, muscular incoordination, and ringing in the ears.

---

Diltiazem (**Cardizem®**, **Cardizem SR®**, **Cardizem CD®**)

Propranolol (**Inderal®**)

[for treatment of high blood pressure, angina pectoris, and irregular heartbeat; also used to prevent migraine headaches]

Diltiazem can increase the amount of propranolol in the blood, and may also produce additive reductions in the blood pressure and slowing of the heart rate. This is usually a favorable interaction that may be used intentionally by your doctor, but occasionally the blood pressure or heart rate may become excessively low.

**Recommendation:** When diltiazem is added to propranolol (or conversely, when propranolol is added to diltiazem), watch for any symptoms of excessive lowering of blood pressure or heart rate (e.g., dizziness, faintness). Diltiazem probably has a similar effect with other beta blockers (antihypertensive medications that are in the same class as propranolol) although the magnitude of the additive effect may be different. Other beta blockers include acebutolol (Sectral®), atenolol (Tenormin®), betaxolol (Kerlone®), carteolol (Cartrol®), esmolol (Brevibloc®), labetalol (Normodyne®, Trandate®), metroprolol (Lopressor®), nadolol (Corgard®), pindolol (Visken®), and timolol (Blocadren®).

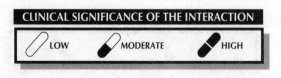

CLINICAL SIGNIFICANCE OF THE INTERACTION

LOW    MODERATE    HIGH

| ANTIHYPERTENSIVE DRUG | INTERACTING DRUG | RESULT |
|---|---|---|

Ethacrynic acid (**Edecrin**®)

Aminoglycosides:

- amikacin (**Amikin**®)
- gentamicin (**Garamycin**®)
- kanamycin (**Kantrex**®)
- netilmicin (**Netromycin**®)
- tobramycin (**Nebcin**®)

[used to treat various bacterial infections]

Aminoglycosides alone can cause hearing loss, and the concurrent use of ethacrynic acid markedly increases the risk (especially if the person has poor kidney function).

**Recommendation:** Combined use of aminoglycosides and ethacrynic acid should generally be avoided. If the combination is used, it should be done only with extreme caution and with careful monitoring for hearing loss.

Furosemide (Lasix®), another diuretic (i.e., medication used to reduce high blood pressure and fluid accumulation), appears to be less likely to interact with aminoglycosides than ethacrynic acid.

---

Ethacrynic acid (**Edecrin**®)

Corticosteroids:

- cortisone (**Cortone**®)
- hydrocortisone (**Cortef**®, **Hydrocortone**®, **Solu-Cortef**®)
- methylprednisolone (**Medrol**®, **Depo-Medrol**®, **Solu-Medrol**®)
- prednisolone (**Delta-Cortef**®, **Hydeltrasol**®, **Pediapred**®, **Prelone**®)
- prednisone (**Deltasone**®, **Liquid-Pred**®, **Meticorten**®)

[for relieving inflammation and suppressing allergic reactions]

Decreased amount of potassium in the body, which may lead to muscle problems (such as weakness, twitching, and pain), nocturia (need to urinate at night), and abnormal sensations, such as feelings of numbness, tingling, or burning.

Corticosteroids can produce potassium depletion if they are given by injection or orally (especially with large doses), but other routes of administration (e.g., inhalation or topical application on the skin or in the eye, ear, etc.) generally have little effect on potassium.

Cortisone and hydrocortisone are more likely than other corticosteroids to lead to these effects.

| ANTIHYPERTENSIVE DRUG | INTERACTING DRUG | RESULT |
|---|---|---|

Ethacrynic acid (**Edecrin**®)

Lithium (**Cibalith-S**®, **Eskalith**®, **Lithane**®, **Lithobid**®, and others)

[for manic-depressive disorder]

May lead to higher levels of lithium in the blood, which could lead to lithium toxicity. Symptoms of lithium toxicity include muscle twitching, dizziness, blurred vision, vomiting or severe nausea, persistent diarrhea, confusion, weakness, coarse trembling of hands or legs, and slurred speech.

---

Furosemide (**Lasix**®)

Corticosteroids:

- cortisone (**Cortone**®)
- hydrocortisone (**Cortef**®, **Hydrocortone**®, **Solu-Cortef**®)
- methylprednisolone (**Medrol**®, **Depo-Medrol**®, **Solu-Medrol**®)
- prednisolone (**Delta-Cortef**®, **Hydeltrasol**®, **Pediapred**®, **Prelone**®)
- prednisone (**Deltasone**®, **Liquid-Pred**®, **Meticorten**®)

[for relieving inflammation and suppressing allergic reactions]

Decreased amount of potassium in the body, which may lead to muscle problems (such as weakness, twitching, and pain), nocturia (need to urinate at night), and abnormal sensations, such as feelings of numbness, tingling, or burning.

Corticosteroids can produce potassium depletion if they are given by injection or orally (especially with large doses), but other routes of administration (e.g., inhalation or topical application) on the skin or in the eye, ear, etc.) generally have little effect on potassium.

Cortisone and hydrocortisone are more likely than other corticosteroids to lead to these effects.

---

Furosemide (**Lasix**®)

Indomethacin (**Indocin**®)

[for reduction of inflammation; used to reduce the pain and swelling associated with arthritis, tendinitis, and bursitis]

Indomethacin may reduce the antihypertensive effect of furosemide.

Some evidence indicates that most other nonsteroidal anti-inflammatory drugs may also decrease the effectiveness of furosemide. These drugs include diclofenac (Voltaren®), diflunisal (Dolobid®), etodolac (Lodine®), fenoprofen (Nalfon®), flurbiprofen (Ansaid®), ibuprofen (Advil®, Motrin®, Nuprin®, Rufen®), ketoprofen (Orudis®), ketorolac (Toradol®), meclofenamate (Meclomen®), nabumetone

| ANTIHYPERTENSIVE DRUG | INTERACTING DRUG | RESULT |
|---|---|---|

*(cont.)*
Furosemide (**Lasix**®) | Indomethacin (**Indocin**®) | (Relafen®), naproxen (Naprosyn®), naproxen sodium (Anaprox®), piroxicam (Feldene®), sulindac (Clinoril®), and tolmetin (Tolectin®).

Large amounts of aspirin may also decrease the effectiveness of furosemide.

Some evidence indicates that sulindac (Clinoril®) is less likely to interfere with the effect of furosemide.

**Recommendation:** Your doctor may want to check your blood pressure if you start, stop, or change the dosage of an NSAID.

Furosemide (**Lasix**®) | Lithium (**Cibalith-S**®, **Eskalith**®, **Lithane**®, **Lithobid**®, and others)

[for manic-depressive disorder] | May lead to higher levels of lithium in the blood, which could lead to lithium toxicity. Symptoms of lithium toxicity include muscle twitching, dizziness, blurred vision, vomiting or severe nausea, persistent diarrhea, confusion, weakness, coarse trembling of hands or legs, and slurred speech.

Guanadrel (**Hylorel**®) | Monoamine oxidase inhibitors:

- isocarboxazid (**Marplan**®)
- phenelzine (**Nardil**®)
- tranylcypromine (**Parnate**®), and others.

[used to treat depression] | May increase blood pressure levels due to reduced antihypertensive effect.

**Recommendation:** The manufacturer of guanadrel states that it should not be used with, or within one week of discontinuing, MAO inhibitors. Some experts recommend waiting two weeks after MAO inhibitors are stopped before starting guanadrel.

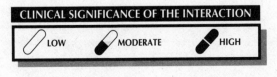

CLINICAL SIGNIFICANCE OF THE INTERACTION

LOW    MODERATE    HIGH

| ANTIHYPERTENSIVE DRUG | INTERACTING DRUG | RESULT |
|---|---|---|

Guanethidine
(**Ismelin**®)

Amphetamines:

- benzphetamine (**Didrex**®)
- dextroamphetamine (**Dexedrine**®)
- fenfluramine (**Pondimin**®)
- mazindol (**Sanorex**®)
- methylphenidate (**Ritalin**®)
- pemoline (**Cylert**®)
- phenmetrazine (**Preludin**®), and others.

[various amphetamines have different uses, such as the management of abnormal and uncontrollable sleeping during the day; another use is to help suppress appetite; methylphenidate is used to treat attention-deficit disorders]

May result in an increase in blood pressure levels due to a reduced antihypertensive effect.

**Recommendation:** It would be best to avoid amphetamines if you are taking guanethidine.

Guanethidine
(**Ismelin**®)

Antidiabetic drugs:

- acetohexamide (**Dymelor**®)
- chlorpropamide (**Diabinese**®)
- glipizide (**Glucotrol**®)
- glyburide (**DiaBeta**®, **Micronase**®)
- insulin (**Humulin**®, **Lente**®, **Novolin**®, and others
- tolazamide (**Tolinase**®)
- tolbutamide (**Orinase**®), and others.

Guanethidine may lower blood sugar levels in diabetics. Symptoms of an excessively low blood sugar level include increased heart rate, cold sweats, trembling, nausea, hunger, mental confusion, and, in severe cases, coma.

**Recommendation:** Persons taking antidiabetic medication should watch for a change in blood sugar levels if guanethidine is started or stopped (i.e., excessively low sugar levels when guanethidine is started, and too high blood sugar levels when guanethidine is stopped).

244

| | | |
|---|---|---|
| Guanethidine (**Ismelin**®)  | Chlorpromazine (**Thorazine**®) [for psychosis-related disorders, such as schizophrenia] | May increase blood pressure levels due to reduced antihypertensive effect. Chlorpromazine is in a class of drug known as phenothiazines. Other phenothiazines may interact similarly. Other phenothiazines include acetophenazine (Tindal®), fluphenazine (Prolixin®), mesoridazine (Serentil®), perphenazine (Trilafon®), thioridazine (Mellaril®), and others. **Recommendation:** It may be necessary for your doctor to adjust the dose of guanethidine if phenothiazines are stopped or started, or if the dosage is changed. (Of course only your doctor should change medication dosage, when appropriate.) |
| Guanethidine (**Ismelin**®)  | Ephedrine (**Primatene**®, **Broncholate**®, **Tedral**®, and others) [for wheezing due to asthma; also for nasal decongestion] | May increase blood pressure due to reduced antihypertensive effect. **Recommendation:** It would be best to avoid this combination. |
| Guanethidine (**Ismelin**®)  | Monoamine oxidase inhibitors: <br> • isocarboxazid (**Marplan**®) <br> • phenelzine (**Nardil**®) <br> • tranylcypromine (**Parnate**®), and others. [for the treatment of depression] | May increase blood pressure due to reduced antihypertensive effect. **Recommendation:** The manufacturer of guanethidine states that it should not be used with, or within one week of discontinuing, MAO inhibitors. Some experts recommend waiting two weeks after MAO inhibitors are stopped before starting guanethidine. |

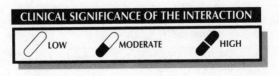

CLINICAL SIGNIFICANCE OF THE INTERACTION

LOW   MODERATE   HIGH

Guanethidine (**Ismelin**®)

Oral contraceptives, such as **Brevicon**®, **Demulen**®, **Enovid**® **Lo/Ovral**®, **Norinyl**®, **Ortho Novum**®, **Ovcon**®, **Ovral**®, **Tri-Norinyl**®, **Triphasil**®, and many others

[for prevention of pregnancy]

May increased blood pressure due to reduced antihypertensive effect.

**Recommendation:** Your doctor may want to check your blood pressure if you start taking oral contraceptives and guanethidine concurrently. Some women with hypertension may need to avoid oral contraceptives.

---

Guanethidine (**Ismelin**®)

Phenylephrine (**Congespirin**®, **Dimetane**® **Decongestant, Dristan**® **Decongestant, 4-Way**® **Fast Acting Nasal Spray, Naldecon**®, **Neo-Synephrine**®, **Pediacof**® **Cough Syrup, Phenergan**® **VC, Robitussin**® **Night Relief, Ru-Tuss**®, **Rynatan**®, and others)

[used as a decongestant to relieve congestion]

Phenylephrine may inhibit the ability of guanethidine to lower the blood pressure. As a result, blood pressure levels may increase.

**Recommendation:** Persons taking guanethidine should probably avoid phenylphrine (and other decongestants).

---

Guanethidine (**Ismelin**®)

Tricyclic antidepressants:

- amitriptyline (**Elavil**®, **Endep**®)
- amoxapine (**Asendin**®)
- desipramine (**Pertofrane**®, **Norpramin**®)
- doxepin (**Adapin**®, **Sinequan**®)
- imipramine (**Janimine**®, **Tofranil**®)
- nortriptyline (**Aventyl**®, **Pamelor**®)
- protriptyline (**Vivactil**®)
- trimipramine (**Surmontil**®)

[for the treatment of depression]

May increase blood pressure due to reduced antihypertensive effect.

**Recommendation:** It may be necessary for your doctor to adjust the dose of guanethidine if tricyclic antidepressants are stopped or started, or if the dosage is changed. (Of course, only your doctor should change medication dosage, when appropriate.)

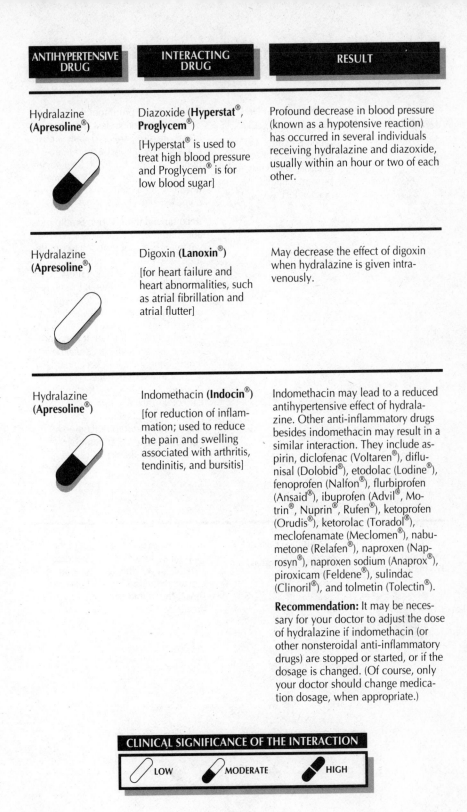

**Hydralazine (Apresoline®)**

Diazoxide (**Hyperstat®, Proglycem®**)

[Hyperstat® is used to treat high blood pressure and Proglycem® is for low blood sugar]

Profound decrease in blood pressure (known as a hypotensive reaction) has occurred in several individuals receiving hydralazine and diazoxide, usually within an hour or two of each other.

---

**Hydralazine (Apresoline®)**

Digoxin (**Lanoxin®**)

[for heart failure and heart abnormalities, such as atrial fibrillation and atrial flutter]

May decrease the effect of digoxin when hydralazine is given intravenously.

---

**Hydralazine (Apresoline®)**

Indomethacin (**Indocin®**)

[for reduction of inflammation; used to reduce the pain and swelling associated with arthritis, tendinitis, and bursitis]

Indomethacin may lead to a reduced antihypertensive effect of hydralazine. Other anti-inflammatory drugs besides indomethacin may result in a similar interaction. They include aspirin, diclofenac (Voltaren®), diflunisal (Dolobid®), etodolac (Lodine®), fenoprofen (Nalfon®), flurbiprofen (Ansaid®), ibuprofen (Advil®, Motrin®, Nuprin®, Rufen®), ketoprofen (Orudis®), ketorolac (Toradol®), meclofenamate (Meclomen®), nabumetone (Relafen®), naproxen (Naprosyn®), naproxen sodium (Anaprox®), piroxicam (Feldene®), sulindac (Clinoril®), and tolmetin (Tolectin®).

**Recommendation:** It may be necessary for your doctor to adjust the dose of hydralazine if indomethacin (or other nonsteroidal anti-inflammatory drugs) are stopped or started, or if the dosage is changed. (Of course, only your doctor should change medication dosage, when appropriate.)

---

**CLINICAL SIGNIFICANCE OF THE INTERACTION**

LOW     MODERATE     HIGH

Isradipine
(**DynaCirc®**)

Propranolol (**Inderal®**)

[for treatment of high blood pressure, angina pectoris, and irregular heartbeat; also used to prevent migraine headaches]

Isradipine and propranolol may have an additive effect in lowering the blood pressure. This is usually a positive effect, and may be used intentionally by your doctor to treat angina or high blood pressure. Occasionally, however, the blood pressure may become excessively low.

**Recommendation:** When isradipine is added to propranolol (or conversely, when propranolol is added to isradipine), watch for any symptoms of excessive lowering of blood pressure (e.g., dizziness, faintness). Isradipine probably has a similar effect with other beta blockers (antihypertensive medications that are in the same class as propranolol) although the magnitude of the additive effect may be different. Other beta blockers include acebutolol (Sectral®), atenolol (Tenormin®), betaxolol (Kerlone®), carteolol (Cartrol®), esmolol (Brevibloc®), labetalol (Normodyne®, Trandate®), metoprolol (Lopressor®), nadolol (Corgard®), pindolol (Visken®), and timolol (Blocadren®).

Labetalol
(**Normodyne®**,
**Trandate®**)

Cimetidine (**Tagamet®**)

[for relief of stomach and intestinal ulcers]

Increased levels of labetalol in the blood may result when cimetidine is also taken, possibly leading to an excessive reduction in blood pressure, slowed heart rate, and difficulty breathing.

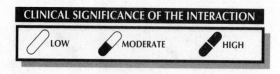

CLINICAL SIGNIFICANCE OF THE INTERACTION

LOW   MODERATE   HIGH

Methyldopa
(**Aldomet**®)

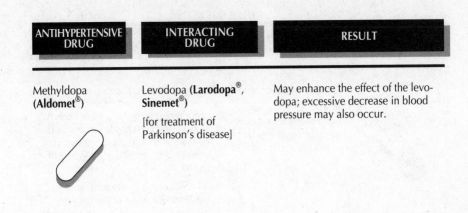

Levodopa (**Larodopa**®, **Sinemet**®)

[for treatment of Parkinson's disease]

May enhance the effect of the levodopa; excessive decrease in blood pressure may also occur.

---

Methyldopa
(**Aldomet**®)

Lithium (**Cibalith-S**®, **Eskalith**®, **Lithane**®, **Lithobid**®, and others)

[for manic-depressive disorder]

Moderate possibility of lithium toxicity. Symptoms of lithium toxicity include muscle twitching, dizziness, blurred vision, vomiting or severe nausea, persistent diarrhea, confusion, weakness, coarse trembling of hands or legs, and slurred speech.

---

Methyldopa
(**Aldomet**®)

Norepinephrine
(**Levophed**®)

[for cardiac arrest, severe low blood pressure (hypotensive crisis), and shock]

May prolong the ability of norepinephrine to increase blood pressure.

---

Methyldopa
(**Aldomet**®)

Oral contraceptives, such as **Brevicon**®, **Demulen**®, **Enovid**®, **Lo/Ovral**®, **Norinyl**®, **Ortho Novum**®, **Ovcon**®, **Ovral**®, **Tri-Norinyl**®, **Triphasil**®, and many others

[for prevention of pregnancy]

Oral contraceptives may decrease the antihypertensive effect of methyldopa.

**Recommendation:** Your doctor may want to check your blood pressure if you start taking oral contraceptives and methyldopa concurrently. Some women with hypertension may need to avoid oral contraceptives.

| ANTIHYPERTENSIVE DRUG | INTERACTING DRUG | RESULT |
|---|---|---|

Metoprolol
**(Lopressor®)**

Amiodarone **(Cordarone®)**

[for treatment of life-threatening ventricular arrhythmias (irregular heartbeat and rhythm)]

In a few cases, combined use of amiodarone with either metoprolol or propranolol (drugs in a class known as beta blockers) has been followed by slowed or irregular heartbeat and even cardiac arrest (i.e., stopping of the heart).

It is not known whether other anti-hypertensive drugs in the beta-blocker class would produce a similar effect, but the beta blockers most likely to be associated with this inter-action are the drugs that are degraded primarily in the liver, such as acebu-tolol (Sectral®), betaxolol (Kerlone®), penbutolol (Levatol®), and pindolol (Viskin®). In one case, atenolol (Tenormin®), another antihypertensive in the beta-blocker class, did not seem to interact with amiodarone.

It is possible that other beta blockers eliminated mainly by the kidneys—such as nadolol (Corgard®)—would also fail to interact.

Metoprolol
**(Lopressor®)**

Antidiabetic drugs:

- acetohexamide **(Dymelor®)**
- chlorpropamide **(Diabinese®)**
- glipizide **(Glucotrol®)**
- glyburide **(DiaBeta®, Micronase®)**
- insulin **(Humulin®, Lente®, Novolin®,** and others)
- tolazamide **(Tolinase®)**
- tolbutamide **(Orinase®),** and others

[for treatment of diabetes mellitus, a condition that results in excessively high amounts of sugar in the blood and urine]

Although the heart typically beats faster (tachycardia) when blood sugar levels are low, this symptom may be absent when metoprolol is given. This effect may occur when antidia-betic agents are combined with any antihypertensive drug in the beta-blocker class, which includes acebu-tolol (Sectral®), atenolol (Tenormin®), betaxolol (Kerlone®), carteolol (Cartrol®), esmolol (Brevibloc®), la-betalol (Normodyne®, Trandate®), nadolol (Corgard®), pindolol (Visken®), propranolol (Inderal®), and timolol (Blocadren®).

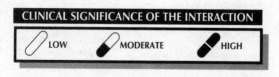

CLINICAL SIGNIFICANCE OF THE INTERACTION

LOW    MODERATE    HIGH

| ANTIHYPERTENSIVE DRUG | INTERACTING DRUG | RESULT |
|---|---|---|

Metoprolol
(**Lopressor**®)

Barbiturates:

- amobarbital (**Amytal**®)
- butabarbital (**Butisol**®)
- butalbital
- pentobarbital (**Nembutal**®)
- phenobarbital (**Luminal**®, **Solfoton**®)
- primidone (**Mysoline**®)
- secobarbital (**Seconal**®), and others

[used to treat insomnia and anxiety; certain barbiturates are used to prevent seizures]

Barbiturates may reduce the concentration of metoprolol, possibly leading to inadequate control of high blood pressure or a worsening of other disorders for which metoprolol is used.

It may be necessary for your doctor to adjust the dose of metoprolol if a barbiturate is started or stopped, or if its dosage is changed. (Of course, only your doctor should change medication dosages, when appropriate).

Metoprolol
(**Lopressor**®)

Cimetidine (**Tagamet**®)

[for relief of stomach and intestinal ulcers]

Increased levels of metoprolol in the blood may result when cimetidine is also taken, possibly leading to an excessive reduction in blood pressure, slowed heart rate, and difficulty breathing.

Metoprolol
(**Lopressor**®)

Lidocaine (**Xylocaine**®, **Anestacon**®, and others)

[used to treat abnormal heart rhythms; for topical anesthesia during minor surgery; also available as an over-the-counter medication for relief of pain, itching, and inflammation, but such topical use is unlikely to interact with metoprolol]

Metoprolol may increase the effect of lidocaine, perhaps to the point of lidocaine toxicity (symptoms of which include dizziness, lethargy, nausea, confusion, agitation, and ringing in ears).

More likely to occur when lidocaine is given intravenously.

251

| ANTIHYPERTENSIVE DRUG | INTERACTING DRUG | RESULT |
|---|---|---|

Metoprolol
(**Lopressor**®)

Oral contraceptives, such as **Brevicon**®, **Demulen**®, **Enovid**®, **Lo/Ovral**®, **Norinyl**®, **Ortho Novum**®, **Ovcon**®, **Ovral**®, **Tri-Norinyl**®, **Triphasil**®, and many others

[for prevention of pregnancy]

Oral contraceptives may increase the concentration of metoprolol in the blood. While it is not known whether this will result in an increased antihypertensive effect, you should have your blood pressure checked regularly to ensure that it is not too low. (This is an unusual interaction because many antihypertensive drugs may interact with oral contraceptives in a way that results in an *increase* in blood pressure levels. When metoprolol was combined with an oral contraceptive, however, the opposite effect—reduced blood pressure—was observed.)

Metoprolol is part of a family of drugs known as beta blockers. It is not known whether oral contraceptives produce a similar interaction with other beta-blocker drugs—such as propranolol (Inderal®)—but such an interaction is likely.

**Recommendation:** Your doctor may want to monitor your blood pressure for any changes if an oral contraceptive is started or stopped in the presence of metoprolol therapy.

---

Metoprolol
(**Lopressor**®)

Propafenone (**Rythmol**®)

[for treatment of life-threatening ventricular arrhythmias (i.e., irregular heartbeat)]

Receiving these drugs together may result in a substantially increased amount of metoprolol in the body, possibly leading to excessive reduction in blood pressure, lethargy, slowed heart rate, difficulty breathing, and cold hands and feet.

---

Metoprolol
(**Lopressor**®)

Propoxyphene
(**Darvocet-N**®, **Darvon**®, **Darvon**® with A.S.A.®, **Dolene**®, and **Wygesic**®)

[for relief of mild to moderate pain]

Can increase the concentration of metoprolol, possibly leading to an excessive reduction in blood pressure, slowed heart rate, difficulty breathing, and cold hands and feet.

**Recommendation:** In most cases, the way to avoid this interaction is to use a pain reliever other than propoxyphene.

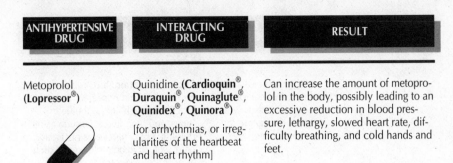

Metoprolol **(Lopressor®)**

Quinidine **(Cardioquin®, Duraquin®, Quinaglute®, Quinidex®, Quinora®)**

[for arrhythmias, or irregularities of the heartbeat and heart rhythm]

Can increase the amount of metoprolol in the body, possibly leading to an excessive reduction in blood pressure, lethargy, slowed heart rate, difficulty breathing, and cold hands and feet.

Metoprolol **(Lopressor®)**

Rifampin **(Rifadin®, Rifamate®, Rimactane®)**

[used in combination with at least one other drug, rifampin is used to treat tuberculosis; also used in the treatment of individuals who are carriers of meningitis]

Rifampin may reduce the concentration of metoprolol, possibly leading to decreased effect (i.e., less control of high blood pressure levels or angina).

Nadolol **(Corgard®)**

Antidiabetic drugs:

- acetohexamide **(Dymelor®)**
- chlorpropamide **(Diabinese®)**
- glipizide **(Glucotrol®)**
- glyburide **(DiaBeta®, Micronase®)**
- insulin **(Humulin®, Lente®, Novolin®,** and others)
- tolazamide **(Tolinase®)**
- tolbutamide **(Orinase®),** and others

Several results have been reported:

1. Secretion of insulin may be inhibited by nadolol, thereby leading to higher blood sugar levels than normal.

2. High blood pressure and markedly slowed heartbeat may result when blood sugar levels are low.

3. Reduced circulation to the hands and feet.

4. Although the heart typically beats faster (tachycardia) when blood sugar levels are low, this symptom may be absent when nadolol is given.

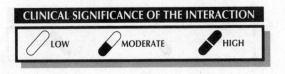

CLINICAL SIGNIFICANCE OF THE INTERACTION

LOW    MODERATE    HIGH

| ANTIHYPERTENSIVE DRUG | INTERACTING DRUG | RESULT |
|---|---|---|

*(cont.)*
Nadolol

[for treatment of diabetes mellitus, a condition that results in excessively high amounts of sugar in the blood and urine]

**Recommendation:** If possible, diabetics should avoid nonselective beta blockers (which act on the heart, lungs, and blood vessels) such as nadolol. If a beta blocker is necessary, cardioselective beta blockers—such as acebutolol (Sectral®), atenolol (Tenormin®), betaxolol (Kerlone®), or metoprolol (Lopressor®)—are usually recommended. These act primarily on the heart.

---

Nadolol (**Corgard**®)

Epinephrine (**Adrenalin**®, **Ana-Kit**®, **AsthmaHaler**®, **Bronkaid**® **Mist**, **Epi-Pen**®, **Primatene**® **Mist**, **Sus-Phrine**®, and others)

[for temporary relief of shortness of breath, and wheezing caused by bronchial asthma; Ana-Kit® and EpiPen® are used for the emergency treatment of allergic reactions to insect stings or bites, food, and other substances that trigger a serious allergic reaction]

The outcome depends on the condition for which the person is being treated, and on how the epinephrine is given.

**Persons with anaphylactic shock:**
Some people develop a severe, possibly life-threatening, allergic reaction (called anaphylactic shock) to insect stings or bites and certain medications or foods. Symptoms of anaphylactic shock include hives, wheezing, difficulty breathing, abdominal pain, incontinence, fever, and loss of consciousness; death may also occur. Epinephrine injections help reverse anaphylactic shock, but in persons taking a specific type of anti-hypertensive drug (i.e., nonselective beta blocker, such as nadolol), the epinephrine may not work very well and other measures often must be taken.

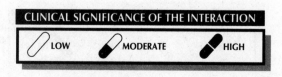

CLINICAL SIGNIFICANCE OF THE INTERACTION

LOW     MODERATE     HIGH

*(cont.)*
Nadolol

**Persons *not* in anaphylactic shock:** People taking nadolol who receive epinephrine for something other than anaphylactic shock are at risk of developing excessively high blood pressure levels. If the epinephrine is injected with the intention of systemic effects (i.e., reaching most of the tissues and organs in the body), the blood pressure may increase dramatically. If, however, the epinephrine is inhaled into the lungs, put in the eye, or injected for only local effects (e.g., by a dentist or dermatologist), the risk of a hypertensive reaction appears to be much less (unless a much larger than usual amount of epinephrine is used).

**Recommendation:** It is best for people who are at risk of anaphylactic shock (e.g., those allergic to beestings) to avoid taking nadolol or other beta blockers.

---

Nadolol (**Corgard®**)

Isoproterenol (**Isuprel®, Duo-Medihaler®**, and others)

[used as a bronchodilator to relieve bronchospasms associated with asthma, bronchitis, and emphysema]

Nadolol may reduce the bronchodilating effect of isoproterenol in asthmatic persons. Bronchodilators other than isoproterenol are probably similarly affected.

**Recommendation:** It is best to avoid this combination; discuss it with your doctor.

---

Nadolol (**Corgard®**)

Lidocaine (**Xylocaine®, Anestacon®**, and others)

[used to treat abnormal heart rhythms; for topical anesthesia during minor surgery; also available as an over-the-counter medication for relief of pain, itching, and inflammation, but such topical use is unlikely to interact with nadolol]

Nadolol may increase the effect of lidocaine, perhaps to the point of lidocaine toxicity (symptoms of which include dizziness, lethargy, nausea, confusion, agitation, ringing in ears).

This interaction is more likely to occur when lidocaine is given intravenously.

255

| ANTIHYPERTENSIVE DRUG | INTERACTING DRUG | RESULT |
|---|---|---|

Nicardipine (**Cardene**®)

Cyclosporine (**Sandimmune**®)

[for immune suppression, which is needed after organ transplantation to prevent rejection of the transplanted organ]

Nicardipine may increase the amount of cyclosporine in the blood. Increased cyclosporine levels have been associated with nephrotoxicity (kidney damage).

**Recommendation:** It may be necessary for your doctor to adjust the dose of cyclosporine if nicardipine is started or stopped, or if its dosage is changed. (Of course only your doctor should change medication dosage, when appropriate.)

Nicardipine (**Cardene**®)

Propranolol (**Inderal**®)

[for treatment of high blood pressure, angina pectoris, and irregular heartbeat; also used to prevent migraine headaches]

Nicardipine and propranolol may have an additive effect in lowering the blood pressure. This is usually a positive effect, and may be used intentionally by your doctor to treat angina or high blood pressure. Occasionally, however, the blood pressure may become excessively low.

**Recommendation:** When nicardipine is added to propranolol (or conversely, when propranolol is added to nicardipine), watch for any symptoms of excessive lowering of blood pressure (e.g., dizziness, faintness). Nicardipine probably has a similar effect with other beta blockers (antihypertensive medications that are in the same class as propranolol) although the magnitude of the additive effect may be different. Other beta blockers include acebutolol (Sectral®), atenolol (Tenormin®), betaxolol (Kerlone®), carteolol (Cartrol®), esmolol (Brevibloc®), labetalol (Normodyne®, Trandate®), metoprolol (Lopressor®), nadolol (Corgard®), pindolol (Visken®), and timolol (Blocadren®).

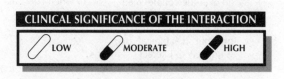

CLINICAL SIGNIFICANCE OF THE INTERACTION

LOW    MODERATE    HIGH

| ANTIHYPERTENSIVE DRUG | INTERACTING DRUG | RESULT |
|---|---|---|

Nifedipine (**Adalat**®, **Procardia XL**®)

Calcium

[a mineral needed for the heart, muscles, and nerves to function properly; also needed for strong bones and teeth]

When large doses of calcium are taken, there is a possible reduced effect of nifedipine. This interaction is not usually significant unless the calcium is given intravenously.

---

Nifedipine (**Adalat**®, **Procardia XL**®)

Cimetidine (**Tagamet**®)

[for relief of stomach and

May increase the amount of nifedipine in the blood, thereby increasing the antihypertensive effect. Possible nifedipine toxicity—evidenced by symptoms such as dizziness, flushing, and headache—may occur.

---

Nifedipine (**Adalat**®, **Procardia XL**®)

Barbiturates:

- amobarbital (**Amytal**®)
- butabarbital (**Butisol**®)
- butalbital
- pentobarbital (**Nembutal**®)
- phenobarbital (**Luminal**®, **Solfoton**®)
- primidone (**Mysoline**®)
- secobarbital (**Seconal**®), and others

[used to treat insomnia and anxiety; certain barbiturates are used to prevent seizures]

Significant decrease in the amount of nifedipine available in the body, possibly leading to a diminished effect of the nifedipine. This effect is particularly likely when nifedipine is taken orally.

Much of the evidence for this interaction comes from studies of phenobarbital, but other barbiturates are expected to interact similarly.

Persons receiving a barbiturate may require higher than usual doses of nifedipine. (Of course, *never* alter the dosage of any medication without your doctor's consent and supervision.)

Nifedipine (**Adalat**®, **Procardia XL**®)

Propranolol (**Inderal**®)

[for treatment of high blood pressure, angina pectoris, and irregular heartbeat; also used to prevent migraine headaches]

Nifedipine and propranolol may have an additive effect in lowering the blood pressure. This is usually a positive effect, and may be used intentionally by your doctor to treat angina or high blood pressure. Occasionally, however, the blood pressure may become excessively low.

**Recommendation:** When nifedipine is added to propranolol (or conversely, when propranolol is added to nifedipine), watch for any symptoms of excessive lowering of blood pressure (e.g., dizziness, faintness). Nifedipine probably has a similar effect with other beta blockers (antihypertensive medications that are in the same class as propranolol) although the magnitude of the additive effect may be different. Other beta blockers include acebutolol (Sectral®), atenolol (Tenormin®), betaxolol (Kerlone®), carteolol (Cartrol®), esmolol (Brevibloc®), labetalol (Normodyne®, Trandate®), metoprolol (Lopressor®), nadolol (Corgard®), pindolol (Visken®), and timolol (Blocadren®).

Nifedipine (**Adalat**®, **Procardia XL**®)

Quinidine (**Cardioquin**®, **Duraquin**®, **Quinaglute**®, **Quinidex**®, **Quinora**®)

[for arrhythmias, or irregularities of the heartbeat and heart rhythm]

Has been known to cause a decrease in quinidine levels and may lead to loss of quinidine efficacy.

Nifedipine (**Adalat**®, **Procardia XL**®)

Ranitidine (**Zantac**®)

[for relief of stomach and intestinal ulcers]

Ranitidine may increase nifedipine levels in the body, but not as much as cimetidine, another drug in the same class as ranitidine (see nifedipine-cimetidine interaction, p.257).

Pindolol (**Visken**®)

Epinephrine (**Adrenalin**®, **Ana-Kit**®, **AsthmaHaler**®, **Bronkaid**® **Mist, Epi-Pen**®, **Primatene**® **Mist, Sus-Phrine**®, and others)

[for temporary relief of shortness of breath, and wheezing caused by bronchial asthma; Ana-Kit® and EpiPen® are used for the emergency treatment of allergic reactions to insect stings of bites, food, and other substances that trigger a serious allergic reaction]

The outcome depends on the condition for which the person is being treated, and on how the epinephrine is given.

**Persons with anaphylactic shock:** Some people develop a severe, possibly life-threatening, allergic reaction (called anaphylactic shock) to insect stings or bites and certain medications or foods. Symptoms of anaphylactic shock include hives, wheezing, difficulty breathing, abdominal pain, incontinence, fever, and loss of consciousness; death may also occur. Epinephrine injections help reverse anaphylactic shock, but in persons taking a specific type of antihypertensive drug (i.e., nonselective beta blocker, such as pindolol), the epinephrine may not work very well and other measures often must be taken.

**Persons not in anaphylactic shock:** People taking pindolol who receive epinephrine for something other than anaphylactic shock are at risk of developing excessively high blood pressure levels. If the epinephrine is injected with the intention of systemic effects (i.e., reaching most of the tissues and organs in the body), the blood pressure may increase dramatically. If, however, the epinephrine is inhaled into the lungs, put in the eye, or injected for only local effects (e.g., by a dentist or dermatologist), the risk of a hypertensive reaction appears to be much less (unless a much larger than usual amount of epinephrine is used).

**Recommendation**: It is best for people who are at risk of anaphylactic shock (e.g., those allergic to bee-stings) to avoid taking pindolol or other beta blockers.

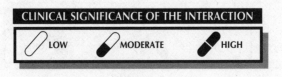

CLINICAL SIGNIFICANCE OF THE INTERACTION

LOW    MODERATE    HIGH

Pindolol (**Visken**®)

Indomethacin (**Indocin**®)

[for reduction of inflammation; used to reduce the pain and swelling associated with arthritis, tendinitis, and bursitis]

Reduction in the antihypertensive or antianginal effect. This effect may occur with other nonsteroidal antiinflammatory agents beside indomethacin, such as piroxicam (Feldene®), naproxen (Naprosyn®), and naproxen sodium (Anaprox®). Sulindac (Clinoril®) appears less likely to interfere with the antihypertensive effect of pindolol.

---

Pindolol (**Visken**®)

Isoproterenol (**Isuprel**®, **Duo-Medihaler**®, and others)

[used as a bronchodilator to relieve bronchospasms associated with asthma, bronchitis, and emphysema]

May reduce the bronchodilating effect of isoproterenol. Bronchodilators other than isoproterenol are probably similarly affected.

**Recommendation:** It is best to avoid this interaction; discuss it with your doctor.

---

Prazosin (**Minipress**®)

Beta blockers:

- acebutolol (**Sectral**®)
- atenolol (**Tenormin**®)
- betaxolol (**Kerlone**®)
- esmolol (**Brevibloc**®)
- metoprolol (**Lopressor**®)
- nadolol (**Corgard**®)
- pindolol (**Visken**®)
- propranolol (**Inderal**®)
- timolol (**Blocadren**®), and others

[for the treatment of high blood pressure]

When prazosin is started in the presence of a beta blocker, there may be an acute, excessive decrease in blood pressure, which may lead to fainting and loss of consciousness.

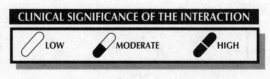

CLINICAL SIGNIFICANCE OF THE INTERACTION

LOW  MODERATE  HIGH

| ANTIHYPERTENSIVE DRUG | INTERACTING DRUG | RESULT |
|---|---|---|

Prazosin **(Minipress®)**

Diazoxide **(Hyperstat®, Proglycem®)**

[Hyperstat® is used to treat high blood pressure and Proglycem® is for low blood sugar]

May result in severely low blood pressure.

---

Prazosin **(Minipress®)**

Nifedipine **(Adalat®, Procardia®, Procardia XL®)**

[for treatment of angina; Procardia XL® is used to treat high blood pressure]

May result in excessive decrease in blood pressure in some persons.

---

Prazosin **(Minipress®)**

Nonsteroidal anti-inflammatory drugs:

- aspirin **(Alka-Seltzer® Antacid and Pain Reliever, Anacin®, Ascriptin®, Bayer®, Bufferin®, Ecotrin®**, and many others)
- diflunisal **(Dolobid®)**
- ibuprofen **(Advil®, Motrin®, Nuprin®, Rufen®)**
- indomethacin **(Indocin®)**
- meclofenamate **(Meclomen®)**
- naproxen **(Naprosyn®)**
- naproxen sodium **(Anaprox®)**, and others

[for reducing inflammation of joints and muscles and pain caused by inflammation]

Nonsteroidal anti-inflammatory drugs (NSAIDs) may reduce the effectiveness of several antihypertensive drugs (such as prazosin, captopril, and thiazide diuretics), resulting in an increase in blood pressure. Although certain studies indicate that specifically ibuprofen and indomethacin can reduce the effectiveness of prazosin, other NSAIDs may interact similarly.

If this interaction occurs, your doctor may adjust your prazosin dosage, switch you to (or add) another antihypertensive medication, or try using a different anti-inflammatory drug.

Some evidence indicates that one NSAID—sulindac (Clinoril®)—is less likely to interfere with the effect of antihypertensive medications.

**Recommendation:** Your doctor may want to check your blood pressure if you start, stop, or change the dose of an NSAID.

| | | |
|---|---|---|
| Prazosin **(Minipress®)**  | Verapamil **(Calan®, Isoptin®, Verelan®)** [for high blood pressure, abnormal heartbeat, and angina] | May result in an excessive decrease in blood pressure in some persons. |

| | | |
|---|---|---|
| Propranolol **(Inderal®)**  | Amiodarone **(Cordarone®)** [for treatment of life-threatening ventricular arrhythmias (irregular heartbeat and rhythm)] | In a few cases, combined use of amiodarone with either propranolol or metoprolol (drugs in a class known as beta blockers) has been followed by slowed or irregular heartbeat and even cardiac arrest (i.e., stopping of the heart).<br><br>It is not known whether other antihypertensive drugs in the beta-blocker class would produce a similar effect, but if so the beta blockers most likely to be associated with this interaction are the drugs that are degraded primarily in the liver, such as acebutolol (Sectral®), betaxolol (Kerlone®), penbutolol (Levatol®), and pindolol (Visken®). In one case, atenolol (Tenormin®), another antihypertensive in the beta-blocker class, did not seem to interact with amiodarone. It is possible that other beta blockers eliminated mainly by the kidneys—such as nadolol (Corgard®)—would also fail to interact. |

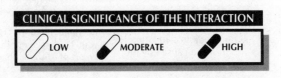

CLINICAL SIGNIFICANCE OF THE INTERACTION

LOW     MODERATE     HIGH

| ANTIHYPERTENSIVE DRUG | INTERACTING DRUG | RESULT |
|---|---|---|

Propranolol
**(Inderal®)**

Antacids that contain aluminum or magnesium, such as **Gaviscon®, Gelusil®, Maalox®, Mylanta®, Phillips' Milk of Magnesia®**, and others

[for relief of acid indigestion, heartburn, and abdominal pain caused by too much acid in the stomach]

The absorption of propranolol may be reduced when taken simultaneously with aluminum- or magnesium-containing antacids.

**Recommendation:** Take the antacid at least four hours before or two hours after propranolol.

Propranolol
-**(Inderal®)**

Antidiabetic drugs:

- acetohexamide **(Dymelor®)**
- chlorpropamide **(Diabinese®)**
- glipizide **(Glucotrol®)**
- glyburide **(DiaBeta®, Micronase®)**
- insulin **(Humulin®, Lente®, Novolin®,** and others)
- tolazamide **(Tolinase®)**
- tolbutamide **(Orinase®)**, and others

[for treatment of diabetes mellitus, a condition that results in excessively high amounts of sugar in the blood and urine]

Several results have been reported:

1. Secretion of insulin may be inhibited by propranolol, thereby leading to higher blood sugar levels than normal.

2. High blood pressure and markedly slowed heartbeat may result when blood sugar levels are low.

3. Reduced circulation to the hands and feet.

4. Although the heart typically beats faster (tachycardia) when blood sugar levels are low, this symptom may be absent when propranolol is given.

**Recommendation:** If possible, diabetics should avoid "nonselective" beta blockers (which act on the heart, lungs, and blood vessels) such as propranolol. If a beta blocker is necessary, cardioselective beta blockers—such as acebutolol (Sectral®), atenolol (Tenormin®), betaxolol (Kerlone®), or metoprolol (Lopressor®)—are usually recommended. These act primarily on the heart.

| ANTIHYPERTENSIVE DRUG | INTERACTING DRUG | RESULT |
|---|---|---|

Propranolol
(**Inderal**®)

Barbiturates:

• butabarbital (**Butisol**®)
• mephobarbital (**Mebaral**®)
• pentobarbital (**Nembutal**®)
• phenobarbital (**Solfoton**®)
• secobarbital (**Seconal**®), and others

[used to treat insomnia and anxiety; certain barbiturates are used to prevent seizures]

Barbiturates may reduce the amount of propranolol in the blood, possibly leading to reduced propranolol effect (i.e., inadequate control of blood pressure or worsening of other conditions for which propranolol is used).

Although this interaction has occurred with the barbiturate phenobarbital, other barbiturates are expected to have a similar effect on propranolol.

It may be necessary for your doctor to adjust the dose of propranolol if a barbiturate is started or stopped, or if its dosage is changed. (Of course, only your doctor should change medication dosages, when appropriate).

Propranolol
(**Inderal**®)

Chlorpromazine (**Thorazine**®)

[for treatment of schizophrenia, mania, and dementia]

Each of these drugs may increase the concentration of the other drug. As a result, increased propranolol levels may lead to an excessive reduction of blood pressure, lethargy, slowed heart rate, difficulty breathing, and cold hands and feet.

An increased amount of chlorpromazine in the body may lead to drowsiness, dry mouth, dizziness, blurred vision, constipation, difficulty urinating, fainting, and involuntary body movements (e.g., tremor, restless movement, facial grimacing).

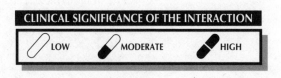

**CLINICAL SIGNIFICANCE OF THE INTERACTION**

LOW    MODERATE    HIGH

Propranolol **(Inderal®)**

Cimetidine **(Tagamet®)**

[for relief of stomach and intestinal ulcers]

The amount of propranolol in the blood may increase when cimetidine is also taken, possibly leading to an excessive reduction in blood pressure, slowed heart rate, difficulty breathing, and cold hands and feet.

**Recommendation:** Be aware of this interaction when taking both cimetidine and propranolol. Use of another antiulcer drug, such as ranitidine (Zantac®), may be preferable when propranolol must be taken.

---

Propranolol **(Inderal®)**

Epinephrine (**Adrenalin®**, **Ana-Kit®**, **AsthmaHaler®**, **Bronkaid® Mist, Epi-Pen®**, **Primatene® Mist, Sus-Phrine®**, and others)

[for temporary relief of shortness of breath, and wheezing caused by bronchial asthma; Ana-Kit® and EpiPen® are used for the emergency treatment of allergic reactions to insect stings or bites, food, and other substances that trigger a serious allergic reaction]

The outcome depends on the condition for which the person is being treated, and on how the epinephrine is given.

**Persons with anaphylactic shock:** Some people develop a severe, possibly life-threatening, allergic reaction (called anaphylactic shock) to insect stings or bites and certain medications or foods. Symptoms of anaphylactic shock include hives, wheezing, difficulty breathing, abdominal pain, incontinence, fever, and loss of consciousness; death may also occur. Epinephrine injections help reverse anaphylactic shock, but in persons taking a specific type of antihypertensive drug (i.e., nonselective beta blocker, such as propranolol), the epinephrine may not work very well and other measures often must be taken.

**Persons *not* in anaphylactic shock:** People taking propranolol who receive epinephrine for something other than anaphylactic shock are at risk of developing excessively high blood pressure levels. If the epinephrine is injected with the intention of systemic effects (i.e., reaching most of the tissues and organs in the body), the blood pressure may increase dramatically. If, however, the epinephrine is inhaled into the lungs, put in

| ANTIHYPERTENSIVE DRUG | INTERACTING DRUG | RESULT |
|---|---|---|

*(cont.)*
**Propranolol** — Epinephrine — the eye, or injected for only local effects (e.g., by a dentist or dermatologist), the risk of a hypertensive reaction appears to be much less (unless a much larger than usual amount of epinephrine is used).

**Recommendation:** It is best for people who are at risk of anaphylactic shock (e.g., those allergic to bee-stings) to avoid taking propranolol or other beta blockers.

---

**Propranolol (Inderal®)**

Furosemide **(Lasix®)**

[for high blood pressure and to reduce fluid accumulation]

May increase the amount of propranolol in the blood, possibly leading to an excessive reduction in blood pressure, slowed heart rate, difficulty breathing, and cold hands and feet. But the combination can be used intentionally for the additive lowering of blood pressure.

---

**Propranolol (Inderal®)**

Indomethacin **(Indocin®)**

[for reduction of inflammation; used to reduce the pain and swelling associated with arthritis, tendinitis, and bursitis]

May be a reduction in the antihypertensive or antianginal effect of propranolol. This effect may occur with other nonsteroidal anti-inflammatory agents, such as piroxicam (Feldene®), naproxen (Naprosyn®), and naproxen sodium (Anaprox®). Sulindac (Clinoril®) appears less likely to interfere with the antihypertensive effect of propranolol.

**Recommendation:** Your doctor may want to check your blood pressure if you start, stop, or change the dose of an NSAID.

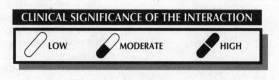

**CLINICAL SIGNIFICANCE OF THE INTERACTION**

LOW      MODERATE      HIGH

Propranolol **(Inderal®)**

Isoproterenol (**Isuprel®**, **Duo-Medihaler®**, and others)

[used as a bronchodilator to relieve bronchospasms associated with asthma, bronchitis, and emphysema]

Propranolol may reduce the bronchodilating effect of isoproterenol (and probably other bronchodilators as well) in asthmatic persons. Other drugs in the same class as propranolol (known as beta blockes) may have a similar effect. Other beta blockers include acebutolol (Sectral®), atenolol (Tenormin®), betaxolol (Kerlone®), carteolol (Cartrol®), esmolol (Brevibloc®), labetalol (Normodyne®, Trandate®), metoprolol (Lopressor®), nadolol (Corgard), pindolol (Visken®), and timolol (Blocadren®).

The nonselective beta blockers (i.e., Blocadren®, Cartrol®, Corgard®, Inderal®, and Visken®) are more likely to reduce the bronchodilating effect of isoproterenol than the selective beta blockers (i.e., Kerlone®, Lopressor®, Sectral®, or Tenormin®).

**Recommendation:** It is best to avoid this combination; discuss it with your doctor.

Propranolol **(Inderal®)**

Lidocaine (**Xylocaine®**, **Anestacon®**, and others)

[used to treat abnormal heart rhythms; for topical anesthesia during minor surgery; also available as an over-the-counter medication for relief of pain, itching, and inflammation, but such topical use is unlikely to interact with propranolol]

Increased lidocaine effect, perhaps to the point of lidocaine toxicity (symptoms of which include dizziness, lethargy, nausea, confusion, agitation, ringing in ears).

This interaction is more likely to occur when lidocaine is given intravenously.

Propranolol **(Inderal®)**

Methyldopa (**Aldomet®**)

[for treatment of high blood pressure]

May result in periods of very high blood pressure in some persons, especially during severe physiologic stress.

| ANTIHYPERTENSIVE DRUG | INTERACTING DRUG | RESULT |
|---|---|---|

Propranolol
(**Inderal**®)

Propoxyphene
(**Darvocet-N**®, **Darvon**®,
**Darvon**® **with A.S.A.**®,
**Dolene**®, and **Wygesic**®)

[for relief of mild to
moderate pain]

Can increase the concentration of
propranolol, possibly leading to an
excessive reduction in blood pressure, slowed heart rate, difficulty
breathing, and cold hands and feet.

---

Propranolol
(**Inderal**®)

Rifampin (**Rifadin**®,
**Rifamate**®, **Rimactane**®)

[used in combination
with at least one other
drug, rifampin is used to
treat tuberculosis; also
used in the treatment of
individuals who are carriers of meningitis]

May result in a reduced propranolol
effect. A larger dose of propranolol
may be needed in the presence of rifampin therapy. (Do *not* change the
dosage of either drug yourself; only
your doctor should do this.)

---

Propranolol
(**Inderal**®)

Theophylline
(**Primatene**® **Tablets,
Slo-bid**®, **Slo-Phyllin**®,
**Theo-Dur**®, **Theo-24**®,
and others)

[used to relieve and/or
prevent symptoms of
asthma bronchospasm as-
sociated with bronchitis
and emphysema]

Increased amount of theophylline in
the blood, possibly leading to toxicity. Symptoms of theophylline toxicity
include nausea, vomiting, diarrhea,
headache, irritability, nervousness,
rapid heartbeat, insomnia, tremor,
and seizure.

**Recommendation:** Since propranolol
(**Inderal**®) and other nonselective beta
blockers (e.g., **Blocadren**®, **Cartrol**®,
**Corgard**®, and **Visken**®) tend to cause
narrowing of the bronchi, they should
generally be avoided in persons with
asthma.

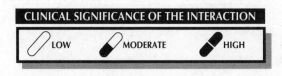

**CLINICAL SIGNIFICANCE OF THE INTERACTION**

LOW    MODERATE    HIGH

| ANTIHYPERTENSIVE DRUG | INTERACTING DRUG | RESULT |
|---|---|---|
| Propranolol **(Inderal®)**  | Thiazide diuretics:<br><br>• chlorothiazide **(Diuril®)**<br>• hydrochlorothiazide **(Esidrix®, HydroDIURIL®, Oretic®**, and others)<br><br>[for treatment of high blood pressure and to reduce fluid retention in persons with congestive heart failure, kidney disorders, and other conditions] | Can increase the concentration of blood glucose (sugar) and triglycerides (fat) in the blood. Other antihypertensive drugs in the beta-blocker class besides propranolol may produce a similar effect. |
| Propranolol **(Inderal®)**  | Thioridazine **(Mellaril®)**<br><br>[for treatment of schizophrenia, mania, and dementia] | Increased concentration of thioridazine, which could lead to side effects such as drowsiness, dizziness, fainting, dry mouth, blurred vision, and constipation. In severe cases, disturbances of heart rhythm could occur. |
| Reserpine **(Serpasil®)**  | Monoamine oxidase inhibitors:<br><br>• isocarboxazid **(Marplan®)**<br>• phenelzine **(Nardil®)**<br>• tranylcypromine **(Parnate®)**, and others<br><br>[for treatment of depression] | Although the evidence is limited, excitation and an increase in blood pressure may occur if reserpine is started in persons already receiving a monoamine-oxidase inhibitor. |

269

Spironolactone **(Aldactone®)**

Lithium **(Cibalith-S®, Eskalith®, Lithane®, Lithobid®,** and others)

[for manic-depressive disorder]

May result in higher levels of lithium in the blood, which could lead to lithium toxicity. Symptoms of this toxicity include muscle twitching, dizziness, blurred vision, vomiting or severe nausea, persistent diarrhea, confusion, weakness, coarse trembling of hands or legs, and slurred speech.

It may be necessary for your doctor to adjust your lithium dose if spironolactone is started or stopped. (Of course, only your doctor should change medication dosages, when appropriate.)

---

Thiazide and thiazide-like diuretics:

- chlorothiazide **(Diuril®)**
- chlorthalidone **(Hygroton®)**
- hydrochlorothiazide **(Esidrix®, HydroDIURIL®, Oretic®,** and others)
- metolazone **(Diulo®, Zaroxolyn®)**

Antidiabetic drugs:

- acetohexamide **(Dymelor®)**
- chlorpropamide **(Diabinese®)**
- glipizide **(Glucotrol®)**
- glyburide **(DiaBeta®, Micronase®)**
- insulin **(Humulin®, Lente®, Novolin®,** and others)
- tolazamide **(Tolinase®)**
- tolbutamide **(Orinase®),** and others

[for treatment of diabetes mellitus, a condition that results in excessively high amounts of sugar in the blood and urine]

Thiazide diuretics may interfere with the effectiveness of antidiabetic drugs.

Thiazide diuretics taken with chlorpropamide (and possibly with other antidiabetic drugs) may cause a deficiency in the amount of sodium in the blood, possibly leading to lethargy, confusion, irritability, headache, nausea, vomiting, and seizures.

| ANTIHYPERTENSIVE DRUG | INTERACTING DRUG | RESULT |
|---|---|---|
| Thiazide and thiazide-like diuretics:<br><br>chlorothiazide **(Diuril®)**<br>• chlorthalidone **(Hygroton®)**<br>• hydrochloro-thiazide **(Esidrix®, HydroDIURIL®, Oretic®**, and others)<br>• metolazone **(Diulo®, Zaroxolyn®)** | Chloestyramine **(Questran®)**<br><br>[for lowering cholesterol levels] | Reduced blood levels of thiazides, possibly leading to a decreased anti-hypertensive effect.<br><br>**Recommendation:** Thiazide diuretics should be taken at least two hours before or four to six hours after taking chloestyramine. |

| | | |
|---|---|---|
| Thiazide and thiazide-like diuretics:<br><br>• chlorothiazide **(Diuril®)**<br>• chlorthalidone **(Hygroton®)**<br>• hydrochloro-thiazide **(Esidrix®, HydroDIURIL®, Oretic®**, and others)<br>• metolazone **(Diulo®, Zaroxolyn®)** | Colestipol **(Colestid®)**<br><br>[for reducing cholesterol levels] | Colestipol may reduce the antihyper-tensive effect of thiazides.<br><br>**Recommendation:** Thiazide diuretics should be taken at least two hours before or four to six hours after taking colestipol. |

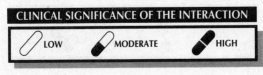

CLINICAL SIGNIFICANCE OF THE INTERACTION

LOW    MODERATE    HIGH

Thiazide and thiazide-like diuretics:

- chlorothiazide (**Diuril**®)
- chlorthalidone (**Hygroton**®)
- hydrochloro-thiazide (**Esidrix**®, **HydroDIURIL**®, **Oretic**®, and others)
- metolazon (**Diulo**® **Zaroxolyn**®)

Corticosteroids:

- cortisone (**Cortone**®)
- hydrocortisone (**Cortef**®, **Hydrocor-tone**®, **Solu-Cortef**®)
- methylprednisolone (**Medrol**®, **Depo-Medrol**®, **Solu-Medrol**®)
- prednisolone (**Delta-Cortef**®, **Hydeltrasol**®, **Pediapred**®, **Prelone**®)
- prednisone (**Delta-sone**®, **Liquid Pred**®, **Meticorten**®)

[for relieving inflammation and suppressing allergic reactions]

May decrease the amount of potassium in the body, which may lead to muscle problems (such as weakness, twitching, and pain), nocturia (need to urinate at night), and abnormal sensations, such as feelings of numbness, tingling, or burning.

Corticosteroids can produce potassium depletion if they are given by injection or orally (especially with large doses), but other routes of administration (e.g., inhalation or topical application on the skin or in the eye, ear, etc.) generally have little effect on potassium.

Cortisone and hydrocortisone are more likely than other corticosteroids to lead to these effects.

Thiazide and thiazide-like diuretics:

- chlorothiazide (**Diuril**®)
- chlorthalidone (**Hygroton**®)
- hydrochloro-thiazide (**Esidrix**®, **HydroDIURIL**®, **Oretic**®, and others)
- metolazone (**Diulo**®, **Zaroxolyn**®)

Digoxin (**Lanoxin**®)

[for heart failure and heart abnormalities, such as atrial fibrillation and atrial flutter]

Certain diuretics can cause a loss of potassium in the body. As the amount of potassium in the body decreases, the likelihood of digoxin toxicity increases. Symptoms of this toxicity include nausea, poor appetite, weakness, lethargy, and visual abnormalities.

**Recommendation:** Your doctor may wish to check your potassium level periodically, especially if you are taking large doses of diuretics and/or if your dietary intake of potassium is low.

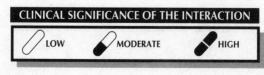

CLINICAL SIGNIFICANCE OF THE INTERACTION

LOW   MODERATE   HIGH

| | | |
| --- | --- | --- |
| Thiazide and thiazide-like diuretics:<br><br>• chlorothiazide **(Diuril®)**<br>• chlorthalidone **(Hygroton®)**<br>• hydrochloro-thiazide **(Esidrix®, HydroDIURIL®, Oretic®**, and others)<br>• metolazone **(Diulo®, Zaroxolyn®)** | Lithium **(Cibalith-S®, Eskalith®, Lithane®, Lithobid®**, and others)<br><br>[for manic-depressive disorder] | May lead to an increased amount of lithium in the blood, possibly to the point of lithium toxicity. Symptoms of this toxicity include muscle twitching, dizziness, blurred vision, vomiting or severe nausea, persistent diarrhea, confusion, weakness, coarse trembling of hands or legs, and slurred speech.<br><br>It may be necessary for your doctor to adjust your lithium dose if a thiazide diuretic is started or stopped, or if its dosage is changed. (Of course, only your doctor should change medication dosages, when appropriate.) |

| | | |
| --- | --- | --- |
| Thiazide and thiazide-like diuretics:<br><br>• chlorothiazide **(Diuril®)**<br>• chlorthalidone **(Hygroton®)**<br>• hydrochloro-thiazide **(Esidrix®, HydroDIURIL®, Oretic®**, and others)<br>• metolazone **(Diulo®, Zaroxolyn®)** | Methotrexate **(Mexate®)**<br><br>[for treatment of certain cancers, such as breast, lung, and certain forms of leukemia; also used in low doses to treat rheumatoid arthritis or psoriasis] | Thiazide diuretics may increase the effect of methotrexate, possibly leading to methotrexate toxicity.<br><br>Enhanced bone marrow suppression has been observed in persons receiving both drugs in combination. |

273

| ANTIHYPERTENSIVE DRUG | INTERACTING DRUG | RESULT |
|---|---|---|

Thiazide and thiazide-like diuretics:

- chlorothiazide (**Diuril**®)
- chlorthalidone (**Hygroton**®)
- hydrochloro-thiazide (**Esidrix**®, **HydroDIURIL**®, **Oretic**®, and others)
- metolazone (**Diulo**®, **Zaroxolyn**®)

Nonsteroidal anti-inflam-matory drugs:

- aspirin (**Alka-Seltzer**® **Antacid and Pain Reliever, Anacin**®, **Ascriptin**®, **Bayer**®, **Bufferin**®, **Ecotrin**®, and many others)
- diflunisal (**Dolobid**®)
- ibuprofen (**Advil**®, **Motrin**®, **Nuprin**®, **Rufen**®)
- indomethacin (**Indocin**®)
- meclofenamate (**Meclomen**®)
- naproxen (**Naprosyn**®)
- naproxen sodium (**Anaprox**®), and others

[for reduction of inflam-mation; used to reduce the pain and swelling associated with arthritis, tendinitis, and bursitis]

May cause a mild reduction in the antihypertensive effect of the thi-azide. This interaction may occur with other nonsteroidal anti-inflam-matory drugs, such as diclofenac (Voltaren®), diflunisal (Dolobid®), etodolac (Lodine®), fenoprofen (Nalfon®), flurbiprofen (Ansaid®), ibuprofen (Advil®, Motrin®, Nuprin®, Rufen®), ketoprofen (Orudis®), ke-torolac (Toradol®), meclofenamate (Meclomen®), nabumetone (Relafen®), naproxen (Naprosyn®), naproxen sodium (Anaprox®), piroxi-cam (Feldene®), sulindac (Clinoril®), and tolmetin (Tolectin®).

**Recommendation:** Although this in-teraction usually does not cause problems, it would be prudent to have your blood pressure checked if you take indomethacin or other non-steroidal anti-inflammatory drugs reg-ularly along with a thiazide diuretic.

Timolol (**Blocadren**®)

Epinephrine (**Adrenalin**®, **Ana-Kit**®, **AsthmaHaler**®, **Bronkaid**® **Mist, Epi-Pen**®, **Primatene**® **Mist, Sus-Phrine**®, and others)

[for temporary relief of shortness of breath, and wheezing caused by bronchial asthma; Ana-Kit® and EpiPen® are used for the emergency treatment of allergic reac-tions to insect stings or bites, food, and other substances that trigger a serious allergic reaction]

The outcome depends on the condi-tion for which the person is being treated, and on how the epinephrine is given.

**Persons with anaphylactic shock:** Some people develop a severe, possi-bly life-threatening, allergic reaction (called anaphylactic shock) to insect stings or bites and certain medica-tions or foods. Symptoms of anaphy-lactic shock include hives, wheezing, difficulty breathing, abdominal pain, incontinence, fever, and loss of con-sciousness; death may also occur. Epinephrine injections help reverse anaphylactic shock, but in persons

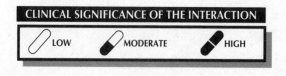

CLINICAL SIGNIFICANCE OF THE INTERACTION

LOW    MODERATE    HIGH

| ANTIHYPERTENSIVE DRUG | INTERACTING DRUG | RESULT |
|---|---|---|

(cont.)
Timolol

Epinephrine

taking a specific type of antihypertensive drug (i.e., nonselective beta blocker, such as timolol), the epinephrine may not work very well and other measures often must be taken.

**Persons *not* in anaphylactic shock:** People taking timolol who receive epinephrine for something other than anaphylactic shock are at risk of developing excessively high blood pressure levels. If the epinephrine is injected with the intention of systemic effects (i.e., reaching most of the tissues and organs in the body), the blood pressure may increase dramatically. If, however, the epinephrine is inhaled into the lungs, put in the eye, or injected for only local effects (e.g., by a dentist or dermatologist), the risk of a hypertensive reaction appears to be much less (unless a much larger than usual amount of epinephrine is used).

**Recommendation:** It is best for people who are at risk of anaphylactic shock (e.g., those allergic to beestings) to avoid taking timolol or other beta blockers.

---

Timolol
(**Blocadren**®)

- guanadrel (**Hylorel**®)
- guanethidine (**Ismelin**®)
- reserpine (**Serpasil**®, **Regroton**®)

[for treatment of high blood pressure]

May result in low blood pressure, which could lead to slowed heartbeat and fainting.

---

Timolol
(**Blocadren**®)

Isoproterenol (**Isuprel**®, **Duo-Medihaler**®, and others)

[used as a bronchodilator to relieve bronchospasms associated with asthma, bronchitis, and emphysema]

May reduce the bronchodilating effect of isoproterenol in asthmatic persons. Bronchodilators other than isoproterenol are probably similarly affected.

**Recommendation:** It is best to avoid this combination; discuss it with your doctor.

| ANTIHYPERTENSIVE DRUG | INTERACTING DRUG | RESULT |
|---|---|---|
| Timolol **(Blocadren®)**  | Quinidine **(Cardioquin®, Duraquin®, Quinaglute®, Quinidex®, Quinora®)** [for arrhythmias, or irregularities of the heartbeat and heart rhythm] | May increase the plasma concentration of timolol, possibly leading to slowed heartbeat and an increased likelihood of the occurrence of side effects, such as cold hands and feet, blurred vision, and headache. |
| Triamterene **(Dyrenium®)** | Indomethacin **(Indocin®)** [for reduction of inflammation; used to reduce the pain and swelling associated with arthritis, tendinitis, and bursitis] | In some persons, this combination can lead to kidney damage, even kidney failure. This interaction may occur with diclofenac (Voltaren®) or ibuprofen (Advil®, Nuprin®, Motrin®), but the evidence is less substantial than that of the indomethacin-triamterene interaction. Until more studies are completed, caution is warranted when any nonsteroidal anti-inflammatory drug is used with triamterene. Other drugs—such as furosemide (Lasix®) and spironolactone (Aldactone®)—that belong to the same class of drug as triamterene have not been associated with kidney damage when given with indomethacin. **Recommendation:** It is best to avoid this combination; discuss it with your doctor. |
| Triamterene **(Dyrenium®)** | Ranitidine **(Zantac®)** [for relief of stomach and intestinal ulcers] | Ranitidine may cause a slight decrease in triamterene blood levels, possibly leading to a reduced ability of triamterene to promote fluid loss and reduce blood pressure. |

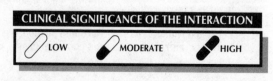

CLINICAL SIGNIFICANCE OF THE INTERACTION

LOW   MODERATE   HIGH

| ANTIHYPERTENSIVE DRUG | INTERACTING DRUG | RESULT |
|---|---|---|

Verapamil **(Calan®, Isoptin®, Verelan®)**

Alcohol

Causes an increased effect of the alcohol. Intoxication may be greater and last longer when verapamil is taken with alcohol.

**Recommendation:** Reduce, or avoid altogether, alcohol while taking verapamil. Check with your doctor.

---

Verapamil **(Calan®, Isoptin®, Verelan®)**

Barbiturates:

- amobarbital **(Amytal®)**
- butabarbital **(Butisol®)**
- butalbital
- pentobarbital **(Nembutal®)**
- phenobarbital **(Luminal®, Solfoton®)**
- primidone **(Mysoline®)**
- secobarbital **(Seconal®)**, and others

[used to treat insomnia and anxiety; certain barbiturates are used to prevent seizures]

Phenobarbital (and probably other barbiturates) substantially reduce the plasma concentration of verapamil, possibly leading to a reduced effect of this antihypertensive. This interaction occurs with oral verapamil, but is unlikely with intravenous verapamil.

Persons receiving phenobarbital or other barbiturates may require higher than usual doses of verapamil. (Of course, *never* alter the dosage of any medication without your doctor's consent and supervision.)

---

Verapamil **(Calan®, Isoptin®, Verelan®)**

Calcium

[a mineral needed for the heart, muscles, and nerves to function properly; also needed for strong bones and teeth]

When large doses of calcium are taken, there is a reduced effect of verapamil. This interaction is not usually significant unless the calcium is given intravenously.

---

Verapamil **(Calan®, Isoptin®, Verelan®)**

Carbamazepine **(Tegretol®)**

[for epilepsy, trigeminal neuralgia (spasms of pain in the face), and other disorders]

May increase carbamazepine concentration in the body, possibly leading to double vision, headaches, abnormal muscle coordination, or dizziness.

Reduced effect of verapamil may also occur.

**Recommendation:** It may be necessary for your doctor to adjust the dose of carbamazepine if verapamil is started or stopped, or if its dosage is changed. (Of course, only your

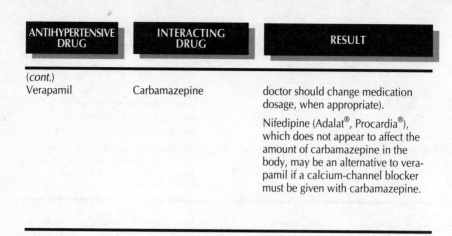
*(cont.)*
Verapamil | Carbamazepine

doctor should change medication dosage, when appropriate).

Nifedipine (Adalat®, Procardia®), which does not appear to affect the amount of carbamazepine in the body, may be an alternative to verapamil if a calcium-channel blocker must be given with carbamazepine.

---

Verapamil (**Calan**®, **Isoptin**®, **Verelan**®)

Cimetidine (**Tagamet**®)

[for relief of stomach and intestinal ulcers]

May increase verapamil levels, possibly leading to toxicity. Symptoms of toxicity include excessive slowing of the heart rate, decreased blood pressure, headache, flushing, and edema (fluid accumulation).

---

Verapamil (**Calan**®, **Isoptin**®, **Verelan**®)

Cyclosporine (**Sandimmune**®)

[for immune suppression, which is needed after organ transplantation to prevent rejection of the transplanted organ]

Verapamil may increase the concentration of cyclosporine in the body. Increased blood levels of cyclosporine have been associated with nephrotoxicity (kidney damage).

**Recommendation:** It may be necessary for your doctor to adjust the dose of cyclosporine if verapamil is started or stopped, or if its dosage is changed. (Of course, only your doctor should change medication dosage, when appropriate.)

---

Verapamil (**Calan**®, **Isoptin**®, **Verelan**®)

Digitoxin (**Crystodigin**®)

[for heart failure and other heart abnormalities]

May increase digitoxin effect, possibly leading to toxicity. Symptoms of digitoxin toxicity include nausea, poor appetite, weakness, lethargy, and visual abnormalities.

**Recommendation:** It may be necessary for your doctor to adjust the dose of digitoxin if verapamil is started or stopped, or if its dosage is changed. (Of course, only your doctor should change medication dosage, when appropriate.)

Verapamil **(Calan®, Isoptin®, Verelan®)**

Digoxin **(Lanoxin®)**

[for heart failure and heart abnormalities, such as atrial fibrillation and atrial flutter]

Verapamil may increase the amount of digoxin in the blood, possibly leading to toxicity. Symptoms of digoxin toxicity include nausea, poor appetite, weakness, lethargy, and visual abnormalities.

Verapamil is in a drug class known as calcium-channel blockers, certain others of which—nifedipine (Adalat®, Procardia®), isradipine (DynaCirc®), and nicardipine (Cardene®)—do not appear to increase digoxin concentrations.

**Recommendation:** It may be necessary for your doctor to adjust the dose of digoxin if verapamil is started or stopped, or if its dosage is changed. (Of course, only your doctor should change medication dosage, when appropriate.)

Verapamil **(Calan®, Isoptin®, Verelan®)**

Lithium **(Cibalith-S®, Eskalith®, Lithane®, Lithobid®, and others)**

[for manic-depressive disorder]

In a few isolated cases, this combination seemed to lead to neurotoxicity. Possible symptoms include nausea, vomiting, muscular incoordination, and ringing in the ears. This interaction may also occur with diltiazem (Cardizem®) and possibly with other calcium-channel blockers (drugs in the same class as Verapamil).

**Recommendation:** Some persons do not seem to have any trouble with the combined use of lithium and verapamil or other calcium-channel blockers. If you are concerned about this unlikely interaction, discuss your concerns with your doctor.

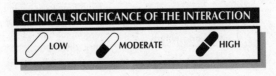

CLINICAL SIGNIFICANCE OF THE INTERACTION

LOW   MODERATE   HIGH

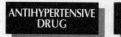

Verapamil (**Calan**®, **Isoptin**®, **Verelan**®)

Prazosin (**Minipress**®)

[for treatment of high blood pressure]

Can result in an excessive decrease in blood pressure levels in some persons.

---

Verapamil (**Calan**®, **Isoptin**®, **Verelan**®)

Propranolol (**Inderal**®)

[for treatment of high blood pressure, angina pectoris, and irregular heartbeat; also used to prevent migraine headaches]

Verapamil can increase the amount of propranolol in the blood, and may also lead to reductions in the blood pressure and slowing of the heart rate. This is usually a favorable interaction that may be used intentionally by your doctor, but occasionally the blood pressure or heart rate may become excessively low.

**Recommendation:** When verapamil is added to propranolol (or conversely, when propranolol is added to verapamil), watch for any symptoms of excessive lowering of blood pressure or heart rate (e.g., dizziness, faintness). Verapamil probably has a similar effect with other beta blockers (antihypertensive medications that are in the same class as propranolol) although the magnitude of the additive effect may be different. Other beta blockers include acebutolol (Sectral®), atenolol (Tenormin®), betaxolol (Kerlone®), carteolol (Cartrol®), esmolol (Brevibloc®), labetalol (Normodyne®, Trandate®), metoprolol (Lopressor®), nadolol (Corgard®), pindolol (Visken®), and timolol (Blocadren®).

---

Verapamil (**Calan**®, **Isoptin**®, **Verelan**®)

Quinidine (**Cardioquin**®, **Duraquin**®, **Quinaglute**®, **Quinidex**®, **Quinora**®)

[for arrhythmias, or irregularities of the heartbeat and heart rhythm]

Can cause increased levels of quinidine in the body, possibly leading to quinidine toxicity. Symptoms of quinidine toxicity include ringing in the ears, nausea, headache, blurred vision, and, in severe cases, psychiatric disorders.

| ANTIHYPERTENSIVE DRUG | INTERACTING DRUG | RESULT |
|---|---|---|

Verapamil **(Calan®, Isoptin®, Verelan®)**

Rifampin **(Rifadin®, Rifamate®, Rimactane®)**

[used in combination with at least one other drug, rifampin is used to treat tuberculosis; also used in the treatment of individuals who are carriers of meningitis]

May cause a large decrease in vera-pamil plasma levels, possibly leading to a diminished antihypertensive effect. This interaction occurs with oral verapamil, but is unlikely with intra-venous verapamil.

**Recommendation:** It may be necessary for your doctor to adjust the dose of verapamil if rifampin is started or stopped, or if its dosage is changed. (Of course, only your doctor should change medication dosage, when appropriate.)

---

Verapamil **(Calan®, Isoptin®, Verelan®)**

Theophylline **(Primatene® Tablets, Slo-bid®, Slo-Phyllin®, Theo-Dur®, Theo-24®,** and others)

[used to relieve and/or prevent symptoms of asthma bronchospasm associated with bronchitis and emphysema]

Verapamil may increase the amount of theophylline in the blood, possibly leading to theophylline toxicity (symptoms of which include nausea, vomiting, diarrhea, headache, irritability, nervousness, rapid heartbeat, insomnia, tremor, and seizure).

Other antihypertensive drugs in this class—diltiazem (Cardizem®) and nifedipine (Adalat®, Procardia®)—are less likely to increase theophylline concentrations, and may do so in only a small percentage of persons.

**Recommendation:** It may be necessary for your doctor to adjust the dose of theophylline if verapamil is started or stopped, or if its dosage is changed. (Of course, only your doctor should change medication dosage, when appropriate.)

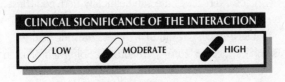

CLINICAL SIGNIFICANCE OF THE INTERACTION

LOW    MODERATE    HIGH

## CHAPTER 8

# HORMONAL DRUGS

Hormones are chemicals secreted into the bloodstream by a particular gland. These chemicals regulate a multitude of events in your body. Hormones are needed for the normal development of virtually all parts of your body—from sexual organs to brain tissue. As a result, it follows that inappropriate amounts of hormone production, either too much or too little, can lead to many different types of disorders. Cells in the pancreas, for example, manufacture the hormone insulin, necessary for just the right amount of sugar to reach cells throughout your body, supplying them with energy. An inadequate amount of insulin in the body results in a disorder known as *diabetes mellitus*.

## The Pituitary: A Master Gland

The pituitary, a gland at the base of the brain, is often dubbed the master gland because it not only produces its own hormones, but also stimulates other organs to manufacture and release their own hormones. For example, women's ovaries are stimulated to release estrogen and progesterone by the pituitary. The male hormone testosterone, produced by the testes, is stimulated by luteinizing hormone, another chemical of the pituitary gland. The pituitary also regulates normal growth by producing growth hormone. An insufficient amount of growth hormone results in dwarfism; an excess supply of this hormone leads to gigantism or acromegaly, a condition marked by abnormally large facial features—such as the nose and jaw—and hands and feet.

The pituitary can also stimulate the production of adrenal corticosteroid hormones, which are manufactured by the adrenal glands (these glands sit on top of each kidney). The adrenal corticosteroid hormones, or corticosteroids as they are often called, have many uses, including the reduction of inflammation (which alleviates swelling, redness, itching, and pain). Reduction of inflammation is important in numerous conditions, from skin rash to rheumatoid arthritis.

Although a naturally occurring corticosteroid is available—cortisone—as a medication, most corticosteroid drugs are synthethically derived. These drugs include betamethasone (Celestone®, Dirolene®, Diprosone®, Valisone®), cortisone (Cortone®), dexamethasone (Decadron®, Hexadrol®), hydrocortisone (Cortef®, Solu-Cortef®), methylprednisolone (Depo-Medrol®, Medrol®, Solu-Medrol®), paramethasone

(Haldrone®), prednisolone (Delta-Cortef®, Hydeltrasol®), prednisone (Deltasone®, Liquid Pred®, Prednicen-M®), triamcinolone (Aristocort®, Kenacort®, Kenalog®), and others. The inhaled form of corticosteroids, which may be used to treat asthma, is discussed in Chapter 4, "Drugs for Asthma and Other Breathing Disorders."

Another gland influenced by the pituitary is the thyroid, a butterfly-shaped organ located in the neck below the Adam's apple. Thydroid hormone is produced by this gland and is absolutely essential for normal metabolism (all of the continuous, energy-generating chemical processes that occur in the body). Major problems may occur when the thyroid gland produces either too little or too much thyroid hormone, and the condition is not corrected.

An insufficient production of thyroid hormone, called hypothyroidism, may lead to symptoms such as fatigue, hoarse voice, slowed speech, apathy, weight gain, and intolerance to cold temperatures. Since some of these symptoms may be falsely attributed to the normal aging process, hypothyroidism is particularly difficult to detect in the elderly. Fortunately, levels of thyroid hormone can be determined, and an inadequate supply of this hormone can then be replaced.

An overactive thyroid producing too much thyroid hormone may lead to a condition known as Graves' disease. Persons who suffer from this disorder may experience nervousness, irritability, heart palpitations, difficulty getting to sleep, and weight loss. One common way of reducing the thyroid gland's hormone production is with radioactive iodine, which destroys thyroid tissue. Other methods of reducing thyroid hormone output is with medication or by surgical removal of part of the thyroid gland.

## The Many Uses of Estrogen

In women, from the time of puberty until menopause, the ovaries manufacture the female sex hormone estrogen. Like other hormones, estrogen has been found to have several functions; this explains, in part, why estrogen drugs have been used to treat many different conditions. In women, estrogen is primarily used for female reproductive tract disorders, prevention of contraception, and treatment of abnormal bleeding from the uterus. In men, certain types of prostate cancer may respond to estrogen therapy. Much evidence indicates that estrogen plays a key role in preventing osteoporosis, a condition in which the bones weaken because they become less dense and more brittle. Estrogen is also prescribed for some women who experience certain unpleasant symptoms at menopause, such as hot flashes, chills, flushing of the face, and vaginal dryness and itching.

Sometimes estrogen can be diagnostic, yielding important information to your doctor. For example, the growth of certain types of breast cancer is stimulated by estrogen; as a result, a drug that blocks the effects of estrogen may be a useful treatment for those women.

Estrogen is available in various forms, such as tablets, skin patches, and cream. Estrogen medications (both natural and synthetic) include chlorotrianisene (TACE®), conjugated estrogen (Premarin®), ethinyl estradiol (Estinyl®), estradiol (Estrace®, Estraderm®), polyestradiol (Estradurin®), quinestrol (Estrovis®), estropipate (Ogen®). Combination products include Menrium® (estrogen with chlordiazepoxide) and PMB 200® (estrogen and meprobamate); both of these drugs combine estrogen with an antianxiety medication.

## Estrogen and Contraception

Oral contraceptives, or birth-control pills, are a widely used form of birth control. Although not all oral contraceptives contain estrogen, the most widely used ones contain estrogen and progestogen, a class of hormone. The combination of those two hormones may be fixed or nonfixed; nonfixed oral contraceptives are usually called biphasic or triphasic. Fixed-combination oral contraceptives contain one of two synthetic estrogens (mestranol or ethinyl estradiol) and one of five synthetic forms of progestogen. The five available progestogens include norethindrone, norethindrone acetate, norethynodrel, norgestrel, or ethynodiol diacetate. The fixed-combination type contains a fixed amount of synthetic estrogen and progestogen.

The biphasic or triphasic oral contraceptives contain varying amounts of estrogen or progesterone, or both. For example, during certain pill-taking days, a woman may be receiving 0.5 milligram of progesterone, whereas on other days she may receive twice that amount. Both the fixed-combination type and the biphasic or triphasic pills are taken for twenty-one consecutive days, followed by seven days off of the active drug.

Although oral contraceptives are considered a relatively safe method of contraception, adverse effects have been reported. These adverse effects typically depend on the dose; that is, oral contraceptives that contain a large amount of estrogen have a higher likelihood of producing adverse effects. That's why your doctor may prescribe an oral contraceptive containing a low dose of estrogen.

## How Oral Contraceptives Work

It's important to understand some basics about how the oral contraceptive works in order to understand some of the drug interactions that you'll learn about in this chapter. Oral contraceptives work by preventing the release of the egg from the ovary, a process called ovulation. While you are taking the active drugs (estrogen and progesterone), the uterus is being toughened; estrogen stimulates the growth and blood supply of the uterine lining, and progesterone thickens its walls.

During the days off the active drug (taking either no pills at all, or a placebo—an inert, inactive pill), the uterine lining is shed as a bloody discharge.

Blood flow, or spotting, should not occur during the days in which you are taking the active drug. On the other hand, it is normal to have a bloody flow during the days you are either not taking the pills or are taking placebo pills. As you'll learn in this chapter, certain drugs can interact with oral contraceptives, possibly leading to decreased efficacy of the oral contraceptive. In fact, one of the signs that an interaction is occurring is experiencing spotting during the days you're taking the active drug. Such a sign may indicate that the oral contraceptive is not working properly. (Of course, it's important to discuss with your doctor any unexpected blood flow that you experience.)

Some of the fixed-combination type of oral contraceptives include Brevicon®, Enovid 5®, Enovid 10®, Loestrin®, Lo/Ovral®, Modicon 28®, Nordette 28®, Norinyl®, Norlestrin®, Ortho Novum®, Ovral®, Ovcon 35®, Ovcon 50®, Ovulen®, and others. Triphasic products include Ortho Novum® 7/7/7, Tri-Levlen®, Tri-Norinyl®, Triphasil®, and others. Several manufacturers of oral contraceptives offer their drug in more than one strength; for example, Loestrin® 1/20 contains 1 milligram of norethindrone and 20 micrograms of ethinyl estradiol, whereas Loestrin® 1.5/30 contains 1.5 milligrams of norethindrone and 30 micrograms of ethinyl estradiol. Currently available oral contraceptives may contain estrogen in a low dose—as little as 20 to 35 micrograms of ethinyl estradiol.

A progesterone-only birth control pill is also available (no estrogen is contained in these). These drugs are taken continuously on a daily basis. Some progesterone-only oral contraceptives include Micronor®, Nor-QD®, Ovrette®, and others.

A relatively new contraceptive device is known as Norplant®, which contains a synthetic progestin hormone. Although this hormone has been around for a while, the method of delivery is different: Norplant® is implanted under the skin of the inner arm, above the elbow. Six flexible silicone tubes (about the size of matchsticks) release a small amount of hormone each day. The device offers effective contraception twenty-four hours after insertion and prevents pregnancy for approximately five years.[1] As is the case with all medications, this drug is not for everyone; your doctor should be able to tell you whether you are a potential candidate for its use.

## Insulin and Diabetes

Insulin is a hormone produced by your pancreas. This hormone allows the glucose (sugar) in your blood to be converted to energy. Persons with *diabetes mellitus,* however, do not produce insulin (or produce an inadequate supply) or the body does not respond to insulin in the usual way (called insulin resistance). The result for the 5 to 10 million diabetics in the United States is an accumulation of sugar in the blood, which often leads to fatigue, weight loss, frequent urination, excessive thirst, and blurred vision.

Persons with diabetes generally are in one of two groups: Type I is insulin-dependent diabetes. These individuals must take a daily injection of insulin to ward off disease (insulin cannot be taken orally because the stomach's corrosive acid would destroy it). Insulin-dependent diabetes is also called juvenile-onset diabetes because it usually begins during childhood or early adolescence.

The other type of diabetes is known as Type II, or adult-onset diabetes; as its name implies, this variation begins in adulthood, usually after age forty. These individuals are far more numerous than their insulin-dependent counterparts (they make up approximately 90 percent of the total diabetic population in the United States). Adult-onset diabetes typically involves an abnormality in the way the body uses or responds to insulin; these diabetics may or may not be deficient in the *amount* of insulin their pancreas produces. Often, they don't need insulin injections. Rather, their symptoms can frequently be controlled through proper diet, exercise, and weight loss if they are overweight (between 70 and 90 percent of adult-onset diabetics are overweight[2]).

# Drug Treatment of Diabetes

Drug treatment of diabetes depends on, among other factors, the type and severity of the diabetes. Insulin-dependent diabetics require insulin as a medication. On the other hand, adult-onset diabetics may take a different type of medication, or perhaps no medication at all. Several insulins are available, and they differ from one another largely in how quickly they work (e.g., rapidly acting, long acting, and intermediate), degree of purity, and source (i.e., beef, pork, beef-pork, or human synthetically derived).

Rapidly acting insulins include Humulin® R, Iletin®, Novolin® R, Semilente Iletin®, Velosulin®, and others. Intermediate-acting insulins include Humulin N®, Humulin® 70/30, Lente Iletin I®, Novolin N®, NPH®, NPH Iletin I®, and others. Long-acting insulins include Protamine, Zinc and Iletin I®, Ultralente®, Ultralente Iletin I®, Ultralente Humulin U®, and others.

Individuals with adult-onset diabetes often receive a medication from a family of drugs called sulfonylureas. These drugs help persons with adult-onset diabetes use insulin more efficiently. In contrast to insulin, these drugs may be taken orally. Sulfonylurea drugs include acetohexamide (Dymelor®), chlorpropamide (Diabinese®), glipizide (Glucotrol®), glyburide (DiaBeta®, Micronase®), tolazamide (Ronase®, Tolinase®), and tolbutamide (Orinase®).

Persons experiencing or suspecting a hormone-related problem should seek the advice of their physician. Doctors who specialize in the management of hormone-related disorders are called endocrinologists.

| HORMONAL DRUG | INTERACTING DRUG | RESULT |
|---|---|---|

Antidiabetic drugs:

- acetohexamide **(Dymelor®)**
- chlorpropamide **(Diabinese®)**
- glipizide **(Glucotrol®)**
- glyburide **(DiaBeta®, Micronase®)**
- insulin **(Humulin®, Lente®, Novolin®,** and others
- tolazamide **(Tolinase®)**
- tolbutamide **(Orinase®),** and others

Acebutolol **(Sectral®)**

[for treatment of high blood pressure and irregular heartbeat and rhythm]

Although the heart typically beats faster (tachycardia) when blood sugar levels are low, this symptom may be absent when acebutolol is given. This effect may occur when antidiabetic agents are combined with other drugs that are in the same class as acebutolol, such as atenolol (Tenormin®), betaxolol (Kerlone®), carteolol (Cartrol®), esmolol (Brevibloc®), labetalol (Normodyne®, Trandate®), metoprolol (Lopressor®), nadolol (Corgard®), pindolol (Visken®), propranolol (Inderal®), and timolol (Blocadren®).

Antidiabetic drugs

- acetohexamide **(Dymelor®)**
- chlorpropamide **(Diabinese®)**
- glipizide **(Glucotrol®)**
- glyburide **(DiaBeta®, Micronase®)**

Alcohol

Alcohol, taken in moderate to large amounts, may lead to a severe drop in the amount of sugar in the blood (i.e., severe hypoglycemia). This is especially a problem if the person also has inadequate food intake. Signs of this severe drop in blood sugar include increased heart rate, cold sweats, trembling, nausea, hunger, mental confusion, and, in severe cases, coma.

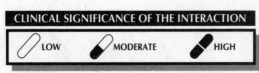

CLINICAL SIGNIFICANCE OF THE INTERACTION

LOW    MODERATE    HIGH

| HORMONAL DRUG | INTERACTING | RESULT |
|---|---|---|

(cont.)
Antidiabetic drugs:

- Insulin (**Humulin**®, **Lente**®, **Novolin**®, and others)
- tolazamide (**Tolinase**®)
- tolbutamide (**Orinase**®), and others

Alcohol

In certain persons one antidiabetic agent in particular, chlorpropamide, when taken with alcohol may occasionally lead to discomforting symptoms such as flushing and headache, nausea, vomiting, sweating, and confusion.

Other oral antidiabetic drugs may produce the same effect with alcohol, but the reaction seems to be rare.

**Recommendation:** Diabetics taking antidiabetic medication should avoid drinking alcohol in moderate to large amounts. Drinking a small amount of alcohol (i.e., one to two drinks), especially during meals, is less problematic; however, you should discuss this with your doctor.

---

Antidiabetic drugs:

- acetohexamide (**Dymelor**®)
- chlorpropamide (**Diabinese**®)
- glipizide (**Glucotrol**®)
- glyburide (**DiaBeta**®, **Micronase**®)
- insulin (**Humulin**®, **Lente**®, **Novolin**®, and others)
- tolazamide (**Tolinase**®)
- tolbutamide (**Orinase**®), and others

Androgens:

- ethylestrenol (**Maxibolin**®)
- fluoxymesterone (**Halotestin**®)
- methandrostenolone
- methyltestosterone (**Metandren**®)
- nandrolone (**Durabolin**®)
- oxandrolone (**Anavar**®)
- oxymetholone (**Androl-50**®)
- stanozolol (**Winstrol**®)
- testosterone

[androgens are male hormones that are given to persons who are deficient in these hormones; also used to treat certain types of breast cancer in women]

Androgens tend to lower blood sugar levels and may enhance the effect of antidiabetic drugs, which could lead to an undesirably low amount of sugar in the blood. Symptoms of excessively low blood sugar levels include increased heart rate, cold sweats, trembling, nausea, hunger, mental confusion, and, in severe cases, coma.

**Recommendation:** Persons taking antidiabetic medication should watch for a change in blood sugar levels if androgens are started or stopped, or if their dosage is changed.

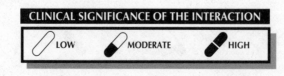

CLINICAL SIGNIFICANCE OF THE INTERACTION

LOW    MODERATE    HIGH

288

| HORMONAL DRUG | INTERACTING DRUG | RESULT |
|---|---|---|

Antidiabetic drugs:

- acetohexamide **(Dymelor®)**
- chlorpropamide **(Diabinese®)**
- glipizide **(Glucotrol®)**
- glyburide **(DiaBeta®, Micronase®)**
- insulin **(Humulin®, Lente®, Novolin®,** and others
- tolazamide **(Tolinase®)**
- tolbutamide **(Orinase®),** and others

Aspirin

[for relief of pain and inflammation]

Reduced blood sugar (hypoglycemic) effect. Symptoms of an excessively low amount of sugar in the blood include increased heart rate, cold sweats, trembling, nausea, hunger, mental confusion, and, in severe cases, coma.

An occasional aspirin has little effect on antidiabetic drugs with the possible exception of chlorpropamide.

Antidiabetic drugs:

- acetohexamide **(Dymelor®)**
- chlorpropamide **(Diabinese®)**
- glipizide **(Glucotrol®)**
- glyburide **(DiaBeta®, Micronase®)**
- insulin **(Humulin®, Lente®, Novolin®,** and others
- tolazamide **(Tolinase®)**
- tolbutamide **(Orinase®),** and others

Atenolol **(Tenormin®)**

[for treatment of high blood pressure and angina]

Although the heart typically beats faster (tachycardia) when blood sugar levels are low, this symptom may be absent when atenolol is given. This effect may occur when antidiabetic agents are combined with other drugs that are in the same class as atenolol, such as acebutolol (Sectral®), betaxolol (Kerlone®), carteolol (Cartrol®), esmolol (Brevibloc®), labetalol (Normodyne®, Trandate®), metoprolol (Lopressor®), nadolol (Corgard®), pindolol (Visken®), propranolol (Inderal®), and timolol (Blocadren®).

| HORMONAL DRUG | INTERACTING DRUG | RESULT |
|---|---|---|

Antidiabetic drugs:

- acetohexamide (**Dymelor**®)
- chlorpropamide (**Diabinese**®)
- glipizide (**Glucotrol**®)
- glyburide (**DiaBeta**®, **Micronase**®)
- insulin (**Humulin**®, **Lente**®, **Novolin**®, and others
- tolazamide (**Tolinase**®)
- tolbutamide (**Orinase**®), and others

Chlorpromazine (**Thorazine**®)

[for treatment of certain mental illnesses such as schizophrenia, mania, and dementia]

Use of chlorpromazine—in doses over 100 mg a day—with insulin may lead to increased blood sugar levels.

Antidiabetic drugs:

- acetohexamide (**Dymelor**®)
- chlorpropamide (**Diabinese**®)
- glipizide (**Glucotrol**®)
- glyburide (**DiaBeta**®, **Micronase**®)
- insulin (**Humulin**®, **Lente**®, **Novolin**®, and others
- tolazamide (**Tolinase**®)
- tolbutamide (**Orinase**®), and others

Corticosteroids:

- betamethasone (**Celestone**®)
- cortisone (**Cortone**®)
- dexamethasone (**Decadron**®, **Dalalone**®)
- hydrocortisone (**Cortef**®, **Hydrocortone**®, **Solu-Cortef**®)
- methylprednisolone (**Medrol**®, **Depo-Medrol**®, **Solu-Medrol**®)
- paramethasone (**Haldrone**®)
- prednisolone (**Delta-Cortef**®, **Hydeltrasol**®)
- prednisone (**Deltasone**®, **Liquid-Pred**®, **Meticorten**®)
- triamcinolone (**Aristocort**®, **Kenacort**®, **Kenalog**®)

[for relieving inflammation and suppressing allergic reactions]

Corticosteroids may increase the amount of sugar in the blood (i.e., hyperglycemic effect). This is most likely to occur when the corticosteroid is taken orally or by injection. Other routes of administration (e.g., inhalation, or topical application on the skin, eye, ear, etc.) usually have little effect on blood sugar.

**Recommendation:** Diabetics should be particularly careful when checking their blood sugar levels if a corticosteroid drug is started or stopped, or if its dosage is changed.

290

| HORMONAL DRUG | INTERACTING DRUG | RESULT |
|---|---|---|

Antidiabetic drugs:

- acetohexamide (**Dymelor**®)
- chlorpropamide (**Diabinese**®)
- glipizide (**Glucotrol**®)
- glyburide (**DiaBeta**®, **Micronase**®)
- insulin (**Humulin**®, **Lente**®, **Novolin**®, and others
- tolazamide (**Tolinase**®)
- tolbutamide (**Orinase**®), and others

Dextrothyroxine (**Choloxin**®)

[for reduction of excessively high serum cholesterol levels]

Dextrothyroxine may increase the amount of sugar in the blood (i.e., hyperglycemic effect).

**Recommendation:** Diabetics should be particularly careful when checking their blood sugar levels if dextrothyroxine is started or stopped, or if its dosage is changed.

Antidiabetic drugs:

- acetohexamide (**Dymelor**®)
- chlorpropamide (**Diabinese**®)
- glipizide (**Glucotrol**®)
- glyburide (**DiaBeta**®, **Micronase**®)
- insulin (**Humulin**®, **Lente**®, **Novolin**®, and others
- tolazamide (**Tolinase**®)
- tolbutamide (**Orinase**®), and others

Epinephrine (**Adrenalin**®, **Ana-Kit**®, **AsthmaHaler**®, **Bronkaid**® **Mist, EpiPen**®, **Primatene**® **Mist, Sus-Phrine**®, and others)

[for temporary relief of shortness of breath and wheezing caused by bronchial asthma; Ana-Kit® and EpiPen® are used for the emergency treatment of allergic reactions to insect stings or bites, food, and other substances that trigger a serious allergic reaction]

Injections of epinephrine can lead to increased blood glucose (sugar) levels in the blood. Inhaled epinephrine is probably less likely to interact unless excessive amounts of epinephrine are used. The epinephrine found in local anesthetic injections would also be unlikely to interact unless large amounts are used.

**Recommendation:** Diabetics should watch for excessive blood sugar levels when epinephrine is being used.

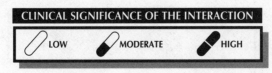

CLINICAL SIGNIFICANCE OF THE INTERACTION

LOW    MODERATE    HIGH

| HORMONAL DRUG | INTERACTING DRUG | RESULT |
|---|---|---|

Antidiabetic drugs:

- acetohexamide **(Dymelor®)**
- chlorpropamide **(Diabinese®)**
- glipizide **(Glucotrol®)**
- glyburide **(DiaBeta®, Micronase®)**
- insulin **(Humulin®, Lente®, Novolin®,** and others
- tolazamide **(Tolinase®)**
- tolbutamide **(Orinase®),** and others

Fenfluramine **(Pondimin®)**

[used for short-term weight loss in obese individuals]

May enhance the effect of antidiabetic drugs, leading to excessively low levels of blood sugar. Symptoms of excessively low blood sugar levels include increased heart rate, cold sweats, trembling, nausea, hunger, mental confusion, and, in severe cases, coma.

---

Antidiabetic drugs:

- acetohexamide **(Dymelor®)**
- chlorpropamide **(Diabinese®)**
- glipizide **(Glucotrol®)**
- glyburide **(DiaBeta®, Micronase®)**
- insulin **(Humulin®, Lente®, Novolin®,** and others
- tolazamide **(Tolinase®)**
- tolbutamide **(Orinase®),** and others

Guanethidine **(Ismelin®)**

[used to treat high blood pressure]

Guanethidine may lower blood sugar levels in diabetics. Symptoms of excessively low blood sugar levels include increased heart rate, cold sweats, trembling, nausea, hunger, mental confusion, and, in severe cases, coma.

**Recommendation:** Persons taking antidiabetic medication should watch for a change in blood sugar levels if guanethidine is started or stopped (i.e., excessively low sugar levels when guanethidine is started, and too high blood sugar levels when guanethidine is stopped).

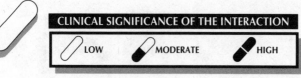

CLINICAL SIGNIFICANCE OF THE INTERACTION

LOW    MODERATE    HIGH

| HORMONAL DRUG | INTERACTING DRUG | RESULT |
| --- | --- | --- |

Antidiabetic drugs:

- acetohexamide (**Dymelor**®)
- chlorpropamide (**Diabinese**®)
- glipizide (**Glucotrol**®)
- glyburide (**DiaBeta**®, **Micronase**®)
- insulin (**Humulin**®, **Lente**®, **Novolin**®, and others
- tolazamide (**Tolinase**®)
- tolbutamide (**Orinase**®), and others

Metoprolol (**Lopressor**®)

[for treatment of high blood pressure and angina]

Although the heart typically beats faster (tachycardia) when blood sugar levels are low, this symptom may be absent when metoprolol is given. This effect may occur when antidiabetic agents are combined with any antihypertensive drug in the beta-blocker class, which includes acebutolol (Sectral®), atenolol (Tenormin®), betaxolol (Kerlone®), carteolol (Cartrol®), esmolol (Brevibloc®), labetalol (Normodyne®, Trandate®), nadolol (Corgard®), pindolol (Visken®), propranolol (Inderal®), and timolol (Blocadren®).

Antidiabetic drugs:

- acetohexamide (**Dymelor**®)
- chlorpropamide (**Diabinese**®)
- glipizide (**Glucotrol**®)
- glyburide (**DiaBeta**®, **Micronase**®)
- insulin (**Humulin**®, **Lente**®, **Novolin**®, and others
- tolazamide (**Tolinase**®)
- tolbutamide (**Orinase**®), and others

Monoamine oxidase inhibitors:

- isocarboxazid (**Marplan**®)
- phenelzine (**Nardil**®)
- tranylcypromine (**Parnate**®), and others

[used to treat depression]

When monoamine oxidase (MAO) inhibitors are taken with antidiabetic medications, blood sugar levels may be reduced excessively. Symptoms of excessively low blood sugar levels include increased heart rate, cold sweats, trembling, nausea, hunger, mental confusion, and, in severe cases, coma.

**Recommendation:** Diabetic individuals should be especially careful in monitoring their blood sugar levels when taking MAO inhibitor drugs, and for three weeks after stopping them.

**Antidiabetic drugs:**

- acetohexamide **(Dymelor®)**
- chlorpropamide **(Diabinese®)**
- glipizide **(Glucotrol®)**
- glyburide **(DiaBeta®, Micronase®)**
- insulin **(Humulin®, Lente®, Novolin®,** and others
- tolazamide **(Tolinase®)**
- tolbutamide **(Orinase®),** and others

Nadolol **(Corgard®)**

[used to treat high blood pressure and angina]

Several results have been reported:

1. Secretion of insulin may be inhibited by nadolol, thereby leading to higher blood sugar levels than normal.

2. High blood pressure and markedly slowed heartbeat may result when blood sugar levels are low.

3. Reduced circulation to the hands and feet.

4. Although the heart typically beats faster (tachycardia) when blood sugar levels are low, this symptom may be absent when nadolol is given.

**Recommendation:** If possible, diabetics should avoid nonselective beta blockers (which act on the heart, lungs, and blood vessels) such as nadolol. If a beta blocker is necessary, cardioselective beta blockers—such as acebutolol (Sectral®), atenolol (Tenormin®), betaxolol (Kerlone®), or metoprolol (Lopressor®)—are usually recommended. These act primarily on the heart.

**Antidiabetic drugs:**

- acetohexamide **(Dymelor®)**
- chlorpropamide **(Diabinese®)**
- glipizide **(Glucotrol®)**
- glyburide. **(DiaBeta®, Micronase®)**
- tolazamide **(Tolinase®)**
- tolbutamide **(Orinase®),** and others

Phenylbutazone **(Azolid®, Butazolidin®)**

[for relief of pain and inflammation]

Phenylbutazone increases the plasma concentration of several antidiabetic drugs, which leads to an enhanced reduction of sugar levels in the blood (a condition known as hypoglycemia). Symptoms of an excessive drop in blood sugar levels include increased heart rate, cold sweats, trembling, nausea, hunger, mental confusion, and, in severe cases, coma.

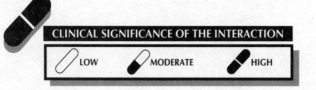

CLINICAL SIGNIFICANCE OF THE INTERACTION

LOW     MODERATE     HIGH

| Hormonal Drug | Interacting Drug | Result |
| --- | --- | --- |
| Antidiabetic drugs:<br><br>• acetohexamide **(Dymelor®)**<br>• chlorpropamide **(Diabinese®)**<br>• glipizide **(Glucotrol®)**<br>• glyburide **(DiaBeta®, Micronase®)**<br>• tolazamide **(Tolinase®)**<br>• tolbutamide **(Orinase®)**, and others<br><br> | Propranolol **(Inderal®)**<br><br>[for treatment of high blood pressure, angina pectoris, and irregular heartbeat; also used to prevent migrane headaches] | Several results have been reported:<br><br>1. Secretion of insulin may be inhibited by propranolol, thereby leading to higher blood sugar levels than normal.<br><br>2. High blood pressure and markedly slowed heartbeat may result when blood sugar levels are low.<br><br>3. Reduced circulation to the hands and feet.<br><br>4. Although the heart typically beats faster (tachycardia) when blood sugar levels are low, this symptom may be absent when propranolol is given.<br><br>**Recommendation:** If possible, diabetics should avoid nonselective beta blockers (which act on the heart, lungs, and blood vessels) such as propranolol. If a beta blocker is necessary, cardioselective beta blockers— such as acebutolol (Sectral®), atenolol (Tenormin®), betaxolol (Kerlone®), or metoprolol (Lopressor®)—are usually recommended. These act primarily on the heart. |
| Antidiabetic drugs:<br><br>• acetohexamide **(Dymelor®)**<br>• chlorpropamide **(Diabinese®)**<br>• glipizide **(Glucotrol®)**<br>• glyburide **(DiaBeta®, Micronase®)**<br>• tolazamide **(Tolinase®)**<br>• tolbutamide **(Orinase®)**, and others<br><br> | Sulfonamides:<br><br>• sulfamethizole **(Thiosulfil®)**<br>• sulfamethoxazole **(Gantanol®)**<br>• sulfisoxazole **(Gantrisin®)**<br>• trimethoprim-sulfamethoxazole **(Bactrim®, Septra®)**, and others<br><br>[used to treat urinary tract infections; has other uses as well] | Some sulfonamides enhance the effect of oral antidiabetic drugs, which may lead to excessively low levels of blood sugar. Symptoms of excessively low blood sugar levels include increased heart rate, cold sweats, trembling, nausea, hunger, mental confusion, and, in severe cases, coma.<br><br>**Recommendation:** Diabetics should be particularly careful when checking their blood sugar levels if a sulfonamide medication is started or stopped, or if its dosage is changed. |

| HORMONAL DRUG | INTERACTING DRUG | RESULT |
|---|---|---|

Antidiabetic drugs:

- acetohexamide **(Dymelor®)**
- chlorpropamide **(Diabinese®)**
- glipizide **(Glucotrol®)**
- glyburide **(DiaBeta®, Micronase®)**
- insulin **(Humulin®, Lente®, Novolin®,** and others
- tolazamide **(Tolinase®)**
- tolbutamide **(Orinase®),** and others

Thiazide and thiazide-like diuretics:

- chlorothiazide **(Diuril®)**
- chlorthalidone **(Hygroton®)**
- hydrochlorothiazide **(Esidrix®, HydroDIURIL®, Oretic®,** and others)
- metolazone **(Diulo®, Zaroxolyn®)**

[for treatment of high blood pressure and relief of excess fluid accumulation]

Thiazide diuretics may interfere with the effectiveness of antidiabetic drugs.

Thiazide diuretics taken with chlorpropamide (and possibly with other antidiabetic drugs) may lead to a deficiency in the amount of sodium in the blood, possibly leading to lethargy, confusion, irritability, headache, nausea, vomiting, and seizures.

Chlorpropamide **(Diabinese®)**

Chloramphenicol **(Chloromycetin®)**

[used to treat various bacterial infections, such as eye and ear infections, Rocky Mountain spotted fever, and typhoid fever]

Chloramphenicol enhances the effect of chlorpropamide, resulting in excessively low blood sugar levels. Symptoms of an excessive drop in blood sugar levels include increased heart rate, cold sweats, trembling, nausea, hunger, mental confusion, and, in severe cases, coma.

Your doctor may need to reduce the dose of chlorpropamide when you are taking chloramphenicol simultaneously.

**Recommendation:** Diabetics should be especially careful when checking their blood sugar levels if they are taking both chloramphenicol and chlorpropamide.

| HORMONAL DRUG | INTERACTING DRUG | RESULT |
|---|---|---|
| Chlorpropamide **(Diabinese®)**  | Dicumarol [for prevention and treatment of blood clots] | Dicumarol may enhance the effect of chlorpropamide, possibly leading to an excessively low amount of sugar in the blood. Symptoms of low blood sugar levels include increased heart rate, cold sweats, trembling, nausea, hunger, mental confusion, and, in severe cases, coma. |
| Coticosteroids:<br><br>• cortisone **(Cortone®)**<br>• hydrocortisone **(Cortef®, Hydrocortone®, Solu-Cortef®)**<br>• methylprednisolone **(Medrol®, Depo-Medrol®, Solu-Medrol®)**<br>• prednisolone **(Delta-Cortef®, Hydeltrasol®)**<br>• prednisone **(Deltasone®, Liquid Pred®, Meticorten®, Prednicen-M®)**, and others | Amphotericin B **(Fungizone®)** [for treatment of a particular type of fungal infection] | Decreased amount of potassium in the body, which may lead to muscle problems (such as weakness, twitching, and pain); nocturia (need to urinate at night); and abnormal sensations, such as feelings of numbness, tingling, or burning.<br><br>Corticosteroids can produce potassium depletion if they are given by injection or orally (especially with large doses), but other routes of administration (e.g., inhalation or topically on the skin or in the eye, ear, etc.) generally have little effect on potassium.<br><br>Cortisone and hydrocortisone are more likely than other corticosteroids to lead to these effects. |

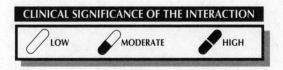

CLINICAL SIGNIFICANCE OF THE INTERACTION

LOW    MODERATE    HIGH

| HORMONAL DRUG | INTERACTING DRUG | RESULT |
|---|---|---|

Corticosteroids:

- betamethasone (**Celestone**®),
- cortisone (**Cortone**®)
- dexamethasone (**Decadron**®)
- hydrocortisone (**Cortef**®, **Hydrocortone**®, **Solu-Cortef**®)
- prednisolone (**Cortalone**® **Delta-Cortef**®)
- prednisone (**Deltasone**®, **Liquid Pred**®, **Prednicen-M**®), and others

Aspirin

[for relief of pain and inflammation]

Corticosteroids (especially when taken orally or by injection) may reduce the concentration of aspirin in the blood, leading to a decrease in the effectiveness of the aspirin.

This interaction may be important in persons taking large amounts of aspirin, such as arthritis sufferers.

Persons taking moderate to high doses of aspirin who are suddenly discontinued from corticosteroid therapy may experience aspirin toxicity; signs of aspirin toxicity include hearing loss, ringing in the ears, rapid breathing, rapid heart rate, nausea, vomiting, agitation, slurred speech, hallucinations, disorientation, and seizures.

Corticosteroids:

- betamethasone (**Celestone**®)
- cortisone (**Cortone**®)
- dexamethasone (**Decadron**®, **Dalalone**®)
- hydrocortisone (**Cortef**®, **Hydrocortone**®, **Solu-Cortef**®)
- methylprednisolone (**Medrol**®, **Depo-Medrol**®, **Solu-Medrol**®)

Barbiturates:

- amobarbital (**Amytal**®)
- butabarbital (**Butisol**®)
- butalbital
- pentobarbital (**Nembutal**®)
- phenobarbital (**Luminal**®, **Solfoton**®)
- primidone (**Mysoline**®)
- secobarbital (**Seconal**®), and others

[used to treat insomnia and anxiety; certain barbiturates are used to prevent seizures]

May cause a reduced amount of corticosteroid in the body, possibly leading to a decreased effect of the corticosteroid. This interaction has been shown to occur with the barbiturate phenobarbital (i.e., decreases the effect of dexamethasone). Other barbiturates and other corticosteroid medications are expected to act similarly.

| HORMONAL DRUG | INTERACTING DRUG | RESULT |
|---|---|---|

(cont.)

**Corticosteroids**

- paramethasone **(Haldrone®)**
- prednisolone **(Delta-Cortef®, Hydeltrasol®)**
- prednisone **(Deltasone®, Liquid-Pred®, Meticorten®)**
- triamcinolone **(Aristocort®, Kenacort®, Kenalog®)**

**Barbiturates**

This interaction is not likely to be a problem if the corticosteroid is inhaled or applied locally to the skin, eye, ear, etc.

**Recommendation:** Your doctor may need to adjust the dose of your corticosteroid if a barbiturate is started or stopped.

---

**Corticosteroids:**

- betamethasone **(Celestone®, Diprolene®, Diprosone®, Valisone)**
- cortisone **(Cortone®)**
- dexamethasone **(Decadron®, Hexadrol®)**
- hydrocortisone **(Cortef®, Hydrocortone®, Solu-Cortef®)**
- methylprednisolone **(Medrol®, Depo-Medrol®, Solu-Medrol®)**
- prednisolone **(Delta-Cortef®, Hydeltrasol®)**
- prednisone **(Deltasone®, Liquid Pred®, Meticorten®, Prednicen-M®)**, and others

Rifampin **(Rifadin®, Rifamate®, Rimactane®)**

[used in combination with at least one other drug, rifampin is used to treat tuberculosis; also used in the treatment of individuals who are carriers of meningitis]

Rifampin may substantially reduce the effectiveness of corticosteroids in some persons.

**Recommendation:** Watch for inadequate control of the condition being treated by the corticosteroid (e.g., asthma, arthritis, etc.). Your doctor may need to use higher than normal doses of corticosteroids during rifampin therapy. (Do *not* change the dosage of either drug yourself; only your doctor should do this.)

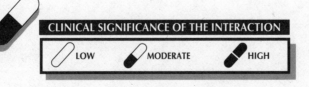

CLINICAL SIGNIFICANCE OF THE INTERACTION

LOW          MODERATE          HIGH

| HORMONAL DRUG | INTERACTING DRUG | RESULT |
|---|---|---|

Corticosteroids:

- cortisone **(Cortone®)**
- hydrocortisone **(Cortef®, Hydrocortone®, Solu-Cortef®)**
- methylpredniso-lone **(Medrol®, Depo-Medrol®, Solu-Medrol®)**
- prednisolone **(Delta-Cortef®, Hydeltrasol®)**
- prednisone **(Deltasone®, Liquid Pred®, Meticorten®, Prednicen-M®),** and others

Thiazide and thiazide-like diuretics:

- chlorothiazide **(Diuril®)**
- chlorthalidone **(Hygroton®)**
- hydrochlorothiazide **(Esidrix®, HydroDIURIL®, Oretic®, and others)**
- metolazone **(Diulo®, Zaroxolyn®)**

[for treatment of high blood pressure and relief of excess fluid accumulation]

Decreased amount of potassium in the body, which may lead to muscle problems (such as weakness, twitching, and pain); nocturia (need to urinate at night); and abnormal sensations, such as feelings of numbness, tingling, or burning.

Corticosteroids can produce potassium depletion if they are given by injection or orally (especially with large doses), but other routes of administration (e.g., inhalation or topical application on the skin or in the eye, ear, etc.) generally have little effect on potassium.

Cortisone and hydrocortisone are more likely than other corticosteroids to lead to these effects.

Dexamethasone **(Decadron®, Hexadrol®)**

Aminoglutethimide **(Cytadren®)**

[used to treat certain patients with Cushing's syndrome, a hormonal disorder]

Aminoglutethimide may greatly reduce one's response to dexamethasone. Someone receiving aminoglutethimide may require an increase in the dosage of dexamethasone to achieve an appropriate response to this medication. (Do *not* change the dosage of either drug yourself; only your doctor should do this.)

Corticosteroids other than dexamethasone may be similarly affected.

| HORMONAL DRUG | INTERACTING DRUG | RESULT |
|---|---|---|

Estrogen

Hydrocortisone **(Cortef®, Hydrocortone®, Solu-Cortef®)**

[for relieving inflammation, particularly of the skin]

Estrogen may increase the amount of hydrocortisone in the blood; thus, a reduction in the dosage of hydrocortisone may be necessary in persons receiving estrogen.

**Recommendation:** When receiving estrogen and hydrocortisone, be alert for signs of excessively high blood levels of hydrocortisone, which could lead to increased blood pressure, increased blood sugar, bone problems (such as osteoporosis, a condition marked by weakened, less dense bones), muscle weakness, insomnia, stomach ulcers, and infections (symptoms of which may include sore throat or fever).

Estrogen

Prednisolone **(Hydeltrasol®, Pediapred®, Prelone®)**

[for treatment of various conditions, including rheumatoid arthritis, skin disorders, bronchial asthma, certain hormone insufficiencies, and other conditions]

Estrogen may increase the amount of prednisolone levels in the blood; thus, a reduction in the dosage of prednisolone may be necessary in persons receiving estrogen.

**Recommendation:** When receiving estrogen and prednisolone, be alert for signs of excessively high blood levels of prednisolone, which could lead to increased blood pressure, increased blood sugar, bone problems (such as osteoporosis, a condition marked by weakened, less dense bones), muscle weakness, insomnia, stomach ulcers, and infections (symptoms of which may include sore throat or fever).

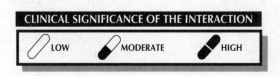

CLINICAL SIGNIFICANCE OF THE INTERACTION

LOW    MODERATE    HIGH

Estrogen-containing oral contraceptives

Alprazolam (**Xanax**®)

[for treatment of anxiety]

Oral contraceptives may increase the concentration of alprazolam in the body, possibly leading to decreased alertness, an impaired ability to concentrate, dizziness, incoordination, forgetfulness, and drowsiness.

**Recommendation:** It may be necessary for your doctor to adjust the dose of alprazolam if oral contraceptives are started or stopped.

---

Estrogen-containing oral contraceptives

Aminopenicillins:

- Ampicillin (**Omnipen**®, **Unasyn**®, and others)
- Amoxicillin (**Amoxil**®, **Larotid**®, and others)
- Bacampicillin (**Spectrobid**®)
- Cyclacillin (**Cyclapen-W**®)

[for treatment of bacterial infections]

Although aminopenicillins may increase the risk of pregnancy in women taking oral contraceptives, this result is probably rare. Menstrual irregularities, such as spotting or breakthrough bleeding, may be a sign that this interaction is occurring. Other types of penicillins and other oral antibiotics in general may produce similar effects.

**Recommendation:** Women wishing to avoid pregnancy would be prudent to institute another form of contraception—in addition to use of their oral contraceptive—while taking aminopenicillins.

---

Estrogen-containing oral contraceptives

Antibiotics (oral)

[for treatment of bacterial infections]

Antibiotics may increase the risk of pregnancy in women taking oral contraceptives. Although most of the cases of unintended pregnancy have occurred with aminopenicillins (see above) or tetracyclines (see p.310), this drug interaction may also occur with other antibiotics.

**Recommendation:** Women wishing to avoid pregnancy would be prudent to institute another form of contraception—in addition to use of their oral contraceptive—while taking antibiotics.

| HORMONAL DRUG | INTERACTING DRUG | RESULT |
|---|---|---|

Estrogen-containing oral contraceptives

Barbiturates:

- amobarbital (**Amytal**®)
- butabarbital (**Butisol**®)
- butalbital
- pentobarbital (**Nembutal**®)
- phenobarbital (**Luminal**®, **Solfoton**®)
- primidone (**Mysoline**®)
- secobarbital (**Seconal**®), and others

[used to treat insomnia and anxiety; certain barbiturates are used to prevent seizures]

Barbiturates may reduce the effectiveness of estrogen-containing oral contraceptives, possibly leading to unintended pregnancy.

Spotting and breakthrough bleeding may be an indication that the oral contraceptive is working at a reduced capacity, although the absence of such menstrual irregularities does not ensure that the oral contraceptive is working.

**Recommendation:** Women taking a barbiturate who wish to avoid becoming pregnant should check with their doctor. Another method of contraception instead of or in addition to an oral contraceptive may be necessary. Or, your doctor may need to adjust the dose of the oral contraceptive in order to overcome the effect of the barbiturate. Of course, only your doctor can make such a dosage adjustment. Similarly, if you are taking an oral contraceptive and a barbiturate is prescribed for you for short-term use, it would be prudent to use alternative methods of contraception in addition to the oral contraceptive during, and for several weeks after, barbiturate use.

Estrogen-containing oral contraceptives

Caffeine (typical sources include caffeinated coffee, tea, and certain carbonated beverages)

Women taking oral contraceptives who also ingest caffeine may experience an enhanced effect of caffeine, symptoms of which include nervousness, anxiety, insomnia, and restlessness.

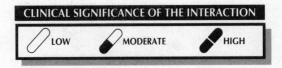

CLINICAL SIGNIFICANCE OF THE INTERACTION

LOW    MODERATE    HIGH

303

| HORMONAL DRUG | INTERACTING DRUG | RESULT |
|---|---|---|

Estrogen-containing oral contraceptives

Carbamazepine **(Tegretol®)**

[for epilepsy, trigeminal neuralgia (spasms of pain in the face), and other disorders]

Carbamazepine may decrease the effectiveness of an estrogen-containing oral contraceptive. The result could be menstrual irregularities and unintended pregnancies (several cases of unintended pregnancies have occurred in epileptic women who were taking oral contraceptives properly).

**Recommendation:** Women taking carbamazepine who wish to avoid becoming pregnant should check with their doctor. Another method of contraception instead of or in addition to an oral contraceptive may be necessary. Or, your doctor may need to adjust the dose of the oral contraceptive in order to overcome the effect of the antiseizure drug. Of course, only your doctor should make such a dosage adjustment.

---

Estrogen-containing oral contraceptives

Chlordiazepoxide **(Librium®)**

[for treatment of anxiety]

Oral contraceptives may increase the concentration of chlordiazepoxide in the body, possibly leading to symptoms such as decreased alertness, an impaired ability to concentrate, dizziness, incoordination, forgetfulness, and drowsiness.

**Recommendation:** It may be necessary for your doctor to adjust the dose of chlordiazepoxide if oral contraceptives are started or stopped.

---

Estrogen-containing oral contraceptives

Clofibrate **(Atromid-S®)**

[for lowering cholesterol and triglyceride levels in the blood]

Oral contraceptives may decrease the effectiveness of clofibrate, resulting in high cholesterol levels.

**Recommendation:** Persons receiving both clofibrate and an oral contraceptive should have their cholesterol levels checked regularly.

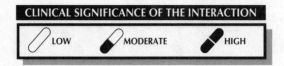

CLINICAL SIGNIFICANCE OF THE INTERACTION

LOW   MODERATE   HIGH

| HORMONAL DRUG | INTERACTING DRUG | RESULT |
|---|---|---|

Estrogen-containing oral contraceptives

Corticosteroids:

- betamethasone (**Celestone**®)
- cortisone (**Cortone**®)
- dexamethasone (**Decadron**®, **Dalalone**®)
- hydrocortisone (**Cortef**®, **Hydrocortone**®, **Solu-Cortef**®)
- methylprednisolone (**Medrol**®, **Depo-Medrol**®, **Solu-Medrol**®)
- paramethasone (**Haldrone**®)
- prednisolone (**Delta-Cortef**®, **Hydeltrasol**®, **Pediapred**®, **Prelone**®)
- prednisone (**Deltasone**®, **Liquid-Pred**®, **Meticorten**®)
- triamcinolone (**Aristocort**®, **Kenacort**®, **Kenalog**®)

[for relieving inflammation and suppressing allergic reactions]

Oral contraceptives—as well as estrogens—may increase the effect of the corticosteroid and may increase the risk of corticosteroid toxicity. Corticosteroid toxicity can result in increased blood pressure, increased blood sugar, thinning of bone (osteoporosis), muscle weakness, insomnia, stomach ulcers, and infections.

Although this interaction has been shown to occur with hydrocortisone and prednisolone, it is likely that other corticosteroids will react in a similar manner.

This interaction is not likely to be a problem if the corticosteroid is inhaled or applied locally to the skin, eye, ear, etc.

**Recommendation:** Your doctor may need to adjust the dose of your corticosteroid if an oral contraceptive is started or stopped.

Estrogen-containing oral contraceptives

Cyclosporine (**Sandimmune**®)

[for prevention of organ rejection after kidney, liver, or heart transplantation]

Could lead to increased plasma levels of cyclosporine.

**Recommendation:** Persons who are receiving both of these drugs should be monitored particularly carefully by their physician. In individuals stabilized on cyclosporine and an oral contraceptive, discontinuation of the oral contraceptive could lead to a decrease in cyclosporine plasma levels, which could possibly lead to rejection of the organ that was transplanted.

| HORMONAL DRUG | INTERACTING DRUG | RESULT |
|---|---|---|

Estrogen-containing oral contraceptives

Diazepam **(Valium®)**

[for treatment of anxiety]

Oral contraceptives may increase the concentration of diazepam in the body, possibly leading to decreased alertness, an impaired ability to concentrate, dizziness, incoordination, forgetfulness, and drowsiness.

**Recommendation:** It may be necessary for your doctor to adjust the dose of diazepam if oral contraceptives are started or stopped. (Of course, only your doctor should make such a dosage adjustment.)

Estrogen-containing oral contraceptives

Griseofulvin **(Fulvicin® P/G, Grisactin®,** and **Gris-PEG®)**

[for treatment of various fungal infections, such as athlete's foot, ringworm of the scalp, and other fungal infections]

Some evidence suggests that griseofulvin may decrease the effectiveness of the oral contraceptive, resulting in unintended pregnancy or menstrual irregularities (such as spotting, breakthrough bleeding, or absence or abnormal stopping of the menses).

**Recommendation:** Women taking griseofulvin who wish to avoid becoming pregnant should check with their doctor. Another method of contraception instead of or in addition to an oral contraceptive may be necessary. Or, your doctor may need to adjust the dose of the oral contraceptive in order to overcome the effect of the griseofulvin. Of course, only your doctor should make such a dosage adjustment.

Estrogen-containing oral contraceptives

Guanethidine **(Ismelin®)**

[for treatment of high blood pressure]

May increase blood pressure due to reduced antihypertensive effect.

**Recommendation:** Your doctor may want to check your blood pressure if you start taking oral contraceptives and guanethidine concurrently. Some women with hypertension may need to avoid oral contraceptives.

Estrogen-containing oral contraceptives

Lorazepam (**Ativan**®)

[for treatment of anxiety]

Oral contraceptives may decrease the concentration of lorazepam in the body, possibly leading to a decreased effect (i.e., inadequate control of anxiety).

**Recommendation:** It may be necessary for your doctor to adjust the dose of lorazepam if oral contraceptives are started or stopped.

Estrogen-containing oral contraceptives

Metoprolol (**Lopressor**®)

[for treatment of high blood pressure]

Oral contraceptives may increase the concentration of metoprolol in the blood. While it is not known whether this will result in an increased antihypertensive effect, you should have your blood pressure checked regularly to ensure that it is not too low. (This is an unusual interaction because many antihypertensive drugs may interact with oral contraceptives in a way that results in an *increase* in blood pressure levels. When metoprolol was combined with an oral contraceptive, however, the opposite effect—reduced blood pressure—was observed.)

Metoprolol is part of a family of drugs known as beta blockers. It is not known whether oral contraceptives produce a similar interaction with other beta-blocker drugs—such as propranolol (Inderal®)—but such an interaction is likely.

**Recommendation:** Your doctor may want to monitor your blood pressure for any changes if an oral contraceptive is started or stopped in the presence of metoprolol therapy.

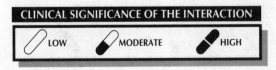

CLINICAL SIGNIFICANCE OF THE INTERACTION

LOW    MODERATE    HIGH

Estrogen-containing oral contraceptives

Oxazepam (**Serax®**)

[for treatment of anxiety]

Oral contraceptives may decrease the concentration of oxazepam in the body, possibly leading to a decreased effect (i.e., inadequate control of anxiety).

**Recommendation:** It may be necessary for your doctor to adjust the dose of oxazepam if oral contraceptives are started or stopped.

---

Estrogen-containing oral contraceptives

Phenytoin (**Dilantin®**)

[for prevention of seizures]

Phenytoin may decrease the effectiveness of an estrogen-containing oral contraceptive. The result could be menstrual irregularities and unintended pregnancies (several cases of unintended pregnancies have occurred in epileptic women who were taking oral contraceptives properly).

**Recommendation:** Women taking phenytoin who wish to avoid becoming pregnant should check with their doctor. Another method of contraception instead of or in addition to an oral contraceptive may be necessary. Or, your doctor may need to adjust the dose of the oral contraceptive in order to overcome the effect of the antiseizure drug. Of course, only your doctor should make such a dosage adjustment.

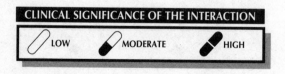

CLINICAL SIGNIFICANCE OF THE INTERACTION

LOW    MODERATE    HIGH

| HORMONAL DRUG | INTERACTING DRUG | RESULT |
|---|---|---|

Estrogen-containing oral contraceptives

Primidone (**Mysoline**®)

[for treatment of various types of epileptic seizures]

Primidone may reduce the effectiveness of estrogen-containing oral contraceptives, possibly leading to unintended pregnancy.

Spotting and breakthrough bleeding may be an indication that the oral contraceptive is working at a reduced capacity, although the absence of such menstrual irregularities does not ensure that the oral contraceptive is working.

**Recommendation:** Women taking primidone who wish to avoid becoming pregnant should check with their doctor. Another method of contraception instead of or in addition to an oral contraceptive may be necessary. Or, your doctor may need to adjust the dose of the oral contraceptive in order to overcome the effect of primidone. Of course, only your doctor should make such a dosage adjustment.

Estrogen-containing oral contraceptives

Rifampin (**Rifadin**®, **Rifamate**®, **Rimactane**®)

[used in combination with at least one other drug, rifampin is used to treat tuberculosis; also used in the treatment of individuals who are carriers of meningitis]

Rifampin significantly increases the likelihood of becoming pregnant while taking an oral contraceptive. Menstrual irregularities—such as spotting, breakthrough bleeding, or absence or abnormal stopping of the menses—may occur while taking these two medications concomitantly.

**Recommendation:** You could use contraceptive methods other than oral contraceptives to avoid this interaction. If the combination is used, your doctor may need to increase the strength of your oral contraceptive. You may also wish to use an additional form of contraception while taking—and for one cycle after finishing—rifampin.

| HORMONAL DRUG | INTERACTING DRUG | RESULT |
|---|---|---|

Estrogen-containing oral contraceptives

Cigarette smoking

Considerable evidence indicates that women who smoke and receive estrogen-containing oral contraceptives are at a significantly greater risk of developing a stroke, heart attack, or blood clots. This risk increases in women over age thirty-five, particularly those who are heavy smokers.

---

Estrogen-containing oral contraceptives

Temazepam (**Restoril**®)

[used in the treatment of insomnia, or difficulty falling or staying asleep]

Oral contraceptives may decrease the concentration of temazepam in the blood, possibly leading to a diminished effect of temazepam.

**Recommendation:** It may be necessary for your doctor to adjust the dose of temazepam if oral contraceptives are started or stopped.

---

Estrogen-containing oral contraceptives

Tetracyclines:

- demeclocycline (**Declomycin**®)
- doxycycline (**Doryx**®, **Vibramycin**®, **Vibra-Tabs**®)
- methacycline (**Rondomycin**®)
- minocycline (**Minocin**®)
- oxytetracycline (**Terramycin**®)
- tetracycline (**Achromycin**®, **Sumycin**®)

[a class of antibiotics used to treat various bacterial infections, such as bronchitis, Lyme disease, gonorrhea, and many others]

Tetracyclines may reduce the effectiveness of oral contraceptives, resulting in unintended pregnancy (probably rare) and menstrual irregularities (such as spotting, breakthrough bleeding, or absence or abnormal stopping of the menses).

**Recommendation:** While taking tetracyclines, additional forms of contraception are advised for women who are taking an oral contraceptive to prevent pregnancy.

**Note:** No oral antibiotic has been proven *not* to affect oral contraceptives, so precautions are warranted even if a different antibiotic is used.

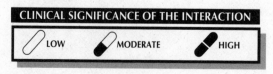

**CLINICAL SIGNIFICANCE OF THE INTERACTION**

LOW   MODERATE   HIGH

Estrogen-containing oral contraceptives

Triazolam **(Halcion®)**

[for induction of sleep]

Oral contraceptives may increase the concentration of triazolam in the body, possibly leading to decreased alertness, an impaired ability to concentrate, forgetfulness, and drowsiness.

**Recommendation:** It may be necessary for your doctor to adjust the dose of triazolam if oral contraceptives are started or stopped.

Glipizide **(Glucotrol®)**

Cimetidine **(Tagamet®)**

[for relief of stomach and intestinal ulcers]

Cimetidine may increase the blood level of glipizide, which may cause an excessively low blood sugar level (an excessive drop in blood sugar levels is undesirable). This may produce symptoms including cold sweats, trembling, and an increased heart rate.

This interaction may be caused by reducing the amount of acid in the stomach, so the same problem may be seen with other antiulcer drugs that decrease stomach acid, such as famotidine (Pepcid®), nizatidine (Axid®), ranitidine (Zantac®), omeprazole (Prilosec®), and antacids.

**Recommendation:** Diabetics taking glipizide should watch for any change in their sugar levels when cimetidine is started or discontinued. Sucralfate (Carafate®) may be a good alternative for diabetics with ulcers because preliminary reports suggest that this medication appears less likely to significantly change blood sugar levels. (Glipizide and sucralfate should be taken at different times to reduce the possibility of sucralfate binding with glipizide in the stomach. Separate doses of these two medications by several hours if possible.)

| HORMONAL DRUG | INTERACTING DRUG | RESULT |
|---|---|---|

Glipizide
(**Glucotrol**®)

Ranitidine (**Zantac**®)

[for relief of stomach and intestinal ulcers]

Ranitidine has been reported to increase the amount of glipizide in the blood, which enhances the effect of lowering the amount of sugar in the blood. (Symptoms of an excessive drop in blood sugar levels include cold sweats, trembling, and an increased heart rate.)

When ranitidine is started or discontinued, diabetics taking glipizide should watch for any change in their sugar levels.

This interaction may be caused by reducing the amount of acid in the stomach, so the same problem may be seen with other antiulcer drugs that decrease stomach acid, such as cimetidine (Tagamet®), famotidine (Pepcid®), nizatidine (Axid®), omeprazole (Prilosec®), and antacids.

**Recommendation:** Diabetics should carefully check their sugar levels after beginning or ending therapy with ranitidine. Sucralfate (Carafate®) may be a good alternative for diabetics with ulcers because preliminary reports suggest that this medication is less likely to significantly change blood sugar levels. (Glipizide and sucralfate should be taken at different times to reduce the possibility of sucralfate binding with glipizide in the stomach. Separate doses of these two medications by several hours if possible.)

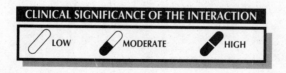

CLINICAL SIGNIFICANCE OF THE INTERACTION

LOW          MODERATE          HIGH

| HORMONAL DRUG | INTERACTING DRUG | RESULT |
|---|---|---|

Glyburide (**DiaBeta®, Micronase®**)

Cimetidine (**Tagamet®**)

[for relief of stomach and intestinal ulcers]

Cimetidine may increase the blood level of glyburide, which may cause an excessively low blood sugar level (an excessive drop in blood sugar levels is undesirable). This may produce symptoms including cold sweats, trembling, and an increased heart rate.

This interaction may be caused by reducing the amount of acid in the stomach, so the same problem may be seen with other antiulcer drugs that decrease stomach acid, such as famotidine (Pepcid®), nizatidine (Axid®), ranitidine (Zantac®), omeprazole (Prilosec®), and antacids.

**Recommendation:** Diabetics taking glyburide should watch for any change in their sugar levels when cimetidine is started or discontinued. Sucralfate (Carafate®) may be a good alternative for diabetics with ulcers because preliminary reports suggest that this medication appears less likely to significantly change blood sugar levels. (Glyburide and sucralfate should be taken at different times to reduce the possibility of sucralfate binding with glyburide in the stomach. Separate doses of these two medications by several hours if possible.)

Insulin (**Humulin®, Lente®, Novolin®,** and others)

Cigarette smoking

Cigarette smoking may make a diabetic less responsive to insulin. As a result, many insulin-dependent diabetics who smoke heavily need more insulin than nonsmokers.

313

| HORMONAL DRUG | INTERACTING DRUG | RESULT |
|---|---|---|

Insulin **(Humulin®, Lente®, Novolin®,** and others)

Clonidine **(Catapres®)**

[for treatment of high blood pressure]

Clonidine may mask symptoms of low blood sugar. Symptoms of low blood sugar levels include increased heart rate, cold sweats, trembling, nausea, hunger, mental confusion, and, in severe cases, coma.

Insulin **(Humulin®, Lente®, Novolin®,** and others)

Oxytetracycline **(Terramycin®)**

[for treatment of several different types of bacterial infections]

Oxytetracycline may enhance the effect of insulin, possibly leading to an excessively low amount of sugar in the blood. Symptoms of low blood sugar levels include increased heart rate, cold sweats, trembling, nausea, hunger, mental confusion, and, in severe cases, coma.

Methylprednisolone **(Medrol®)**

Ketoconazole **(Nizoral®)**

[used to treat various fungal infections]

Ketoconazole may increase the amount of methylprednisolone in the blood, possibly leading to methylprednisolone toxicity. Symptoms of methylprednisolone toxicity include increased blood pressure, increased blood sugar, thinning of the bones (osteoporosis), muscle weakness, insomnia, stomach ulcers, and infection.

The effect of ketoconazole on other corticosteroids is not well established, but prednisolone may not be affected.

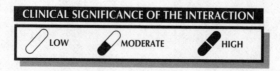

CLINICAL SIGNIFICANCE OF THE INTERACTION

LOW     MODERATE     HIGH

314

| HORMONAL DRUG | INTERACTING DRUG | RESULT |
|---|---|---|

Methylprednisolone **(Medrol®)**

Troleandomycin **(TAO®)**

[for treatment of upper and lower respiratory tract infections]

Troleandomycin significantly enhances the effect of methylprednisolone, possibly leading to methylprednisolone toxicity. Symptoms of methylprednisolone toxicity include increased blood pressure, increased blood sugar, thinning of the bones (osteoporosis), muscle weakness, insomnia, stomach ulcers, and infection (symptoms of infection include sore throat and fever).

Prednisolone **(Delta-Cortef®, Hydeltrasol®)**

Carbamazepine **(Tegretol®)**

[for epilepsy, trigeminal neuralgia (spasms of pain in the face), and other disorders]

Carbamazepine reduces the amount of prednisolone in the body, leading to a decreased effect of this corticosteroid.

This effect has been shown to occur with another corticosteroid (i.e., dexamethasone) and probably occurs with other corticosteroid drugs as well.

Thyroid replacement hormone:

- **Armour® Thyroid Tablets**
- levothyroxine (**Levothroid®, Synthroid®**)
- liothyronine (**Cytomel®**)
- liotrix (**Euthroid®, Thyrolar®**)

Cholestyramine **(Questran®)**

[for reduction of elevated cholesterol levels; also used to relieve severe itching associated with partial biliary obstruction]

Cholestyramine may reduce the amount of thyroxine hormone in the body.

**Recommendation:** Persons receiving thyroid replacement hormone should not take their hormone therapy with cholestyramine. At least four hours should elapse between taking these two drugs.

Tolbutamide
(**Orinase**®)

Chloramphenicol
(**Chloromycetin**®)

[used to treat various bacterial infections, such as eye and ear infections, Rocky Mountain spotted fever, and typhoid fever]

Chloramphenicol enhances the effect of tolbutamide, possibly resulting in excessively low blood sugar levels. Symptoms of low blood sugar levels include increased heart rate, cold sweats, trembling, nausea, hunger, mental confusion, and, in severe cases, coma.

Your doctor may need to reduce the dose of tolbutamide when you are taking chloramphenicol simultaneously.

**Recommendation:** Diabetics should be especially careful when checking their blood sugar levels if they are taking both chloramphenicol and tolbutamide.

Tolbutamide
(**Orinase**®)

Cimetidine (**Tagamet**®)

[for relief of stomach and intestinal ulcers]

Cimetidine can increase the serum concentration of tolbutamide. It is not known whether this enhances the blood sugar–lowering effect of tolbutamide.

**Recommendation:** Diabetics taking tolbutamide should watch for any change in their sugar levels when cimetidine is started or discontinued. Sucralfate (Carafate®) may be a good alternative for diabetics with ulcers because preliminary reports indicate that this medication appears less likely to significantly change blood sugar levels.

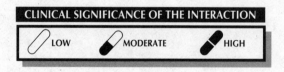

CLINICAL SIGNIFICANCE OF THE INTERACTION

LOW    MODERATE    HIGH

| HORMONAL DRUG | INTERACTING DRUG | RESULT |
|---|---|---|

Tolbutamide
**(Orinase®)**

Dicumarol

[for prevention and treatment of blood clots]

Dicumarol enhances the effect of tolbutamide, possibly leading to an excessively low amount of sugar in the blood. Symptoms of low blood sugar levels include increased heart rate, cold sweats, trembling, nausea, hunger, mental confusion, and, in severe cases, coma.

---

Tolbutamide
**(Orinase®)**

Oxytetracycline
**(Terramycin®)**

[for treatment of several different types of bacterial infections]

Oxytetracycline may enhance the effect of tolbutamide, possibly leading to an excessively low amount of sugar in the blood. Symptoms of low blood sugar levels include increased heart rate, cold sweats, trembling, nausea, hunger, mental confusion, and, in severe cases, coma.

---

Tolbutamide
**(Orinase®)**

Rifampin **(Rifadin®, Rifamate®, Rimactane®)**

[used in combination with at least one other drug, rifampin is used to treat tuberculosis; also used in the treatment of individuals who are carriers of meningitis]

Rifampin reduces the amount of tolbutamide in the body and may reduce the sugar-lowering effect of tolbutamide. The result may be an unexpected increase in the amount of sugar in the blood.

**Recommendation:** It may be necessary for your doctor to adjust the dose of tolbutamide if rifampin is started or stopped, or if its dosage is changed. (Of course, only your doctor should change medication dosages, when appropriate.)

Tolbutamide
**(Orinase®)**

Sulfinpyrazone
**(Anturane®)**

[used to treat gouty arthritis]

Sulfinpyrazone may enhance the effect of tolbutamide, possibly leading to excessively low amounts of sugar in the blood. Symptoms of an excessive drop in blood sugar levels include increased heart rate, cold sweats, trembling, nausea, hunger, mental confusion, and, in severe cases, coma.

**Recommendation:** It may be necessary for your doctor to adjust the dose of tolbutamide if sulfinpyrazone is started or stopped, or if its dosage is changed. (Of course, only your doctor should change medication dosages, when appropriate.)

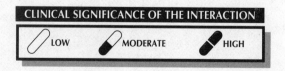

CLINICAL SIGNIFICANCE OF THE INTERACTION

LOW     MODERATE     HIGH

CHAPTER 9

# ANTIDEPRESSANT DRUGS

All of us become depressed during certain periods of our lives. Occasional bouts of sadness that result from losing a job or arguing with a spouse are normal. A period of grief is also to be expected after the loss of a relative or close friend. *Major* depression, however, is another matter. Individuals who suffer from major depression experience a debilitating condition that prevents them from having an interest in or getting pleasure from their daily activities. In short, major depression interferes with a person's normal functioning.

Symptoms of major depression include sleep disturbances such as insomnia (difficulty falling or staying asleep) or excessive sleep. The depressed individual may feel nervous and agitated. Weight loss or gain is common. Depressed people often experience several physical symptoms, such as headache, visual disturbances, and fatigue. Psychological components of depression include feelings of worthlessness, lack of motivation, inappropriate feelings of guilt, and social withdrawal. In extreme cases, the depressed person seriously contemplates suicide. Some people with major depression may have one long episode, lasting months, or even years; others may experience several "attacks" of major depression during their lifetime.

## Medications Used to Treat Depression

The drugs most commonly used to treat depression are a class of antidepressants known as tricyclics—named after their three-ringed chemical structure. Several tricyclic drugs are available, such as amitriptyline (Elavil®, Endep®), amoxapine (Asendin®), desipramine (Pertofrane®, Norpramin®), doxepin (Adapin®, Sinequan®), imipramine (Janimine®, Tofranil®), nortriptyline (Aventyl®, Pamelor®), protriptyline (Vivactil®), trimipramine (Surmontil®), and others. Maprotiline (Ludiomil®) is an antidepressant medication related to the tricyclics.

If you require a tricyclic antidepressant, your doctor will choose one, in part, based on your symptoms. For example, certain tricyclics (such as amitriptyline or doxepin) have a sedative effect, which usually provides prompt relief to persons who have difficulty sleeping. Other tricyclics (such as desipramine or protriptyline) are less sedating; these antidepressants are often prescribed for individuals who feel sluggish and apathetic.

Tricyclic antidepressants often must be taken for several weeks before the depressed person feels much better. More than one quarter of the patients in controlled trials of several antidepressant drugs feel better only after four weeks of treatment.[1,2] Certain symptoms, such as insomnia, may improve much earlier than others.

Tricyclic antidepressants vary in the degree to which they induce side effects known as *anticholinergic* effects; these side effects include dry mouth, constipation, blurred vision, rapid heartbeat, and difficulty urinating. In addition, light-headedness, dizziness, or fainting may also occur. In high doses, tricyclic antidepressants may disturb the heart's normal rhythm; as a result, physicians must closely monitor patients with heart problems, especially the elderly, who take these drugs.

Another "family" of antidepressant medication is the monoamine oxidase inhibitor, or MAO inhibitors for short. These drugs are usually prescribed for depressed persons who do not respond to tricyclic antidepressants or for whom the tricyclics cannot be given. The MAO inhibitors used to treat depression include isocarboxazid (Marplan®), phenelzine (Nardil®), and tranylcypromine (Parnate®). A newer MAO inhibitor, moclobemide, is a more selective inhibitor of monoamine oxidase and is less likely to interact with certain foods, but it may have some of the same interactions with drugs as do the older MAO inhibitors. Other antidepressants—not tricyclics nor monoamine oxidase inhibitors—include bupropion (Wellbutrin®), fluoxetine (Prozac®), sertraline (Zoloft®), and trazodone (Desyrel®).

# How Do Antidepressant Medications Work?

Antidepressant drugs work by affecting the amount of certain chemicals—called amines—in the brain. Although the causes of major depression are complex and multiple, many experts have reported that a substantial part of the problem is not enough amines in the right places in the brain. Antidepressant medications are thought to increase the amount of these amines, either by keeping the amines at their sites of action longer (tricyclic antidepressants) or by blocking the enzymes that break down the amines (MAO inhibitors).

# Manic-Depression Disorder

A disorder related to depression is a condition known as *manic-depression disorder* (also called bipolar-mood disorder). Individuals who suffer from this disorder experience bouts of depression at certain times and episodes of another mood change—known as mania—at other times. Mania is characterized by feelings of elation, increased energy levels, excessive and rapid talking, and disconnected and racing thoughts. Lithium is a drug used to control this disorder. Most persons who suffer from manic-depression experience recurrent episodes of both phases of this disorder. Lithium tends to stabilize mood so that these extremes are avoided. Although lithium is the preferred medication for treating mania alone, it is occasionally used to treat the depression phase of manic-depression disorder.

| ANTIDEPRESSANT DRUG | INTERACTING DRUG | RESULT |
|---|---|---|

Amitriptyline (**Elavil**®, **Endep**®)

Alcohol

May result in a greater than expected impairment of psychomotor skills—such as those necessary to drive a car or operate machinery—especially during the first week of treatment.

When combining alcohol with other tricyclic antidepressants, the same result may occur. Other tricyclic antidepressants include amoxapine (Asendin®), desipramine (Pertofrane®, Norpramin®), doxepin (Adapin®, Sinequan®), imipramine (Janimine®, Tofranil®), nortriptyline (Aventyl®, Pamelor®), protriptyline (Vivactil®), and trimipramine (Surmontil®).

**Recommendation:** Limit or avoid alcohol intake if you are taking tricyclic antidepressants. Discuss this interaction with your doctor.

Amitriptyline (**Elavil**®, **Endep**®)

Cimetidine (**Tagamet**®)

[for stomach and intestinal ulcers]

Can result in an increased blood concentration of amitriptyline, possibly to a toxic level. Symptoms of amitriptyline toxicity include severe dry mouth, blurred vision, fast heartbeat, difficulty or inability to urinate, and constipation.

Other tricyclic antidepressants may be similarly affected by cimetidine. They include amoxapine (Asendin®), desipramine (Pertofrane®, Norpramin®), doxepin (Adapin®, Sinequan®), imipramine (Janimine®, Tofranil®), nortriptyline (Aventyl®, Pamelor®), protriptyline (Vivactil®), and trimipramine (Surmontil®).

**Recommendation:** It may be necessary for your doctor to adjust the dose of amitriptyline if cimetidine is started or stopped, or if its dosage is changed. (Of course, only your doctor should change medication dosages, when appropriate).

Your doctor may choose to use ranitidine (Zantac®), famotidine (Pepcid®), or nizatidine (Axid®) instead of cimetidine, because they are less likely to interact.

Amitriptyline
(**Elavil®, Endep®**)

Clonidine (**Catapres®**)

[for treatment of high blood pressure]

Reduced antihypertensive effect has been reported in persons taking amitriptyline and clonidine. Other tricyclic antidepressants—amoxapine (Asendin®), doxepin (Adapin®, Sinequan®), nortriptyline (Aventyl®, Pamelor®), protriptyline (Vivactil®), and trimipramine (Surmontil®)—probably interact with clonidine in the same way, but little data are available.

Tricyclic antidepressants may also increase the risk of hypertensive reaction—symptoms of which include elevated blood pressure levels, flushing of the face, pounding of the heart, and lightheadedness—if clonidine is discontinued too rapidly.

**Recommendation:** It is best to avoid this combination; discuss it with your doctor.

Desipramine
(**Pertofrane®, Norpramin®**)

Cimetidine (**Tagamet®**)

[for stomach and intestinal ulcers]

Can result in an increased blood concentration of desipramine, possibly to a toxic level. Symptoms of desipramine toxicity include severe dry mouth, blurred vision, fast heartbeat, difficulty or inability to urinate, and constipation.

Other tricyclic antidepressants may be similarly affected by cimetidine. They include amitriptyline (Elavil®, Endep®), amoxapine (Asendin®), doxepin (Adapin®, Sinequan®), imipramine (Janimine®, Tofranil®), nortriptyline (Aventyl®, Pamelor®), protriptyline (Vivactil®), and trimipramine (Surmontil®).

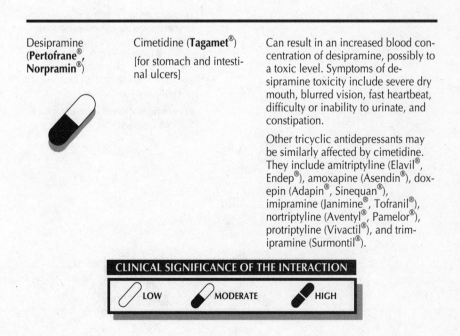

CLINICAL SIGNIFICANCE OF THE INTERACTION

LOW    MODERATE    HIGH

| ANTIDEPRESSANT DRUG | INTERACTING DRUG | RESULT |
|---|---|---|

*(cont.)*

**Desipramine** — **Cimetidine**

**Recommendation:** It may be necessary for your doctor to adjust the dose of desipramine if cimetidine is started or stopped, or if its dosage is changed. (Of course, only your doctor should change medication dosages, when appropriate.)

Your doctor may choose to use ranitidine (Zantac®), famotidine (Pepcid®), or nizatidine (Axid®) instead of cimetidine, because they are less likely to interact.

---

Desipramine
(**Pertofrane®, Norpramin®**)

Clonidine (**Catapres®**)

[for treatment of high blood pressure]

Reduced antihypertensive effect has been reported in persons taking desipramine and clonidine. Other tricyclic antidepressants—amoxapine (Asendin®), doxepin (Adapin®, Sinequan®), nortriptyline (Aventyl®, Pamelor®), protriptyline (Vivactil®), and trimipramine (Surmontil®)—probably interact with clonidine in the same way, but little data are available.

Tricyclic antidepressants may also increase the risk of hypertensive reaction—symptoms of which include elevated blood pressure levels, flushing of the face, pounding of the heart, and lightheadedness—if clonidine is discontinued too rapidly.

**Recommendation:** It is best to avoid this combination; discuss it with your doctor.

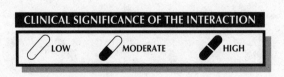

CLINICAL SIGNIFICANCE OF THE INTERACTION

LOW      MODERATE      HIGH

324

| ANTIDEPRESSANT DRUG | INTERACTING DRUG | RESULT |
|---|---|---|
| Desipramine (**Pertofrane®, Norpramin®**) | Quinidine (**Cardioquin®, Duraquin®, Quinaglute®, Quinidex®, Quinora®**)<br><br>[for arrhythmias, or irregularities of the heartbeat and heart rhythm] | Quinidine may cause an increased amount of desipramine in the blood, possibly leading to side effects such as severe dry mouth, blurred vision, fast heartbeat, difficulty or inability to urinate, and constipation. Tricyclic antidepressants other than desipramine may also interact with quinidine.<br><br>It may be necessary for your doctor to adjust the dose of desipramine if quinidine is started or stopped, or if its dosage is changed. (Of course, only your doctor should change medication dosages, when appropriate). |
| Doxepin (**Adapin®, Sinequan®**) | Alcohol | Doxepin combined with alcohol may result in a greater than expected impairment of psychomotor skills—such as those needed to drive a car or operate machinery—especially during the first week of treatment. (This result is even more pronounced with the tricyclic antidepressant amitriptyline, which has a sedative effect by itself.)<br><br>When combining alcohol with other tricyclic antidepressants, the same result may occur. Other tricyclic antidepressants include amitriptyline (Elavil®, Endep®), amoxapine (Asendin®), desipramine (Pertofrane®, Norpramin®), imipramine (Janimine®, Tofranil®), nortriptyline (Aventyl®, Pamelor®), protriptyline (Vivactil®), and trimipramine (Surmontil®).<br><br>**Recommendation:** Limit or avoid alcohol intake if you are taking tricyclic antidepressants. Discuss this interaction with your doctor. |

| ANTIDEPRESSANT DRUG | INTERACTING DRUG | RESULT |
| --- | --- | --- |
| Doxepin (**Adapin**®, **Sinequan**®)  | Cimetidine (**Tagamet**®)<br><br>[for stomach and intestinal ulcers] | Can result in an increased blood concentration of doxepin, possibly to a toxic level. Symptoms of doxepin toxicity include severe dry mouth, blurred vision, fast heartbeat, difficulty or inability to urinate, and constipation.<br><br>Other tricyclic antidepressants may be similarly affected by cimetidine. They include amitriptyline (Elavil®, Endep®), amoxapine (Asendin®), desipramine (Pertofrane®, Norpramin®), imipramine (Janimine®, Tofranil®), nortriptyline (Aventyl®, Pamelor®), protriptyline (Vivactil®), and trimipramine (Surmontil®).<br><br>**Recommendation:** It may be necessary for your doctor to adjust the dose of doxepin if cimetidine is started or stopped, or if its dosage is changed. (Of course, only your doctor should change medication dosages, when appropriate).<br><br>Your doctor may choose to use ranitidine (Zantac®), famotidine (Pepcid®), or nizatidine (Axid®) instead of cimetidine, because they are less likely to interact. |
| Doxepin (**Adapin**®, **Sinequan**®)  | Propoxyphene (**Darvocet-N**®, **Darvon**®, **Darvon**® **with A.S.A.**®, **Dolene**®, and **Wygesic**®)<br><br>[for relief of mild to moderate pain] | Increased blood concentration of doxepin (and possibly other tricyclic antidepressants), leading to an enhanced effect of the doxepin. Possible symptoms of excessive doxepine effect include lethargy, dry mouth, blurred vision, and constipation. |
| Doxepin (**Adapin**®, **Sinequan**®)  | Tolazamide (**Tolinase**®)<br><br>[for treatment of diabetes mellitus, a condition that results in excessively high amounts of sugar in the blood and urine] | May lead to excessively low blood sugar levels in certain persons.<br><br>**Recommendation:** Individuals who have diabetes should monitor their blood sugar levels even more carefully when taking—and for two weeks after discontinuing—a tricyclic antidepressant (such as doxepin). |

Fluoxetine (**Prozac**®)

Carbamazepine (**Tegretol**®)

[for epilepsy, trigeminal neuralgia (spasms of pain in the face), and other disorders]

Fluoxetine increases the amount of carbamazepine in the blood, possibly to toxic levels. Symptoms of carbamazepine toxicity include nausea, vomiting, ringing in the ears, vertigo (a sensation in which you feel as if you are revolving in space or your surroundings are revolving around you), blurred vision, and tremor.

**Recommendation:** It may be necessary for your doctor to adjust the dose of carbamazepine if fluoxetine is started or stopped, or if its dosage is changed. (Of course, only your doctor should change medication dosages, when appropriate).

---

Fluoxetine (**Prozac**®)

Monoamine oxidase inhibitors:

- isocarboxazid (**Marplan**®)
- phenelzine (**Nardil**®)
- tranylcypromine (**Parnate**®), and others

[for treatment of depression]

Severe or fatal reactions have developed in persons receiving fluoxetine shortly after they began taking tranylcypromine concomitantly.

Since fluoxetine stays in the body for a relatively long period of time, fluoxetine interactions could occur days, even weeks, after fluoxetine is discontinued.

The effect of combining fluoxetine with monoamine oxidase (MAO) inhibitors other than tranylcypromine is not known, but a similar interaction may occur.

**Recommendation:** Avoid combined use of fluoxetine and antidepressants from the MAO inhibitor family. One should wait two weeks after stopping an MAO inhibitor before starting fluoxetine, and six weeks after stopping fluoxetine before starting an MAO inhibitor.

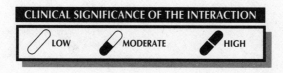

CLINICAL SIGNIFICANCE OF THE INTERACTION

LOW    MODERATE    HIGH

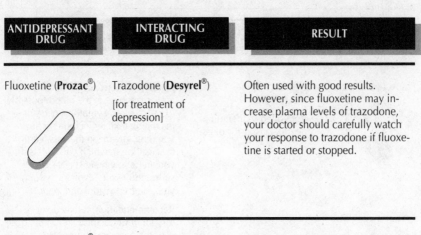

Fluoxetine (**Prozac**®)

Trazodone (**Desyrel**®)

[for treatment of depression]

Often used with good results. However, since fluoxetine may increase plasma levels of trazodone, your doctor should carefully watch your response to trazodone if fluoxetine is started or stopped.

---

Fluoxetine (**Prozac**®)

Tricyclic antidepressants:

- amitriptyline (**Elavil**®, **Endep**®)
- amoxapine (**Asendin**®)
- desipramine (**Pertofrane**®, **Norpramin**®)
- doxepin (**Adapin**®, **Sinequan**®)
- imipramine (**Janimine**®, **Tofranil**®)
- nortriptyline (**Aventyl**®, **Pamelor**®)
- protriptyline (**Vivactil**®)
- trimipramine (**Surmontil**®)

[for treatment of depression]

Markedly increased plasma levels of the tricyclic antidepressant have been shown when given in combination with fluoxetine. This can lead to antidepressant toxicity, signs of which include severe lethargy, fatigue, severe dry mouth, blurred vision, fast heartbeat, difficulty or inability to urinate, and constipation.

**Recommendation:** It may be necessary for your doctor to adjust the dose of a tricyclic antidepressant if fluoxetine is started or stopped, or if its dosage is changed. (Of course, only your doctor should change medication dosages, when appropriate.)

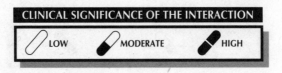

CLINICAL SIGNIFICANCE OF THE INTERACTION

LOW    MODERATE    HIGH

| ANTIDEPRESSANT DRUG | INTERACTING DRUG | RESULT |
|---|---|---|

Imipramine (**Janimine®, Tofranil®**)

Carbamazepine (**Tegretol®**)

[for epilepsy, trigeminal neuralgia (spasms of pain in the face), and other disorders]

Some evidence indicates that carbamazepine can decrease the effect of imipramine. A decreased effect may also occur with the use of other tricyclic antidepressants, namely amitriptyline (Elavil®, Endep®), amoxapine (Asendin®), desipramine (Pertofrane®, Norpramin®), doxepin (Adapin®, Sinequan®), nortriptyline (Aventyl®, Pamelor®), protriptyline (Vivactil®), and trimipramine (Surmontil®).

Individuals taking carbamazepine regularly may require a larger than expected dose of imipramine or other tricyclics for an adequate antidepressant effect. (Of course, only your doctor should change medication dosages, when appropriate.)

Imipramine (**Janimine®, Tofrani®**)

Cimetidine (**Tagamet®**)

[for stomach and intestinal ulcers]

Can result in an increased blood concentration of the imipramine, possibly to a toxic level. Symptoms of imipramine toxocity include severe dry mouth, blurred vision, fast heartbeat, difficulty or inability to urinate, and constipation.

Other tricyclic antidepressants may be similarly affected by cimetidine. They include amitriptyline (Elavil®, Endep®), amoxapine (Asendin®), desipramine (Pertofrane®, Norpramin®), doxepin (Adapin®, Sinequan®), nortriptyline (Aventyl®, Pamelor®), protriptyline (Vivactil®), and trimipramine (Surmontil®).

It may be necessary for your doctor to adjust the dose of imipramine if cimetidine is started or stopped, or if its dosage is changed. (Of course, only your doctor should change medication dosages, when appropriate).

Your doctor may choose to use ranitidine (Zantac®), famotidine (Pepcid®), or nizatidine (Axid®) instead of cimetidine, because they are less likely to interact.

Imipramine (**Janimine®**, **Tofranil®**)

Clonidine (**Catapres®**)

[for treatment of high blood pressure]

Reduced antihypertensive effect has been reported in persons taking imipramine and clonidine. Other tricyclic antidepressants—amoxapine (Asendin®), doxepin (Adapin®, Sinequan®), nortriptyline (Aventyl®, Pamelor®), protriptyline (Vivactil®), and trimipramine (Surmontil®)—probably interact with clonidine in the same way, but little data are available.

Tricyclic antidepressants may also increase the risk of hypertensive reaction—symptoms of which include elevated blood pressure levels, flushing of the face, pounding of the heart, and lightheadedness—if clonidine is discontinued too rapidly.

**Recommendation:** It is best to avoid this combination; discuss it with your doctor.

Imipramine (**Janimine®**, **Tofranil®**)

Norepinephrine (**Levophed®**)

[for cardiac arrest, severe low blood pressure (hypotensive crisis), and shock]

Imipramine, when taken with norepinephrine in an intravenous form, may cause a marked increase in blood pressure and the force with which the heart contracts. Symptoms associated with an acute increase in blood pressure include headache, nausea, vomiting, sleepiness, irritability, confusion, visual disturbances, and chest pain.

Although this interaction has been shown to occur with imipramine (Janimine®, Tofranil®), other tricyclic antidepressants are expected to act similarly when combined with norepinephrine. These include amitriptyline (Elavil®, Endep®), amoxapine (Asendin®), desipramine (Pertofrane®, Norpramin®), doxepin (Adapin®, Sinequan®), nortriptyline (Aventyl®, Pamelor®), protriptyline (Vivactil®), and trimipramine (Surmontil®).

| ANTIDEPRESSANT DRUG | INTERACTING DRUG | RESULT |
|---|---|---|

Imipramine
(**Janimine®**,
**Tofranil®**)

Phenylephrine (**Neo-Synephrine®** Injection)

[for increasing blood pressure level when it is too low]

Imipramine, when taken with phenylephrine in an intravenous form, may lead to an increase in blood pressure and the force with which the heart contracts. Symptoms associated with an acute increase in blood pressure include headache, nausea, vomiting, sleepiness, irritability, confusion, visual disturbances, and chest pain.

This interaction is based on phenylephrine given intravenously; it is not known whether this result occurs when phenylephrine is taken orally. However, one should be alert to the reactions mentioned above when an oral form of phenylephrine is taken with imipramine and other tricyclic antidepressants. (Oral forms of phenylephrine include Dristan®, Neo-Synephrine® Nasal Spray, Dimetane®, Novahistine® Elixir, Robitussin® Night Relief, and others.)

Although this interaction has been shown to occur with imipramine, other tricyclic antidepressants are expected to act similarly when combined with phenylephrine. These include amitriptyline (Elavil®, Endep®), amoxapine (Asendin®), desipramine (Pertofrane®, Norpramin®), doxepin (Adapin®, Sinequan®), nortriptyline (Aventyl®, Pamelor®), protriptyline (Vivactil®), and trimipramine (Surmontil®).

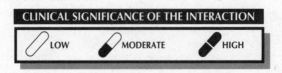

CLINICAL SIGNIFICANCE OF THE INTERACTION

LOW    MODERATE    HIGH

| ANTIDEPRESSANT DRUG | INTERACTING DRUG | RESULT |
|---|---|---|

Imipramine (**Janimine**®, **Tofranil**®)

Phenytoin (**Dilantin**®)

[for prevention of seizures]

Increased concentration of phenytoin in the blood, which may lead to rapid involuntary movement of the eyes, muscular incoordination, dizziness, confusion, double vision, sleepiness, and, in severe cases, seizures and coma.

This interaction may also result in a reduced concentration of imipramine, leading to decreased imipramine effect (i.e., inadequate control of depression). Phenytoin may produce a similar effect with other tricyclic antidepressants, including amitriptyline (Elavil®, Endep®), amoxapine (Asendin®), desipramine (Pertofrane®, Norpramin®), doxepin (Adapin®, Sinequan®), nortriptyline (Aventyl®, Pamelor®), protriptyline (Vivactil®), and trimipramine (Surmontil®).

Imipramine (**Janimine**®, **Tofranil**®)

Quinidine (**Cardioquin**®, **Duraquin**®, **Quinaglute**®, **Quinidex**®, **Quinora**®)

[for arrhythmias, or irregularities of the heartbeat and heart rhythm]

Quinidine may cause an increased amount of imipramine in the blood, possibly leading to side effects such as severe dry mouth, blurred vision, fast heartbeat, difficulty or inability to urinate, and constipation.

Lithium (**Cibalith-S**®, **Eskalith**®, **Lithane**®, **Lithobid**®, and others)

Bumetanide (**Bumex**®)

[for high blood pressure and to reduce fluid accumulation]

May lead to higher levels of lithium in the blood, which could lead to lithium toxicity. Symptoms of this toxicity include muscle twitching, dizziness, blurred vision, vomiting or severe nausea, persistent diarrhea, confusion, weakness, coarse trembling of hands or legs, and slurred speech.

| ANTIDEPRESSANT DRUG | INTERACTING DRUG | RESULT |
|---|---|---|

Lithium (**Cibalith-S**®, **Eskalith**®, **Lithane**®, **Lithobid**®, and others)

Carbamazepine (**Tegretol**®)

[for epilepsy, trigeminal neuralgia (spasms of pain in the face), and other disorders]

Lithium and carbamazepine are commonly used together without any problems. However, carbamazepine tends to increase the effect of lithium, producing lithium toxicity in some persons. Symptoms of this toxicity include muscle twitching, dizziness, blurred vision, vomiting or severe nausea, persistent diarrhea, confusion, weakness, coarse trembling of hands or legs, and slurred speech.

**Recommendation:** If you are taking lithium, watch for signs of lithium toxicity if carbamazepine is started.

Lithium (**Cibalith-S**®, **Eskalith**®, **Lithane**®, **Lithobid**®, and others)

Diclofenac (**Voltaren**®)

[for reduction of inflammation; used to reduce the pain and swelling associated with arthritis, tendinitis, and bursitis]

May produce higher levels of lithium in the blood, which could lead to lithium toxicity. Symptoms of this toxicity include muscle twitching, dizziness, blurred vision, vomiting or severe nausea, persistent diarrhea, confusion, weakness, coarse trembling of hands or legs, and slurred speech.

**Recommendation:** If you are taking lithium, do not start or stop taking diclofenac without consulting with your doctor. Sulindac (Clinoril®), a drug in the same class as diclofenac, appears to produce a slight decrease in the amount of lithium in the body, and does not seem to cause difficulties in people taking lithium. However, your doctor may wish to monitor your lithium levels when *any* nonsteroidal anti-inflammatory drug is started or stopped.

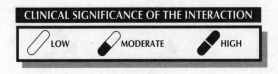

CLINICAL SIGNIFICANCE OF THE INTERACTION

LOW · MODERATE HIGH

| ANTIDEPRESSANT DRUG | INTERACTING DRUG | RESULT |
|---|---|---|
| Lithium (**Cibalith-S**®, **Eskalith**®, **Lithane**®, **Lithobid**®, and others) | Diltiazem (**Cardizem**® **Cardizem SR**®, **Cardizem CD**®)<br><br>[used to treat angina] | Could lead to neurotoxicity, possible symptoms of which include nausea, vomiting, muscular incoordination, and ringing in the ears. |
| Lithium (**Cibalith-S**®, **Eskalith**®, **Lithane**®, **Lithobid**®, and others) | Ethacrynic acid (**Edecrin**®)<br><br>[for high blood pressure and to reduce fluid accumulation] | May produce higher levels of lithium in the blood, which could lead to lithium toxicity. Symptoms of this toxicity include muscle twitching, dizziness, blurred vision, vomiting or severe nausea, persistent diarrhea, confusion, weakness, coarse trembling of hands or legs, and slurred speech. |
| Lithium (**Cibalith-S**®, **Eskalith**®, **Lithane**®, **Lithobid**®, and others) | Furosemide (**Lasix**®)<br><br>[for high blood pressure and to reduce fluid accumulation] | May produce higher levels of lithium in the blood, which could lead to lithium toxicity. Symptoms of this toxicity include muscle twitching, dizziness, blurred vision, vomiting or severe nausea, persistent diarrhea, confusion, weakness, coarse trembling of hands or legs, and slurred speech. |

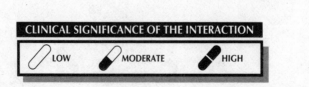

CLINICAL SIGNIFICANCE OF THE INTERACTION

LOW    MODERATE    HIGH

| ANTIDEPRESSANT DRUG | INTERACTING DRUG | RESULT |
|---|---|---|

Lithium (**Cibalith-S®, Eskalith®, Lithane®, Lithobid®,** and others)

Haloperidol (**Haldol®**)

[for relieving symptoms of schizophrenia and mania]

Some persons are thought to be more susceptible to developing severe reactions, particularly when one or both of these drugs are given in large amounts. Reactions include fever, confusion, and lethargy.

When lithium is combined with haloperidol, some persons may have an increased likelihood of developing what are known as extrapyramidal symptoms; these severe side effects are involuntary body movements, such as facial grimacing; abnormal posturing of the head, neck, and eyes; restlessness; rigidity; and tremor at rest.

This combination should be used only by physicians experienced in the combined use of these drugs.

---

Lithium (**Cibalith-S®, Eskalith®, Lithane®, Lithobid®,** and others)

Ibuprofen (**Advil®, Medipren®, Midol®, Motrin®, Nuprin®,** and **Rufen®**)

[for reduction of inflammation; used to reduce the pain and swelling associated with arthritis, tendinitis, and bursitis]

May produce higher levels of lithium in the blood, which could lead to lithium toxicity. Symptoms of this toxicity include muscle twitching, dizziness, blurred vision, vomiting or severe nausea, persistent diarrhea, confusion, weakness, coarse trembling of hands or legs, and slurred speech.

**Recommendation:** If you are taking lithium, do not start or stop taking ibuprofen without consulting with your doctor. Sulindac (Clinoril®), a drug in the same class as ibuprofen, appears to produce a slight decrease in the amount of lithium in the body, and does not seem to cause difficulties in people taking lithium. However, your doctor may wish to monitor your lithium levels when *any* nonsteroidal anti-inflammatory drug is started or stopped.

| ANTIDEPRESSANT DRUG | INTERACTING DRUG | RESULT |
| --- | --- | --- |
| Lithium (**Cibalith-S®, Eskalith®, Lithane®, Lithobid®**, and others)  | Indomethacin (**Indocin®**) [for reduction of inflammation; used to reduce the pain and swelling associated with arthritis, tendinitis, and bursitis] | May produce higher levels of lithium in the blood, which could lead to lithium toxicity. Symptoms of this toxicity include muscle twitching, dizziness, blurred vision, vomiting or severe nausea, persistent diarrhea, confusion, weakness, coarse trembling of hands or legs, and slurred speech. **Recommendation:** If you are taking lithium, do not start or stop taking indomethacin without consulting with your doctor. Sulindac (Clinoril®), a drug in the same class as indomethacin, appears to produce a slight decrease in the amount of lithium in the body, and does not seem to cause difficulties in people taking lithium. However, your doctor may wish to monitor your lithium levels when *any* nonsteroidal anti-inflammatory drug is started or stopped. |
| Lithium (**Cibalith-S®, Eskalith®, Lithane®, Lithobid®**, and others)  | Methyldopa (**Aldomet®**) [for the reduction of high blood pressure] | There is a moderate possibility of lithium toxicity. Symptoms of this toxicity include muscle twitching, dizziness, blurred vision, vomiting or severe nausea, persistent diarrhea, confusion, weakness, coarse trembling of hands or legs, and slurred speech. |

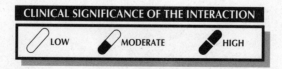

CLINICAL SIGNIFICANCE OF THE INTERACTION

LOW    MODERATE    HIGH

Lithium (**Cibalith-S**®, **Eskalith**®, **Lithane**®, **Lithobid**®, and others)

Naproxen (**Anaprox**®, **Naprosyn**®)

[for reduction of inflammation; used to reduce the pain and swelling associated with arthritis, tendinitis, and bursitis]

May produce higher levels of lithium in the blood, which could lead to lithium toxicity. Symptoms of this toxicity include muscle twitching, dizziness, blurred vision, vomiting or severe nausea, persistent diarrhea, confusion, weakness, coarse trembling of hands or legs, and slurred speech.

**Recommendation:** If you are taking lithium, do not start or stop taking naproxen without consulting with your doctor. Sulindac (Clinoril®), a drug in the same class as naproxen, appears to produce a slight decrease in the amount of lithium in the body, and does not seem to cause difficulties in people taking lithium. However, your doctor may wish to monitor your lithium levels when *any* nonsteroidal anti-inflammatory drug is started or stopped.

Lithium (**Cibalith-S**®, **Eskalith**®, **Lithane**®, **Lithobid**®, and others)

Phenylbutazone (**Azolid**®, **Butazolidin**®)

[for reduction of inflammation; used to reduce the pain and swelling associated with arthritis, tendinitis, and bursitis]

May produce higher levels of lithium in the blood, which could lead to lithium toxicity. Symptoms of this toxicity include muscle twitching, dizziness, blurred vision, vomiting or severe nausea, persistent diarrhea, confusion, weakness, coarse trembling of hands or legs, and slurred speech.

**Recommendation:** If you are taking lithium, do not start or stop taking phenylbutazone without consulting with your doctor. Sulindac (Clinoril®), a drug in the same class as phenylbutazone, appears to produce a slight decrease in the amount of lithium in the body, and does not seem to cause difficulties in people taking lithium. However, your doctor may wish to monitor your lithium levels when *any* nonsteroidal anti-inflammatory drug is started or stopped.

| ANTIDEPRESSANT DRUG | INTERACTING DRUG | RESULT |
|---|---|---|
| Lithium (**Cibalith-S**®, **Eskalith**®, **Lithane**®, **Lithobid**®, and others)  | Piroxicam (**Feldene**®) <br><br>[for reduction of inflammation; used to reduce the pain and swelling associated with arthritis, tendinitis, and bursitis] | May produce higher levels of lithium in the blood, which could lead to lithium toxicity. Symptoms of this toxicity include muscle twitching, dizziness, blurred vision, vomiting or severe nausea, persistent diarrhea, confusion, weakness, coarse trembling of hands or legs, and slurred speech. <br><br>**Recommendation:** If you are taking lithium, do not start or stop taking piroxicam without consulting with your doctor. Sulindac (Clinoril®), a drug in the same class as piroxicam, appears to produce a slight decrease in the amount of lithium in the body, and does not seem to cause difficulties in people taking lithium. However, your doctor may wish to monitor your lithium levels when *any* nonsteroidal anti-inflammatory drug is started or stopped. |
| Lithium (**Cibalith-S**®, **Eskalith**®, **Lithane**®, **Lithobid**®, and others)  | Potassium iodide (**Pima**® **Syrup** and **SSKI**®; also found in various preparations, such as **Elixophyllin-KI**®, **Iodo-Niacin**®, **Mudrane**®, **Pediacof**® **Cough Syrup**, **Quadrinal**®, and others) <br><br>[used in the management of thyroid disease] | Could lead to hypothyroidism, a condition in which the activity of the thyroid gland is decreased. Symptoms include tiredness, lethargy, weakness, headache, dry skin, constipation, sensitivity to cold; also, menstrual disturbances in women. |

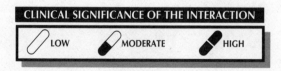

CLINICAL SIGNIFICANCE OF THE INTERACTION

LOW    MODERATE    HIGH

| ANTIDEPRESSANT DRUG | INTERACTING DRUG | RESULT |
|---|---|---|

Lithium (**Cibalith-S®, Eskalith®, Lithane®, Lithobid®**, and others)

Sodium bicarbonate (**Alka-Seltzer®, Arm & Hammer®Pure Baking Soda, Citrocarbonate®**, and others)

[for relief of acid indigestion and heartburn]

Sodium bicarbonate may lower the concentration of lithium in the blood, thereby leading to a decreased lithium effect.

An occasional dose of sodium bicarbonate probably would not cause difficulty, but more than a few doses a week may begin to reduce lithium levels.

**Recommendation:** If you are on lithium, avoid more than a few doses a week of products containing sodium bicarbonate. If you take more than that, consult with your doctor.

---

Lithium (**Cibalith-S®, Eskalith®, Lithane®, Lithobid®**, and others)

Salt (sodium chloride)

Salt has a marked effect on the amount of lithium in the blood. If the body becomes salt-depleted (for example, on a low-salt diet), the kidneys get rid of lithium more slowly and the concentration of lithium in the body increases. In these cases, symptoms of lithium toxicity may occur, such as muscle twitching, dizziness, blurred vision, vomiting or severe nausea, persistent diarrhea, confusion, weakness, coarse trembling of hands or legs, and slurred speech.

**Recommendation:** Avoid extremely large or extremely small intakes of salt. Inform your doctor before you begin any new diet, particularly a low-salt diet.

339

| ANTIDEPRESSANT DRUG | INTERACTING DRUG | RESULT |
| --- | --- | --- |
| Lithium (**Cibalith-S**®, **Eskalith**®, **Lithane**®, **Lithobid**®, and others)  | Spironolactone (**Aldactone**®) <br><br>[for treatment of high blood pressure and to reduce fluid accumulation in persons with congestive heart failure, liver or kidney disease] | May result in higher levels of lithium in the blood, which could lead to lithium toxicity. Symptoms of this toxicity include muscle twitching, dizziness, blurred vision, vomiting or severe nausea, persistent diarrhea, confusion, weakness, coarse trembling of hands or legs, and slurred speech. <br><br>It may be necessary for your doctor to adjust your lithium dose if spironolactone is started or stopped. (Of course, only your doctor should change medication dosages, when appropriate.) |
| Lithium (**Cibalith-S**®, **Eskalith**®, **Lithane**®, **Lithobid**®, and others)  | Theophylline (**Bronkaid**®, **Primatene**®, **Slo-bid**®, **Theo-24**®, **Theobid**®, **Theo-Dur**®, **Uniphyl**®, and others) <br><br>[for relief and/or prevention of asthma attacks and bronchospasm associated with emphysema and bronchitis] | May be a reduced effect of the lithium in some persons. If you take these drugs concurrently, your doctor may need to increase the dosage of your lithium. (Do *not* change the dosage of either drug yourself; only your doctor should do this.) <br><br>This interaction is also important in individuals on long-term lithium therapy who intermittently use theophylline preparations. |
| Lithium (**Cibalith-S**®, **Eskalith**®, **Lithane**®, **Lithobid**®, and others)  | Thiazide and related diuretics: <br><br>• chlorothiazide (**Diuril**®) <br>• chlorthalidone (**Hygroton**®) <br>• hydrochlorothiazide (**Esidrix**®, **HydroDIURIL**®, **Oretic**®, and others) <br>• indapamide (**Lozol**®) <br>• metolazone (**Diulo**®, **Zaroxolyn**®) <br><br>[for the treatment of high blood pressure and fluid accumulation] | May lead to an increased amount of lithium in the blood, possibly to the point of lithium toxicity. Symptoms of this toxicity include muscle twitching, dizziness, blurred vision, vomiting or severe nausea, persistent diarrhea, confusion, weakness, coarse trembling of hands or legs, and slurred speech. <br><br>It may be necessary for your doctor to adjust your lithium dose if a thiazide diuretic is started or stopped. (Of course, only your doctor should change medication dosages, when appropriate.) |

Lithium (**Cibalith-S**®, **Eskalith**®, **Lithane**®, **Lithobid**®, and others)

Thioridazine (**Mellaril**®)

[for relieving symptoms of schizophrenia and mania]

Some persons are more susceptible to developing severe reactions, particularly when one or both of these drugs are given in large amounts. Reactions include fever, confusion, and lethargy.

When lithium is combined with antipsychotic medications known as phenothiazines (especially thioridazine), some persons may have an increased likelihood of developing what are known as extrapyramidal symptoms; these severe side effects include involuntary body movements, such as facial grimacing; abnormal posturing of the head, neck, and eyes; restlessness; rigidity; and tremor at rest.

Lithium (**Cibalith-S**®, **Eskalith**®, **Lithane**®, **Lithobid**®, and others)

Verapamil (**Calan**®; **Isoptin**®)

[for treatment of high blood pressure]

In a few isolated cases, this combination seemed to lead to certain disturbances of the nervous system. Possible symptoms include nausea, vomiting, muscular incoordination, and ringing in the ears. This interaction may also occur with diltiazem (Cardizem®) and possibly other calcium-channel blockers (a particular class of medication used to treat hypertension and angina).

Some persons do not seem to have any trouble with combined use of lithium and verapamil or other calcium-channel blockers. If you are concerned about this unlikely interaction, discuss your concerns with your doctor.

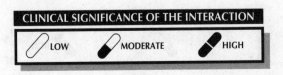

CLINICAL SIGNIFICANCE OF THE INTERACTION

LOW    MODERATE    HIGH

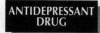
Lithium (**Cibalith-S**®, **Eskalith**®, **Lithane**®, **Lithobid**®, and others)

Zidovudine (**Retrovir**®)

[for managing the symptoms of adults with human immunodeficiency virus (HIV)]

Lithium has been used to help maintain an adequate number of neutrophils (a particular type of white blood cell, needed to ward off infection) in persons receiving zidovudine. However, some evidence indicates that this combination results in a high incidence of lithium toxicity.

Monoamine oxidase inhibitors:

- . isocarboxazid (**Marplan**®)
- phenelzine (**Nardil**®)
- tranylcypromine (**Parnate**®),and others

Alcohol

Can pose a threat to health when MAO inhibitors are taken with alcohol that contains tyramine, a chemical found in wine (particularly chianti wine) and some types of beer. Normally, the body converts tyramine to harmless chemicals, but in the presence of an MAO inhibitor, tyramine causes the release of norepinephrine, a chemical that causes blood vessels to narrow. As a result, blood pressure rises dramatically, and the person may develop dizziness, headaches, and nausea. In extreme cases, brain hemorrhage and death can result.

**Recommendation:**Even though some alcoholic beverages (e.g., vodka, gin, whiskey) are unlikely to contain a substantial amount of tyramine, it would be prudent to avoid all alcoholic beverages while taking, or within two weeks after stopping, MAO inhibitors. See also the MAO inhibitor-food entry on pp. 345–46.

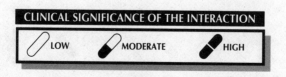

CLINICAL SIGNIFICANCE OF THE INTERACTION

LOW     MODERATE     HIGH

| ANTIDEPRESSANT DRUG | INTERACTING DRUG | RESULT |
|---|---|---|

Monoamine oxidase inhibitors:

- isocarboxazid (**Marplan**®)
- phenelzine (**Nardil**®)
- tranylcypromine (**Parnate**®), and others

Amphetamines:

- benzphetamine (**Didrex**®)
- dextroamphetamine (**Dexedrine**®)
- fenfluramine (**Pondimin**®)
- mazindol (**Sanorex**®)
- methylphenidate (**Ritalin**®)
- pemoline (**Cylert**®)
- phenmetrazine (**Preludin**®) and others

[for abnormal and uncontrollable sleeping during the day; also used to help suppress appetite; methylphenidate is also used to treat attention-deficit disorders]

Can be a deadly combination (fatalities and near-fatalities have occurred). This interaction may lead to an extreme rise in blood pressure and bleeding around the brain (i.e., cerebral hemorrhage). Although tranylcypromine appears to be the riskiest antidepressant in this regard, use of other antidepressants that are MAO inhibitors may also lead to this effect.

Some evidence indicates that methylphenidate (Ritalin®), which has amphetamine-like characteristics, reacts less severely with MAO inhibitors than other amphetamines. But severe reactions may occur, especially with larger doses of methylphenidate.

**Recommendation:** Avoid using antidepressants of the MAO inhibitor class with amphetamines. Also, amphetamines should not be used within two weeks after stopping MAO inhibitors.

Monoamine oxidase inhibitors:

- isocarboxazid (**Marplan**®)
- phenelzine (**Nardil**®)
- tranylcypromine (**Parnate**®), and others

Antidiabetic drugs:

- acetohexamide (**Dymelor**®)
- chlorpropamide (**Diabinese**®)
- glipizide (**Glucotrol**®)
- glyburide (**DiaBeta**®, **Micronase**®)
- insulin (**Humulin**®, **Lente**®, **Novolin**®, and others)
- tolazamide (**Tolinase**®)
- tolbutamide (**Orinase**®), and others

[for treatment of diabetes mellitus, a condition that results in excessively high amounts of sugar in the blood and urine]

When monoamine oxidase (MAO) inhibitors are taken with antidiabetic medications, blood sugar levels may be reduced excessively. Symptoms of excessively low blood sugar levels include increased heart rate, cold sweats, trembling, nausea, hunger, mental confusion, and, in severe cases, coma.

**Recommendation:** Diabetic individuals should be especially careful in monitoring their blood sugar levels when taking MAO inhibitor drugs, and for three weeks after stopping them.

Monoamine oxidase inhibitors:

- isocarboxazid (**Marplan**®)
- phenelzine (**Nardil**®)
- tranylcypromine (**Parnate**®), and others

Barbiturates:

- amobarbital (**Amytal**®)
- butabarbital (**Butisol**®)
- butalbital
- pentobarbital (**Nembutal**®)
- phenobarbital (**Luminal**®, **Solfoton**®)
- primidone (**Mysoline**®)
- secobarbital, (**Seconal**®) and others

[used to treat insomnia and anxiety; certain barbiturates are used to prevent seizures]

Antidepressants in the monoamine oxidase inhibitor class may prolong the effect of the barbiturate, causing the person to become oversedated. Although this interaction has been reported with one particular monoamine oxidase inhibitor (tranylcypromine) and one specific barbiturate (amobarbital), a similar effect may be seen with other combinations of MAO inhibitors and barbiturates.

---

Monoamine oxidase inhibitors:

- isocarboxazid (**Marplan**®)
- phenelzine (**Nardil**®)
- tranylcypromine (**Parnate**®), and others

Dextromethorphan (**Benylin**® DM, **Delsym**®, **Hold**® Cough Suppressant Lozenges, **Sucret**® Cough Control Lozenges)

[used as a cough suppressant]

Preliminary data indicate that this combination may be serious, possibly leading to dizziness, nausea, tremor, fever, and coma.

**Recommendation:** Until more is known about this possible interaction, people taking monoamine oxidase inhibitors should avoid taking dextromethorphan.

---

Monoamine oxidase inhibitors:

- isocarboxazid (**Marplan**®)
- phenelzine (**Nardil**®)
- tranylcypromine (**Parnate**®), and others

Doxapram (**Dopram**®)

[used to stimulate breathing after surgery in which anesthesia was used and breathing is depressed]

Monoamine oxidase inhibitors may enhance certain cardiovascular effects of doxapram, such as increased blood pressure levels and the development of arrhythmias (irregularities of the heartbeat and heart rhythm).

| ANTIDEPRESSANT DRUG | INTERACTING DRUG | RESULT |
|---|---|---|

Monoamine oxidase inhibitors:

- isocarboxazid (**Marplan**®)
- phenelzine (**Nardil**®)
- tranylcypromine (**Parnate**®), and others

Ephedrine (**Primatene**®, **Broncholate**®, **Tedral**®, and others

[for wheezing due to asthma]

Can result in severe high blood pressure.

**Recommendation:** Avoid using these two medications together. Also, ephedrine should not be used within two weeks after stopping an MAO inhibitor.

---

Monoamine oxidase inhibitors:

- isocarboxazid (**Marplan**®)
- phenelzine (**Nardil**®)
- tranylcypromine (**Parnate**®), and others

Foods that contain a large amount of tyramine

A serious reaction may ensue in persons taking an MAO inhibitor and eating tyramine-containing foods. Tyramine is a chemical found in various foods. Normally, the body converts tyramine to harmless chemicals, but in the presence of an MAO inhibitor, tyramine causes the release of norepinephrine, a chemical that causes blood vessels to narrow. As a result, blood pressure rises dramatically, and the person may develop dizziness, headaches, and nausea. In extreme cases, brain hemorrhage and death can result.

Foods that may be rich in tyramine (or other similar substances) include cheese—particularly strong or aged cheese such as Cheddar, Camembert, and Stilton—sour cream, wine (especially chianti), beer, liver (especially chicken liver), raisins, avocados (especially if overripe), caviar, pickled herring, canned figs, fermented or spoiled meats (including salami, pepperoni, summer sausage), fava beans, yeast extracts, and chocolate.

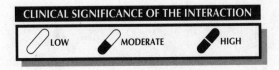

CLINICAL SIGNIFICANCE OF THE INTERACTION

LOW   MODERATE   HIGH

*(cont.)*

| ANTIDEPRESSANT DRUG | INTERACTING DRUG | RESULT |
| --- | --- | --- |
| Monoamine oxidase inhibitors | Foods that contain a large amount of tyramine | **Recommendation:** Avoid the above-mentioned foods while taking, or within two weeks after stopping, MAO inhibitors, particularly tranylcypromine. Consult your doctor or dietician for a complete list of tyramine-containing foods. See also the MAO inhibitor–alcohol entry on p. 342. |
| Monoamine oxidase inhibitors:<br>• isocarboxazid (**Marplan**®)<br>• phenelzine (**Nardil**®)<br>• tranylcypromine (**Parnate**®), and others | Guanadrel (**Hylorel**®)<br>[used to reduce high blood pressure] | May increase blood pressure due to a reduced antihypertensive effect.<br>**Recommendation:** The manufacturer of guanadrel states that it should not be used with, or within one week of discontinuing, MAO inhibitors. Some experts recommend waiting two weeks after MAO inhibitors are stopped before starting guanadrel. |

| Monoamine oxidase inhibitors:<br>• isocarboxazid (**Marplan**®)<br>• phenelzine (**Nardil**®)<br>• tranylcypromine (**Parnate**®), and others | Guanethidine (**Ismelin**®)<br>[used to reduce high blood pressure] | May increase blood pressure due to a reduced antihypertensive effect.<br>**Recommendation:** The manufacturer of guanethidine states that it should not be used with, or within one week of discontinuing, MAO inhibitors. Some experts recommend waiting two weeks after MAO inhibitors are stopped before starting guanethidine. |

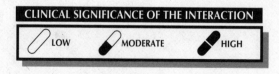

CLINICAL SIGNIFICANCE OF THE INTERACTION

LOW    MODERATE    HIGH

| ANTIDEPRESSANT DRUG | INTERACTING DRUG | RESULT |
|---|---|---|

Monoamine oxidase inhibitors:

- isocarboxazid (**Marplan**®)
- phenelzine (**Nardil**®)
- tranylcypromine (**Parnate**®), and others

Levodopa (**Larodopa**®)

[for treatment of Parkinson's disease]

Taking levodopa with a monoamine oxidase inhibitor may lead to a hypertensive reaction, which results in elevated blood pressure levels, flushing of the face, pounding of the heart, and lightheadedness.

Some evidence also indicates that when levodopa is taken with a monoamine oxidase inhibitor, there is a worsening of certain symptoms, such as tremor and akathisia (a feeling of restlessness and a compelling need to be in constant movement), in persons who suffer from these symptoms.

**Recommendation:** Combined use of levodopa and this family of antidepressants is generally to be avoided. However, if the drugs must be taken together, the evidence indicates that use of carbidopa along with the levodopa (the brand name is Sinemet®) can prevent the hypertensive reactions mentioned above.

**Note:** Selegeline (Eldepryl®), a different kind of monoamine oxidase inhibitor, is often used with levodopa with good results.

Monoamine oxidase inhibitors:

- isocarboxazid (**Marplan**®)
- phenelzine (**Nardil**®)
- tranylcypromine (**Parnate**®), and others

Meperidine (**Demerol**®, **Mepergan**®)

[for relief of moderate to severe pain]

Can be very dangerous interaction. Some individuals receiving meperidine and a monoamine oxidase inhibitor may develop severe side effects, such as extreme alterations in blood pressure (both excessively high blood pressure in some persons, and excessively low blood pressure in others), respiratory depression, rigidity, convulsions, coma, and death. Less severe side effects include excitation and sweating.

**Recommendation:** Avoid this combination. Also, do not use meperidine for three weeks following the cessation of an antidepressant from the monoamine oxidase inhibitor class.

| ANTIDEPRESSANT DRUG | INTERACTING DRUG | RESULT |

Monoamine oxidase inhibitors:

- isocarboxazid (**Marplan**®)
- phenelzine (**Nardil**®)
- tranylcypromine (**Parnate**®), and others

Metaraminol (**Aramine**®)

[given to increase blood pressure levels]

Evidence indicates that pargyline (Eutonyl®)—a MAO inhibitor used to treat hypertension and rarely used today—given with metaraminol may lead to dangerously high blood pressure levels. However, other antidepressants in the monoamine oxidase inhibitor family are expected to lead to a similar result when given with metaraminol.

**Recommendation:** Avoid this combination. Also, do not use metaraminol for three weeks following the cessation of an antidepressant from the monoamine oxidase inhibitor class.

---

Monoamine oxidase inhibitors:

- isocarboxazid (**Marplan**®)
- phenelzine (**Nardil**®)
- tranylcypromine (**Parnate**®), and others

Phenylephrine, which is found in several medications, such as **Congespirin**®, **Dimetane**®, **Dristan**®, **4-Way**® **Fast Acting Nasal Spray, NeoSynephrine**®, **Pediacof**® **Cough Syrup, Phenergan**® **VC, Robitussin**® **Night Relief,** and others

[used as a decongestant; also used to treat low blood pressure levels]

Oral phenylephrine taken with antidepressants in the monoamine oxidase inhibitor family can cause an increase in blood pressure levels, rapid heartbeat, and hypertensive reaction, symptoms of which include headache, palpitations, visual disturbances, and chest pain.

The effect of phenylephrine-containing nasal sprays in persons receiving MAO inhibitors is not established, but such nasal sprays should probably be avoided until more is known about this interaction.

**Recommendation:** Phenylephrine should not be taken by persons who are using an antidepressant in the monoamine oxidase inhibitor family, or within two weeks after stopping an MAO inhibitor.

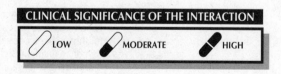

CLINICAL SIGNIFICANCE OF THE INTERACTION

LOW     MODERATE     HIGH

| ANTIDEPRESSANT DRUG | INTERACTING DRUG | RESULT |
|---|---|---|

Monoamine oxidase inhibitors:

- isocarboxazid (**Marplan**®)
- phenelzine (**Nardil**®)
- tranylcypromine (**Parnate**®), and others

Phenylpropranolamine (**Acutrim**®, **Allerest**®, **Comtrex**® **Multi-Symptom Cold Reliever, Contac**® **Continuous Action Decongestant, Coricidin "D"**®, **Dexatrim**®, **Dimetapp**®, **Naldecon**®, **Ornade**®, **Ru-Tuss**®, **Sinarest**® **Regular and Extra Strength, Tavist-D**®, **Triaminic**®, and others)

[used as a decongestant; also used to dilate the bronchioles for symptomatic relief of certain allergies]

Can result in severe hypertensive reactions, which include symptoms such as elevated blood pressure levels, flushing of the face, pounding of the heart, and lightheadedness. Persons taking medications containing phenylpropanolamine with a monoamine oxidase inhibitor have also experienced other symptoms, such as headache, vomiting, and irregularities of the heartbeat and heart rhythm.

**Recommendation:** Phenylpropanolamine should not be taken by persons who are using an antidepressant in the monoamine oxidase inhibitor family, or within two weeks after stopping an MAO inhibitor.

---

Monoamine oxidase inhibitors:

- isocarboxazid (**Marplan**®)
- phenelzine (**Nardil**®)
- tranylcypromine (**Parnate**®), and others

Pseudoephedrine (**Actifed**®, **Benadryl**®, **Bromfed**®, **Contac**® **Nighttime Cold Medicine, Deconamine**®, **Deconsal**® **L.A., Fedahist**®, **Novahistine**®**DMX, Robitussin-DAC**®, **Sine-Aid**®, **Sine-Off**®, **Sinutab**®, **Sudafed**®, **Tylenol**® **Cold Medication, Vicks Formula 44D**®, **Vicks Nyquil**®, and others)

[for nasal decongestion and to dilate the bronchial tubes]

Severe high blood pressure may result when taking medications that contain pseudoephedrine with an antidepressant in the monoamine oxidase inhibitor class. Symptoms may include headache, palpitations, visual disturbances, and chest pain.

**Recommendation:** Persons taking an antidepressant that is in the monoamine oxidase inhibitor family (or who have taken such a drug within the past two weeks) should avoid taking pseudoephedrine and medications containing pseudoephedrine.

| ANTIDEPRESSANT DRUG | INTERACTING DRUG | RESULT |
|---|---|---|

Monoamine oxidase inhibitors:

- isocarboxazid (**Marplan**®)
- phenelzine (**Nardil**®)
- tranylcypromine (**Parnate**®), and others

Reserpine (**Serpasil**®)

[for treatment of high blood pressure]

Although the evidence is limited, excitation and an increase in blood pressure may occur if reserpine is started in persons already receiving a monoamine oxidase inhibitor.

**Recommendation:** It is best to avoid this combination; discuss it with your doctor.

Monoamine oxidase inhibitors:

- isocarboxazid (**Marplan**®)
- phenelzine (**Nardil**®)
- tranylcypromine (**Parnate**®), and others

L-Tryptophan

[formerly used for persons who have mild difficulty falling asleep. No longer commercially available in the United States]

L-Tryptophan is an amino acid, a building block of proteins, that has been advertised as an aid to falling asleep. (Note: L-Tryptophan is no longer commercially available in the United States.) L-Tryptophan is normally present in the diet and is necessary for the formation of serotonin, a chemical that has been shown to play a role in normal sleep. The safety of taking repeated, high doses of L-tryptophan has not been established.

Use of L-Tryptophan with an antidepressant in the monoamine oxidase inhibitor class can lead to certain disturbances of the nervous system, symptoms of which include agitation, disorientation, confusion, incoordination, shivering, and seizures. L-Tryptophan combined with an MAO inhibitor may also lead to hypomania—a moderate form of mania, which involves elation, excessive irritability, and excessive talking.

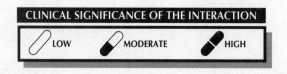

CLINICAL SIGNIFICANCE OF THE INTERACTION

LOW    MODERATE    HIGH

| ANTIDEPRESSANT DRUG | INTERACTING DRUG | RESULT |
| --- | --- | --- |

Nortriptyline (**Aventyl**®, **Pamelor**®)

Chlorpropamide (**Diabinese**®)

[for treatment of diabetes mellitus, a condition that results in excessively high amounts of sugar in the blood and urine]

May lead to excessively low blood sugar levels in certain persons. Symptoms of low blood sugar include increased heart rate, cold sweats, trembling, nausea, hunger, mental confusion, and, in severe cases, coma.

**Recommendation:** Individuals who have diabetes should monitor their blood sugar levels even more carefully when taking—and for two weeks after discontinuing—a tricyclic antidepressant, such as nortriptyline.

Nortriptyline (**Aventyl**®, **Pamelor**®)

Cimetidine (**Tagamet**®)

[for stomach and intestinal ulcers]

Can result in an increased blood concentration of nortriptyline, even to a toxic level. Symptoms of nortriptyline toxicity include severe dry mouth, blurred vision, fast heartbeat, difficulty or inability to urinate, and constipation.

Other tricyclic antidepressants may be similarly affected by cimetidine. They include amitriptyline (Elavil®, Endep®), amoxapine (Asendin®), desipramine (Pertofrane®, Norpramin®), doxepin (Adapin®, Sinequan®), imipramine (Janimine®, Tofranil®), protriptyline (Vivactil®), and trimipramine (Surmontil®).

It may be necessary for your doctor to adjust the dose of nortriptyline if cimetidine is started or stopped, or if its dosage is changed. (Of course, only your doctor should change medication dosages, when appropriate.)

Your doctor may choose to use ranitidine (Zantac®), famotidine (Pepcid®), or nizatidine (Axid®) instead of cimetidine, because they are less likely to interact.

| ANTIDEPRESSANT DRUG | INTERACTING DRUG | RESULT |
|---|---|---|

Trazodone (**Desyrel**®)

Phenytoin (**Dilantin**®)

[for the prevention of seizures]

Increased concentration of phenytoin in the blood, which may lead to rapid involuntary movement of the eyes, muscular incoordination, dizziness, confusion, double vision, sleepiness, and, in, severe cases, seizures and coma.

**Recommendation:** It may be necessary for your doctor to adjust the dose of phenytoin if trazodone is started or stopped, or if its dosage is changed. (Of course, only your doctor should change medication dosages, when appropriate.)

---

Tricyclic antidepressants:

- amitriptyline (**Elavil**®, **Endep**®)
- amoxapine (**Asendin**®)
- desipramine (**Pertofrane**®, **Norpramin**®)
- doxepin (**Adapin**®, **Sinequan**®)
- imipramine (**Janimine**®, **Tofranil**®)
- nortriptyline (**Aventyl**®, **Pamelor**®)
- protriptyline (**Vivactil**®)
- trimipramine (**Surmontil**®)

Anticholinergic drugs:

- atropine
- belladonna
- benztropine (**Cogentin**®)
- biperiden (**Akineton**®)
- clidinium (**Quarzan**®)
- dicyclomine (**Bentyl**®)
- ethopropazine (**Parsidol**®)
- glycopyrrolate (**Robinul**®)
- hexocyclium (**Tral**®)
- isopropamide (**Darbid**®)
- methantheline (**Banthine**®)
- methscopolamine (**Pamine**®)
- orphenadrine (**Disipal**®)
- oxyphencyclimine (**Daricon**®)
- propantheline (**Pro-Banthine**®)
- trihexyphenidyl (**Artane**®)

[used for gastrointestinal diseases, Parkinson's disease, and other disorders]

May lead to an enhanced anticholinergic effect, such as dry mouth, constipation, blurred vision, rapid heartbeat, and difficulty or inability to urinate.

| ANTIDEPRESSANT DRUG | INTERACTING DRUG | RESULT |
|---|---|---|

Tricyclic antidepressants:

- amitriptyline (**Elavil**®, **Endep**®)
- amoxapine (**Asendin**®)
- desipramine (**Pertofrane**®, **Norpramin**®)
- doxepin (**Adapin**®, **Sinequan**®)
- imipramine (**Janimine**®, **Tofranil**®)
- nortriptyline (**Aventyl**®, **Pamelor**®)
- protriptyline (**Vivactil**®)
- trimipramine (**Surmontil**®)

Barbiturates:

- amobarbital (**Amytal**®)
- butabarbital (**Butisol**®)
- butalbital
- pentobarbital (**Nembutal**®)
- phenobarbital (**Luminal**®, **Solfoton**®)
- primidone (**Mysoline**®)
- secobarbital (**Seconal**®), and others

[used to treat insomnia and anxiety; certain barbiturates are used to prevent seizures]

Decreased blood concentration of the tricyclic antidepressant, possibly leading to a reduced effect (i.e., inadequate control of depression).

Although studies have shown that barbiturates can decrease the effect of three specific tricyclic antidepressants (desipramine, nortriptyline, and protriptyline), other tricyclic antidepressants (see list at left) are expected to be affected similarly by barbiturates.

It may be necessary for your doctor to adjust the dose of an antidepressant if a barbiturate is started or stopped, or if its dosage is changed. (Do *not* change the dosage of either drug yourself; only your doctor should do this.)

Tricyclic antidepressants:

- amitriptyline (**Elavil**®, **Endep**®)
- amoxapine (**Asendin**®)
- desipramine (**Pertofrane**®, **Norpramin**®)
- doxepin (**Adapin**®, **Sinequan**®)

Epinephrine (**Adrenalin**®, **Ana-Kit**®, **AsthmaHaler**®, **Bronkaid**® Mist, **EpiPen**®, **Primatene**® Mist, **Sus-Phrine**®, and others)

[for temporary relief of shortness of breath, and wheezing caused by bronchial asthma; Ana-Kit® and EpiPen® are used for the emergency treatment of allergic reactions

Can lead to excessively high blood pressure levels, rapid heartbeat, or irregular heartbeat if the epinephrine is injected. This effect may also occur when epinephrine is injected into the subcutaneous tissues (e.g., for severe allergic reactions). Epinephrine that is inhaled or used as eye drops is probably less likely to interact unless excessive epinephrine doses are used.

Although this interaction has been shown to occur with imipramine

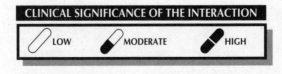

CLINICAL SIGNIFICANCE OF THE INTERACTION

LOW    MODERATE    HIGH

353

| ANTIDEPRESSANT DRUG | INTERACTING DRUG | RESULT |
|---|---|---|

*(cont.)*

Tricyclic antidepressants:

- imipramine (**Janimine**®, **Tofranil**®)
- nortriptyline (**Aventyl**®, **Pamelor**®)
- protriptyline (**Vivactil**®)
- trimipramine (**Surmontil**®)

Epinephrine

to insect stings or bites, food, and other substances that trigger a serious allergic reaction]

(Janimine®, Tofranil®), other tricyclic antidepressants are expected to act similarly when combined with epinephrine.

---

Tricyclic antidepressants:

- amitriptyline (**Elavil**®, **Endep**®)
- amoxapine (**Asendin**®)
- desipramine (**Pertofrane**®, **Norpramin**®)
- doxepin (**Adapin**®, **Sinequan**®)
- imipramine (**Janimine**®, **Tofranil**®)
- nortriptyline (**Aventyl**®, **Pamelor**®)
- protriptyline (**Vivactil**®)
- trimipramine (**Surmontil**®)

Guanethidine (**Ismelin**®)

[used to reduce high blood pressure]

May increase blood pressure due to reduced antihypertensive effect.

**Recommendation:** It may be necessary for your doctor to adjust the dose of guanethidine if a tricyclic antidepressant is started or stopped, or if its dosage is changed. (Of course, only your doctor should change medication dosages, when appropriate.)

| ANTIDEPRESSANT DRUG | INTERACTING DRUG | RESULT |
|---|---|---|

Tricyclic antidepressants:

- amitriptyline (**Elavil®, Endep®**)
- amoxapine (**Asendin®**)
- desipramine (**Pertofrane®, Norpramin®**)
- doxepin (**Adapin®, Sinequan®**)
- imipramine (**Janimine®, Tofranil®**)
- nortriptyline (**Aventyl®, Pamelor®**)
- protriptyline (**Vivactil®**)
- trimipramine (**Surmontil®**)

Monoamine oxidase inhibitors:

- isocarboxazid (**Marplan®**)
- phenelzine (**Nardil®**)
- tranylcypromine (**Parnate®**), and others

Caution is advised when taking a tricyclic antidepressant together with a monoamine oxidase (MAO) inhibitor. Reactions such as excitation, fever, agitated delirium, dizziness, mania, and convulsions have been reported in persons taking both of these classes of antidepressants together. These reactions occur much more often when a tricyclic medication is given to persons who are already taking an MAO drug.

**Recomendation:** The combination of MAO inhibitors and tricyclic antidepressants should be used only under special circumstances and by physicians experienced in the use of these types of antidepressants. Some experts feel that when this combination is used, imipramine and clomipramine should be avoided.

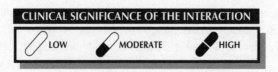

CLINICAL SIGNIFICANCE OF THE INTERACTION

LOW    MODERATE    HIGH

## CHAPTER 10

# ANTIANXIETY AND SLEEP-INDUCING DRUGS

## ˙Anxiety

Fear is a feeling experienced by all of us at times. Certain situations warrant a response of fear: seeing a car racing toward you, for instance, or being threatened by a mugger. Fear, in these cases, leads to a desirable physical effect—rapid heartbeat so more blood can be pumped to the brain for quick thinking and to the muscles for a speedy escape, if necessary. These responses are the body's way of preparing for anticipated danger.

In many circumstances, fear or worry, in moderate amounts, can be an excellent motivator. However, a persistent feeling of tension or fear, often when no concrete problem, stress, or danger can be identified, is known as *anxiety*. Once again, feelings of fear and distress elicit physical symptoms, such as shakiness, pounding heartbeat, restlessness, sweating, rapid breathing, lightheadedness, headache, and others. The intensity of these symptoms can vary greatly.

When the symptoms are particularly intense, often accompanied by a feeling of impending doom, the person is said to be suffering from *panic*. Because these typically brief episodes—called panic attacks—may be accompanied by symptoms such as palpitations, accelerated heart rate, chest pain, trembling, and shortness of breath, panic-attack sufferers sometimes mistakenly think they are having a heart attack.

When a fear is particularly intense and disproportionate to the object or circumstance that evokes it, the fear becomes a *phobia*. Persons who suffer from a phobia avoid the feared object or situation. The fear may be of a specific object or group of objects, such as spiders (arachnophobia), heights (acrophobia), or strangers (xenophobia).

Various anxiety-related conditions are well described by their names; for instance, "performance" anxiety is marked by extreme, often incapacitating, fear of performing an act, such as presenting a speech to an audience. "Situational" anxiety involves fear of a particular situation but only immediately before or during the event; on the other hand, "anticipatory" anxiety makes an individual anxious just thinking about the situation.

Obsessive-compulsive disorder is a particular type of anxiety disorder. Obsessions are unwanted, recurrent thoughts that intrude on a person's consciousness. Compulsions are repetitive behaviors performed intentionally, often in response to an obsession. Compulsive behavior typically involves a ritual that is repeated many times. Locking the doors to one's house or apartment is a reasonable behavior in many American neighborhoods; however, checking and rechecking them a dozen times to ensure they are locked is a compulsive ritual.

Individuals who feel anxious in the presence of dirt (real or imagined) may be affected by a cleaning ritual. Washing the hands excessively and spending several hours in the shower before one feels clean are examples of an obsessive-compulsive disorder.

# Medications Used to Treat Anxiety

Medications used to relieve anxiety are also called *anxiolytics* or *minor tranquilizers.* Your doctor will select an antianxiety agent based on several factors, such as your general health, family history, and particular type of anxiety disorder. The most commonly used antianxiety medication is a group of drugs known as *benzodiazepines.* (Some benzodiazepines are used to relieve insomnia, as described below.)

The benzodiazepines used to treat anxiety include alprazolam (Xanax®), chlordiazepoxide (Librium®), clorazepate (Tranxene®), diazepam (Valium®), halazepam (Paxipam®), lorazepam (Ativan®), oxazepam (Serax®), and prazepam (Centrax®). It's important to note that one particular benzodiazepine may work more effectively in a given person. A side effect sometimes associated with the use of benzodiazepines is oversedation, that is, a feeling of tiredness and grogginess.

Other drugs that are not benzodiazepines are also used to treat anxiety. One such drug is buspirone (BuSpar®). Although buspirone is unlikely to cause sedation, it does not act as rapidly as a benzodiazepine (it may take one to two weeks to exert an antianxiety effect). Also, the effectiveness of buspirone may be decreased in people who have previously taken benzodiazepines.[1]

Another antianxiety drug, meprobamate (Equanil®, Meprospan®, Miltown®), while still available, is no longer widely used since the advent of benzodiazepines. Clomipramine (Anafranil®) and fluoxetine (Prozac®) are drugs used to treat obsessive-compulsive disorder as well as panic disorder. Pharmacologically, clomipramine belongs to the same class of drug as many of the medications used to treat depression, that of the tricyclic antidepressants (see Chapter 9 for more information on tricyclic antidepressants). The monoamine oxidase (MAO) inhibitors have also been used effectively to treat panic disorder and a particular type of phobia, known as "social" phobia (a condition in which the individual experiences extreme discomfort in social situations).

# Sleep

A good night's sleep is another part of life that is often taken for granted. But for 35 million Americans who have *insomnia*—difficulty falling or staying asleep—a restful night of sleep is only a dream. Lack of sound sleep shows up in diminished physical and mental performance. Although insomnia is not usually thought of as a life-threatening condition, individuals who suffer from disturbed sleep are more likely to make more mistakes and be involved in—if not cause—more accidents than those who experience no such disorders.

Nearly everyone suffers from insomnia occasionally. It may be caused by a physical condition or by anxiety. Insomnia may be traced to too much nicotine, caffeine, or use of certain medications, such as thyroid preparations, theophylline, various antihypertensive agents, and others. Disturbance of the body's biological clock—as occurs with jet lag or a work-shift change—may lead to sleeplessness. When mild insomnia hits, most persons have their own way of finding a way to get to sleep—perhaps reading a book, watching television, or drinking a warm glass of milk. However, when your sleep-inducing techniques are not working and insomnia occurs repeatedly, you may need to see your doctor. Your doctor may prescribe sleeping pills for you, especially if the sleepless nights are beginning to interfere with your health or your ability to function during the day.

## Medications to Help You Sleep Better

Sleep-inducing drugs are known as *sedative-hypnotics.* Various over-the-counter as well as prescription products are available.

### Over-the-Counter Medications

Some common over-the-counter medications used to promote sleep are Nytol®, Sleep-ettes-D®, Sleep-eze-3®, Sleepinal®, Sominex®, and Unisom®. With the exception of Unisom®, the active ingredient in all of these products is the antihistamine diphenhydramine; Unisom®, which contains doxylamine, is also an antihistamine. Although antihistamines are usually promoted to relieve symptoms of allergy (diphenhydramine is the active ingredient in Benadryl®, for example), certain antihistamines induce drowsiness as an unwanted side effect. Diphenhydramine and doxylamine are highly sedating; thus, their usefulness as sleep-inducing agents. (To review other antihistamines, see Chapter 3.)

### Prescription Medications

Barbiturates are a group of prescription drugs used to treat insomnia. Although these drugs were commonly prescribed for insomnia in the past, they are used much less frequently today because the risk of addiction (a physical and psychological dependence to the medication) is high. Another drawback of barbiturate use is that high doses may lead to unwanted and dangerous adverse effects; too high a dose can be lethal. Furthermore, certain barbiturates may produce a "residual" effect: the desired drowsiness that a barbiturate elicits when taken at bedtime may persist into the next day.

Some of the barbiturates used include amobarbital (Amytal®), butabarbital (Butisol®), butalbital, pentobarbital (Nembutal®), phenobarbital (Luminal®, Solfoton®), primidone (Mysoline®), secobarbital (Seconal®), and others. Thiopental (Pentothal®) is a barbiturate that is given to persons by intravenous injection to induce a short period of sleep—about fifteen minutes—during which time brief surgical procedures can be performed.

Another drug used to relieve insomnia is chloral hydrate (Noctec®). This medication also relaxes persons who are tense and nervous. Chloral hydrate may make you feel lightheaded and unsteady on your feet. Other nonbarbiturate prescription hypnotic agents include ethchlorvynol (Placidyl®) and ethinamate (Valmid®), but these medications are rarely used today.

## Modern Prescription Hypnotics: The Benzodiazepines

The use of barbiturates and chloral hydrate as sleep-inducing drugs has waned considerably since the introduction of a family of drugs known as *benzodiazepines*. There are several medications in the benzodiazepine group; your doctor may select one appropriate for you. Benzodiazepine drugs used to relieve sleep disorders include estazolam (ProSom®), flurazepam (Dalmane®), quazepam (Doral®), temazepam (Restoril®), and triazolam (Halcion®). Some individuals taking certain benzodiazepines may experience daytime drowsiness; if this happens, be sure to tell your doctor, who may lower the dose of your medication or adjust your treatment to resolve this problem.

Benzodiazepine sleeping pills are often effective for only a few days; after that, the person may return to the same sleep pattern that was established before taking the sleeping pills. Therefore, sleeping pills are typically justified for only a temporary period in one's life, particularly when one is going through a highly emotional—but recognizably temporary—period, such as bereavement or hospitalization. If your doctor determines that you need a hypnotic for short-term insomnia for a slightly longer period of time, many sleep experts recommend using the smallest effective dose for the shortest necessary period of time.[2]

Do not stop taking prescription hypnotics without first checking with your doctor. Stopping certain medications abruptly may lead to symptoms of withdrawal, such as anxiety, shaking, and even difficulty falling asleep.[3] Your doctor may wish to reduce the dose gradually before stopping the drug.

A particular word of caution should be noted for alcohol. Do *not* take alcohol with any sleep-inducing medication. Such a combination increases the likelihood that you will experience severe drowsiness, decreased alertness (including re-duced ability to concentrate and think clearly), and slowed reaction time. This re-action may be very dangerous. Taking alcohol with a sedative-hypnotic could interfere with normal breathing and may lead to coma. This interaction may be fatal, so avoid alcohol while taking any sleep-inducing medication.

| ANTIANXIETY OR SLEEP DRUG | INTERACTING DRUG | RESULT |
| --- | --- | --- |

Alprazolam (**Xanax**®)

Alcohol

Alprazolam combined with alcohol may result in the enhanced effect of the alcohol, such as decreased alertness, an impaired ability to concentrate, dizziness, incoordination, forgetfulness, and drowsiness.

If either one or both agents is taken in large amounts, the combination can be very dangerous, leading to impaired breathing, coma, and, in severe cases, heart failure.

Individuals on this combination should be warned not to operate heavy machinery or drive a car.

**Recommendation:** Do not drink alcoholic beverages when taking alprazolam or any other benzodiazepine drug.

---

Alprazolam (**Xanax**®)

Cimetidine (**Tagamet**®)

[for relief of stomach and intestinal ulcers]

Cimetidine may increase the plasma concentration of alprazolam, which could lead to an increased effect as evidenced by decreased alertness, an impaired ability to concentrate, dizziness, incoordination, forgetfulness, and drowsiness.

**Recommendation:** If you must take a benzodiazepine (i.e., a type of drug such as alprazolam) for the treatment of anxiety while you are taking cimetidine, your doctor may need to monitor your response to the antianxiety medication more carefully than usual. Two antianxiety benzodiazepines that do not appear to be affected by cimetidine are lorazepam (Ativan®) and oxazepam (Serax®).

Another way to reduce the risk of this interaction is to use ranitidine (Zantac®) or famotidine (Pepcid®) rather than cimetidine; they are probably less likely to interact with benzodiazepines than cimetidine.

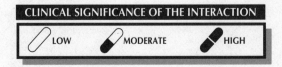

CLINICAL SIGNIFICANCE OF THE INTERACTION

LOW    MODERATE    HIGH

| ANTIANXIETY OR SLEEP DRUG | INTERACTING DRUG | RESULT |
|---|---|---|
| Alprazolam (**Xanax**®)  | Oral contraceptives; such as **Brevicon**®, **Demulen**®, **Enovid**®, **Lo/Ovral**®, **Norinyl**®, **Ortho Novum**®, **Ovcon**®, **Ovral**®, **Tri-Norinyl**®, **Triphasil**®, and many others<br><br>[for prevention of pregnancy] | Oral contraceptives may increase the concentration of alprazolam in the body, possibly leading to symptoms such as decreased alertness, an impaired ability to concentrate, dizziness, incoordination, forgetfulness, and drowsiness.<br><br>**Recommendation:** It may be necessary for your doctor to adjust the dose of alprazolam if oral contraceptives are started or stopped. |
| Barbiturates:<br>• amobarbital (**Amytal**®)<br>• butabarbital (**Butisol**®)<br>• butalbital<br>• pentobarbital (**Nembutal**®)<br>• phenobarbital (**Luminal**®, **Solfoton**®)<br>• primidone (**Mysoline**®)<br>• secobarbital (**Seconal**®), and others<br><br> | Acetaminophen (**Anacin-3**®, **Panadol**®, **Tempra**®, **Tylenol**®, and others); also found in many combination products. | In persons who regularly take barbiturates, the effect of the acetaminophen may be reduced. In addition, when too much acetaminophen is taken, this interaction may increase the likelihood of toxicity and the risk of liver damage. Symptoms of toxicity include nausea, vomiting, diarrhea, sweating, loss of appetite, and abdominal pain.<br><br>**Recommendation:** If you are taking barbiturates, be sure not to take more than the recommended amount of acetaminophen per day. It would also be wise to avoid taking acetaminophen for prolonged periods unless your doctor has advised you to do so. |
| Barbiturates:<br>• amobarbital (**Amytal**®)<br>• butabarbital (**Butisol**®)<br>• butalbital<br>• pentobarbital (**Nembutal**®)<br>• phenobarbital (**Luminal**®, **Solfoton**®)<br>• primidone (**Mysoline**®)<br>• secobarbital | Alcohol | Taken individually, barbiturates or alcohol may decrease alertness. Taken together, they have an additive effect; this means that they can cause severe drowsiness, decreased alertness (including a reduced ability to concentrate and think clearly), and slowed reaction time. Respiratory depression and coma may also occur.<br><br>This interaction is very dangerous; several fatalities have been reported. |

362

| ANTIANXIETY OR SLEEP DRUG | INTERACTING DRUG | RESULT |
|---|---|---|

(cont.)
**Barbiturates**
(**Seconal**®),
and others

Alcohol

Operating dangerous machinery (including driving a car) may be hazardous when taking this combination of medications.

**Recommendation:** Avoid drinking alcoholic beverages while taking barbiturates.

---

Barbiturates:

- amobarbital (**Amytal**®)
- butabarbital (**Butisol**®)
- butalbital
- pentobarbital (**Nembutal**®)
- phenobarbital (**Luminal**®, **Solfoton**®)
- primidone (**Mysoline**®)
- secobarbital (**Seconal**®), and others

Anticoagulants (oral), such as dicumarol and warfarin (**Coumadin**®, **Panwarfin**®)

[for the prevention of blood clots]

Barbiturates can accelerate the metabolism of certain oral anticoagulants, which leads to a decreased amount of the oral anticoagulant in the blood and a resultant decrease in therapeutic effect. Importantly, fatal bleeding has occurred in persons on oral anticoagulant therapy when they *stopped* taking their barbiturate (causing a significant increase in the amount of oral anticoagulant available in the body).

**Recommendation:** It is best to avoid this combination; discuss it with your doctor.

---

Barbiturates:

- amobarbital (**Amytal**®)
- butabarbital (**Butisol**®)
- butalbital

Central nervous system depressants, such as narcotics (e.g., codeine, morphine), antianxiety drugs, sleeping pills, and many antihistamines

Taking barbiturates and medications that depress the central nervous system may result in excessive drowsiness, decreased alertness (including a reduced ability to concentrate and think clearly), and slowed reaction time. Respiratory depression and

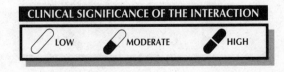

CLINICAL SIGNIFICANCE OF THE INTERACTION

LOW    MODERATE    HIGH

| ANTIANXIETY OR SLEEP DRUG | INTERACTING DRUG | RESULT |
|---|---|---|

*(cont.)*
Barbiturates:
- pentobarbital (**Nembutal**®)
- phenobarbital (**Luminal**®, **Solfoton**®)
- primidone (**Mysoline**®)
- secobarbital (**Seconal**®), and others

Central nervous system depressants

coma may also occur, depending on the doses of the drugs used.

Individuals with chronic lung disease are especially susceptible to respiratory depression.

Operating dangerous machinery (including driving a car) may be hazardous when taking this combination of medications.

**Recommendation:** Persons taking a barbiturate should avoid taking another central nervous system depressant unless instructed to do so by their doctor.

**Note**: (See also the entry on barbiturate-alcohol interaction, p. 362–63.)

---

Barbiturates:
- amobarbital (**Amytal**®)
- butabarbital (**Butisol**®)
- butalbital
- pentobarbital (**Nembutal**®)
- phenobarbital (**Luminal**®, **Solfoton**®)
- primidone (**Mysoline**®)
- secobarbital (**Seconal**®), and others

Chloramphenicol (**Chloromycetin**®)

[for the treatment of certain bacterial infections]

May increase the amount of barbiturate in the blood, increasing the risk of adverse effects (such as increased sedation).

In addition, barbiturates may reduce the amount of chloramphenicol in the blood, possibly decreasing the bacteria-fighting ability of chloramphenicol.

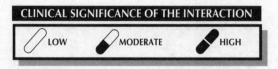

CLINICAL SIGNIFICANCE OF THE INTERACTION

LOW    MODERATE    HIGH

| ANTIANXIETY OR SLEEP DRUG | INTERACTING DRUG | RESULT |
|---|---|---|

Barbiturates:

- amobarbital (**Amytal**®)
- butabarbital (**Butisol**®)
- butalbital
- pentobarbital (**Nembutal**®)
- phenobarbital (**Luminal**®, **Solfoton**®)
- primidone (**Mysoline**®)
- secobarbital (**Seconal**®), and others

Corticosteroids:

- betamethasone (**Celestone**®)
- cortisone (**Cortone**®)
- dexamethasone (**Decadron**®, **Dalalone**®)
- hydrocortisone (**Cortef**®, **Hydrocortone**®, **Solu-Cortef**®)
- methylprednisolone (**Medrol**®, **Depo-Medrol**®, **Solu-Medrol**®)
- paramethasone (**Haldrone**®)
- prednisolone (**Delta-Cortef**®, **Hydeltrasol**®)
- prednisone (**Deltasone**®, **Liquid-Pred**®, **Meticorten**®)•
- triamcinolone (**Aristocort**®, **Kenacort**®, **Kenalog**®)

[for relieving inflammation and suppressing allergic reactions]

May cause a reduced amount of corticosteroid in the body, possibly leading to a decreased effect of the corticosteroid. This interaction has been shown to occur with the barbiturate phenobarbital (i.e., it decreases the effect of dexamethasone). Other barbiturates and other corticosteroid medications are expected to act similarly.

This interaction is not likely to be a problem if the corticosteroid is inhaled or applied locally to the skin, eye, ear, etc.

**Recommendation:** Your doctor may need to adjust the dose of your corticosteroid if a barbiturate is started or stopped.

---

Barbiturates:

- amobarbital (**Amytal**®)
- butabarbital (**Butisol**®)
- butalbital
- pentobarbital (**Nembutal**®)
- phenobarbital (**Luminal**®, **Solfoton**®)
- primidone (**Mysoline**®)
- secobarbital (**Seconal**®), and others

Cyclosporine (**Sandimmune**®)

[for the prevention of rejection in kidney, liver, and heart transplantation]

Phenobarbital may reduce the effect of the cyclosporine, thus increasing the risk of rejection of the transplanted organ. Although this interaction has been reported with phenobarbital, it probably occurs with other barbiturates as well.

If barbiturates cannot be avoided, it may be necessary for your doctor to adjust the dose of cyclosporine if a barbiturate is started or stopped, or if the dosage is changed. (Do *not* change the dosage of either drug yourself; only your doctor should do this.)

| ANTIANXIETY OR SLEEP DRUG | INTERACTING DRUG | RESULT |
|---|---|---|

Barbiturates:

- amobarbital (**Amytal**®)
- butabarbital (**Butisol**®)
- butalbital
- pentobarbital (**Nembutal**®)
- phenobarbital (**Luminal**®, **Solfoton**®)
- primidone (**Mysoline**®)
- secobarbital (**Seconal**®), and others

Digitoxin (**Crystodigin**®)

[for heart failure and other heart abnormalities]

Phenobarbital may reduce the amount of digitoxin in the blood, thereby reducing the effect of the digitoxin. (Other barbiturates are expected to act similarly.)

It may be necessary for your doctor to adjust the dose of digitoxin if a barbiturate is started or stopped, or if its dosage is changed. (Do *not* change the dosage of either drug yourself; only your doctor should do this.)

Barbiturates:

- amobarbital (**Amytal**®)
- butabarbital (**Butisol**®)
- butalbital
- pentobarbital (**Nembutal**®)
- phenobarbital (**Luminal**®, **Solfoton**®)
- primidone (**Mysoline**®)
- secobarbital (**Seconal**®), and others

Disopyramide (**Norpace**®, **Norpace CR**®)

[for arrhythmias, or irregularities of the heartbeat and heart rhythm]

Phenobarbital may decrease the effectiveness of disopyramide, even to the point of increasing the likelihood of arrhythmias occurring.

**Recommendation:** Your doctor should monitor the concentration of disopyramide (he or she does this with a blood test) when phenobarbital—or another barbiturate—is prescribed for you (or when you are told to stop taking a barbiturate).

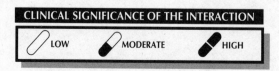

CLINICAL SIGNIFICANCE OF THE INTERACTION

LOW     MODERATE     HIGH

| ANTIANXIETY OR SLEEP DRUG | INTERACTING DRUG | RESULT |
|---|---|---|

Barbiturates:

- amobarbital (**Amytal**®)
- butabarbital (**Butisol**®)
- butalbital
- pentobarbital (**Nembutal**®)
- phenobarbital (**Luminal**®, **Solfoton**®)
- primidone (**Mysoline**®)
- secobarbital (**Seconal**®), and others

Meperidine (**Demerol**®, **Mepergan**®)

[for relief of moderate to severe pain]

Barbiturates may increase the sedative effect of merperidine, leading to prolonged sedation, dizziness, drowsiness, or visual disturbances. Although much of the documentation on this interaction has been done on one barbiturate in particular, phenobarbital, other barbiturates are likely to act in the same way.

Barbiturates:

- amobarbital (**Amytal**®)
- butabarbital (**Butisol**®)
- butalbital
- pentobarbital (**Nembutal**®)
- phenobarbital (**Luminal**®, **Solfoton**®)•
  primidone (**Mysoline**®)
- secobarbital (**Seconal**®), and others

Methadone (**Dolophine**®)

[used to relieve pain]

Barbiturates may cause the concentration of methadone in the blood to drop, possibly leading to a decreased effect of the methadone and sometimes to symptoms of methadone withdrawal.

| ANTIANXIETY OR SLEEP DRUG | INTERACTING DRUG | RESULT |
|---|---|---|

Barbiturates:

- amobarbital (**Amytal**®)
- butabarbital (**Butisol**®)
- butalbital
- pentobarbital (**Nembutal**®)
- phenobarbital (**Luminal**®, **Solfoton**®)
- primidone (**Mysoline**®)
- secobarbital (**Seconal**®), and others

Metoprolol (**Lopressor**®)

[for the treatment of high blood pressure]

Barbiturates may reduce the concentration of metoprolol, possibly leading to inadequate control of high blood pressure or a worsening of other disorders for which metoprolol is used.

It may be necessary for your doctor to adjust the dose of metoprolol if a barbiturate is started or stopped, or if its dosage is changed. (Of course, only your doctor should change medication dosages, when appropriate).

Barbiturates:

- amobarbital (**Amytal**®)
- butabarbital (**Butisol**®)
- butalbital
- pentobarbital (**Nembutal**®)
- phenobarbital (**Luminal**®, **Solfoton**®)
- primidone (**Mysoline**®)
- secobarbital (**Seconal**®), and others

Monoamine oxidase inhibitors:

- isocarboxazid (**Marplan**®)
- phenelzine (**Nardil**®)
- tranylcypromine (**Parnate**®), and others

[used to treat depression]

Antidepressants in the monoamine oxidase inhibitor class may prolong the effect of the barbiturate, causing the person to become oversedated. Although this interaction has been reported with one particular monoamine oxidase inhibitor (tranylcypromine) and one specific barbiturate (amobarbital), a similar effect may be seen with other combinations of MAO inhibitors and barbiturates.

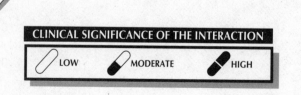

CLINICAL SIGNIFICANCE OF THE INTERACTION

LOW    MODERATE    HIGH

Barbiturates:

- amobarbital (**Amytal**®)
- butabarbital (**Butisol**®)
- butalbital
- pentobarbital (**Nembutal**®)
- phenobarbital (**Luminal**®, **Solfoton**®)
- primidone (**Mysoline**®)
- secobarbital (**Seconal**®), and others

Nifedipine (**Adalat**®, **Procardia**®)

[for the treatment of angina and high blood pressure]

Barbiturates may cause a significant decrease in the amount of nifedipine available in the body, possibly leading to a decreased effect of the nifedipine. This effect is particularly likely when nifedipine is taken orally.

Much of the evidence for this interaction comes from studies of phenobarbital, but other barbiturates are expected to interact similarly.

Persons receiving a barbiturate may require higher than usual doses of nifedipine. (Of course, *never* alter the dosage of any medication without your doctor's consent and supervision.)

Barbiturates:

- amobarbital (**Amytal**®)
- butabarbital (**Butisol**®)
- butalbital
- pentobarbital (**Nembutal**®)
- phenobarbital (**Luminal**®, **Solfoton**®)
- primidone (**Mysoline**®)
- secobarbital (**Seconal**®), and others

Oral contraceptives, such as **Brevicon**®, **Demulen**®, **Enovid**®, **Lo/Ovral**®, **Norinyl**®, **Ortho Novum**®, **Ovcon**®, **Ovral**®, **Tri-Norinyl**®, **Triphasil**®, and many others

[for prevention of pregnancy]

Barbiturates may reduce the effectiveness of estrogen-containing oral contraceptives, possibly leading to unintended pregnancy.

Spotting and breakthrough bleeding may be an indication that the oral contraceptive is working at a reduced capacity, although the absence of such menstrual irregularities does not ensure that the oral contraceptive is working.

**Recommendation:** Women taking a barbiturate who wish to avoid becoming pregnant should check with their doctor. Another method of contraception instead of or in addition to an oral contraceptive may be necessary. Or, your doctor may need to adjust the dose of the oral contraceptive in order to overcome the effect of the barbiturate. Of course, only your doctor should make such a dosage adjustment. Similarly, if you are taking an oral contraceptive and a barbiturate is prescribed for you for short-term use, it would be prudent to use alternative

| ANTIANXIETY OR SLEEP DRUG | INTERACTING DRUG | RESULT |
|---|---|---|

(*cont.*)
Barbiturates

Oral contraceptives

methods of contraception in addition to the oral contraceptive during, and for several weeks after, barbiturate use.

---

Barbiturates:

- amobarbital (**Amytal**®)
- butabarbital (**Butisol**®)
- butalbital
- pentobarbital (**Nembutal**®)
- phenobarbital (**Luminal**®, **Solfoton**®)
- primidone (**Mysoline**®)
- secobarbital (**Seconal**®), and others

Propranolol (**Inderal**®)

[for the treatment of high blood pressure]

Barbiturates may reduce the amount of propranolol in the blood, possibly leading to reduced propranolol effect (i.e., inadequate control of blood pressure or worsening of other conditions for which propranolol is used).

Although this interaction has occurred with the barbiturate phenobarbital, other barbiturates are expected to have a similar effect on propranolol.

It may be necessary for your doctor to adjust the dose of propranolol if a barbiturate is started or stopped, or if its dosage is changed. (Of course, only your doctor should change medication dosages, when appropriate.)

---

Barbiturates:

- amobarbital (**Amytal**®)
- butabarbital (**Butisol**®)
- butalbital
- pentobarbital (**Nembutal**®)
- phenobarbital (**Luminal**®, **Solfoton**®)
- primidone (**Mysoline**®)
- secobarbital (**Seconal**®), and others

Quinidine (**Cardioquin**®, **Duraquin**®, **Quinaglute**®, **Quinidex**®, **Quinora**®)

[for arrhythmias, or irregularities of the heartbeat and heart rhythm]

Barbiturates may reduce the amount of quinidine in the blood, possibly leading to decreased effectiveness of quinidine.

Your doctor may need to change the dose of quinidine if he or she prescribes a barbiturate for you or discontinues you from barbiturate therapy. (Do *not* change the dosage of either drug yourself; only your doctor should do this.)

| ANTIANXIETY OR SLEEP DRUG | INTERACTING DRUG | RESULT |
|---|---|---|

Barbiturates:

- amobarbital (**Amytal**®)
- butabarbital (**Butisol**®)
- butalbital
- pentobarbital (**Nembutal**®)
- phenobarbital (**Luminal**®, **Solfoton**®)
- primidone (**Mysoline**®)
- secobarbital (**Seconal**®), and others

Theophylline (**Theo-Dur**®, **Theo-24**®, **Slo-bid**®, **Slo-Phyllin**®, **Uniphyl**®, and others)

[for relief of asthma]

Barbiturates may reduce the effectiveness of theophylline.

It may be necessary for your doctor to adjust the dose of theophylline if a barbiturate is started or stopped, or if its dosage is changed. (Of course, only your doctor should change medication dosages, when appropriate.)

---

Barbiturates:

- amobarbital (**Amytal**®)
- butabarbital (**Butisol**®)
- butalbital
- pentobarbital (**Nembutal**®)
- phenobarbital (**Luminal**®, **Solfoton**®)
- primidone (**Mysoline**®)
- secobarbital (**Seconal**®), and others

Tricyclic antidepressants:

- amitriptyline (**Elavil**®, **Endep**®)
- amoxapine (**Asendin**®)
- desipramine (**Pertofrane**®, **Norpramin**®)
- doxepin (**Adapin**®, **Sinequan**®)
- imipramine (**Janimine**®, **Tofranil**®)
- nortriptyline (**Aventyl**®, **Pamelor**®)
- protriptyline (**Vivactil**®)
- trimipramine (**Surmontil**®)

[for treatment of depression]

Decreased blood concentration of the tricyclic antidepressant, possibly leading to a reduced effect (i.e., inadequate control of depression).

Although studies have shown that barbiturates can decrease the effect of three specific tricyclic antidepressants (desipramine, nortriptyline, and protriptyline), other tricyclic antidepressants (see list at left) are expected to be affected similarly by barbiturates.

It may be necessary for your doctor to adjust the dose of an antidepressant if a barbiturate is started or stopped, or if its dosage is changed. (Do *not* change the dosage of either drug yourself; only your doctor should do this.)

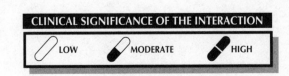

CLINICAL SIGNIFICANCE OF THE INTERACTION

LOW          MODERATE          HIGH

| ANTIANXIETY OR SLEEP DRUG | INTERACTING DRUG | RESULT |
|---|---|---|

Barbiturates:

- amobarbital (**Amytal**®)
- butabarbital (**Butisol**®)
- butalbital
- pentobarbital (**Nembutal**®)
- phenobarbital (**Luminal**®, **Solfoton**®)
- primidone (**Mysoline**®)
- secobarbital (**Seconal**®), and others

Verapamil (**Calan**®, **Isoptin**®)

[for the treatment of angina and high blood pressure]

Phenobarbital (and probably other barbiturates) substantially reduces the plasma concentration of verapamil, possibly leading to a reduced effect of this antihypertensive. This effect is particularly likely when verapamil is taken orally.

Persons receiving phenobarbital or other barbiturates may require higher than usual doses of verapamil. (Of course *never* alter the dosage of any medication without your doctor's consent and supervision.)

---

Chloral hydrate (**Noctec**®)

Alcohol

Chloral hydrate taken alone often results in reduced alertness. Taken with alcohol, this combination results in a severe reduction in alertness. This combination also may lead to a reduced ability to concentrate, dizziness, incoordination, forgetfulness, and drowsiness.

**Recommendation:** Do not drink alcoholic beverages when taking chloral hydrate.

| ANTIANXIETY OR SLEEP DRUG | INTERACTING DRUG | RESULT |
|---|---|---|

Chloral hydrate
(**Noctec**®)

Warfarin (**Coumadin**®, **Panwarfin**®)

[for the prevention of blood clots]

Chloral hydrate may result in a temporary increase in the anticoagulant effect. Your doctor may wish to use a sleep-inducing drug other than chloral hydrate. If chloral hydrate is used with warfarin, the increased anti-coagulant effect usually lasts only for the first several days of chloral hydrate use.

Chlordiazepoxide
(**Librium**®)

Alcohol

Enhanced effect of the alcohol, such as decreased alertness, an impaired ability to concentrate, dizziness, incoordination, forgetfulness, and drowsiness.

If either one or both agents is taken in large amounts, the combination can be very dangerous (e.g., impaired breathing, coma, and, in severe cases, heart failure).

Individuals on this combination should be warned not to operate heavy machinery, including driving a car.

**Recommendation:** Do not drink alcoholic beverages when taking chlordiazepoxide or any other benzodiazepine drug.

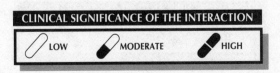

CLINICAL SIGNIFICANCE OF THE INTERACTION

LOW    MODERATE    HIGH

| ANTIANXIETY OR SLEEP DRUG | INTERACTING DRUG | RESULT |
|---|---|---|

Chlordiazepoxide (**Librium**®)

Cimetidine (**Tagamet**®)

[for relief of stomach and intestinal ulcers]

Cimetidine may increase the plasma concentration of chlordiazepoxide, which could lead to an increased effect as evidenced by decreased alertness, an impaired ability to concentrate, dizziness, incoordination, forgetfulness, and drowsiness.

This interaction may be more severe in elderly persons or in individuals with liver disease, who are more sensitive to the action of chlordiazepoxide.

**Recommendation:** If you must take a benzodiazepine (i.e., a type of drug such as chlordiazepoxide) for the treatment of anxiety while you are taking cimetidine, your doctor may need to monitor your response to the antianxiety medication more carefully than usual. Two antianxiety benzodiazepines that do not appear to be affected by cimetidine are lorazepam (Ativan®) and oxazepam (Serax®).

Another way to reduce the risk of this interaction is to use ranitidine (Zantac®) or famotidine (Pepcid®) rather than cimetidine; they are probably less likely to interact with benzodiazepines than cimetidine.

Chlordiazepoxide (**Librium**®)

Ketoconazole (**Nizoral**®)

[used to treat fungal infections]

Ketoconazole may increase the amount of chlordiazepoxide in the blood, possibly enhancing the sedative effect of chlordiazepoxide. This enhanced effect could lead to decreased alertness, an impaired ability to concentrate, forgetfulness, and drowsiness.

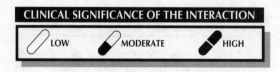

CLINICAL SIGNIFICANCE OF THE INTERACTION

LOW    MODERATE    HIGH

| ANTIANXIETY OR SLEEP DRUG | INTERACTING DRUG | RESULT |
|---|---|---|

Chlordiazepoxide (**Librium**®)

Oral contraceptives, such as **Brevicon**®, **Demulen**®, **Enovid**®, **Lo/Ovral**®, **Norinyl**®, **Ortho Novum**®, **Ovcon**®, **Ovral**®, **Tri-Norinyl**®, **Triphasil**®, and many others

[for prevention of pregnancy]

Oral contraceptives may increase the concentration of chlordiazepoxide in the body, possibly leading to symptoms such as decreased alertness, an impaired ability to concentrate, dizziness, incoordination, forgetfulness, and drowsiness.

**Recommendation:** It may be necessary for your doctor to adjust the dose of chlordiazepoxide if oral contraceptives are started or stopped.

Clorazepate (**Tranxene**®)

Alcohol

Enhanced effect of the alcohol, such as decreased alertness, an impaired ability to concentrate, dizziness, incoordination, forgetfulness, and drowsiness.

If either one or both agents is taken in large amounts, the combination can be very dangerous, leading to impaired breathing, coma, and, in severe cases, heart failure.

Individuals on this combination should be warned not to operate heavy machinery or drive a car.

**Recommendation:** Do not drink alcoholic beverages when taking clorazepate or any other benzodiazepine drug.

Clorazepate (**Tranxene**®)

Cimetidine (**Tagamet**®)

[for relief of stomach and intestinal ulcers]

Cimetidine may increase the plasma concentration of clorazepate, which could lead to an increased effect, such as decreased alertness, an impaired ability to concentrate, forgetfulness, and drowsiness.

This interaction may be more severe in elderly persons, who are more sensitive to the action of clorazepate.

**Recommendation:** If you must take a benzodiazepine (i.e., a type of drug such as clorazepate) for the treatment of anxiety while you are taking cimetidine, your doctor may need to monitor your response to the antianxiety

| ANTIANXIETY OR SLEEP DRUG | INTERACTING DRUG | RESULT |
|---|---|---|

*(cont.)*

| Clorazepate | Cimetidine | medication more carefully than usual. Two antianxiety benzodiazepines that do not appear to be affected by cimetidine are lorazepam (Ativan®) and oxazepam (Serax®). |
|---|---|---|

Another way to reduce the risk of this interaction is to use ranitidine (Zantac®) or famotidine (Pepcid®) rather than cimetidine; they are probably less likely to interact with benzodiazepines than cimetidine.

| Clorazepate (**Tranxene®**) | Rifampin (**Rifadin®, Rimactane®**) | Rifampin may decrease the effect of clorazepate (i.e., inadequately control the anxiety). |
|---|---|---|

[used in combination with at least one other drug, rifampin is used to treat tuberculosis; also used in the treatment of individuals who are carriers of meningitis]

| Diazepam (**Valium®**) | Alcohol | Enhanced effect of the alcohol, such as decreased alertness, an impaired ability to concentrate, dizziness, incoordination, forgetfulness, and, drowsiness. |
|---|---|---|

If either one or both agents is taken in large amounts, the combination can be very dangerous, leading to impaired breathing, coma, and, in severe cases, heart failure.

Individuals on this combination should be warned not to operate heavy machinery or drive a car.

**Recommendation:** Do not drink alcoholic beverages when taking diazepam or any other benzodiazepine drug.

| ANTIANXIETY OR SLEEP DRUG | INTERACTING DRUG | RESULT |
|---|---|---|

Diazepam (**Valium**®)

Cimetidine (**Tagamet**®)

[for relief of stomach and intestinal ulcers]

Cimetidine may increase the plasma concentration of diazepam, which could lead to an increased effect as evidenced by decreased alertness, an impaired ability to concentrate, dizziness, incoordination, forgetfulness, and drowsiness.

This interaction may be more severe in elderly persons or in individuals with liver disease, who are more sensitive to the action of diazepam.

**Recommendation:** If you must take a benzodiazepine (a type of drug such as diazepam) for the treatment of anxiety while you are taking cimetidine, your doctor may need to monitor your response to the antianxiety medication more carefully than usual. Two antianxiety benzodiazepines that do not appear to be affected by cimetidine are lorazepam (Ativan®) and oxazepam (Serax®).

Another way to reduce the risk of this interaction is to use ranitidine (Zantac®) or famotidine (Pepcid®) rather than cimetidine; they are probably less likely to interact with benzodiazepines than cimetidine.

Diazepam (**Valium**®)

Isoniazid (**INH**®)

[used to treat tuberculosis]

Isoniazid may increase the amount of diazepam in the blood, possibly leading to drowsiness, impaired ability to concentrate, and forgetfulness.

Little is known regarding the effect of isoniazid on other drugs in the same class as diazepam, known as benzodiazepines.

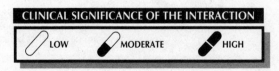

CLINICAL SIGNIFICANCE OF THE INTERACTION

LOW    MODERATE    HIGH

Diazepam (**Valium**®)

Oral contraceptives, such as **Brevicon**®, **Demulen**®, **Enovid**®, **Lo/Ovral**®, **Norinyl**®, **Ortho Novum**®, **Ovcon**®, **Ovral**®, **Tri-Norinyl**®, **Triphasil**®, and many others

[for prevention of pregnancy]

Oral contraceptives may increase the concentration of diazepam in the body, possibly leading to decreased alertness, an impaired ability to concentrate, forgetfulness, and drowsiness.

**Recommendation:** It may be necessary for your doctor to adjust the dose of diazepam if oral contraceptives are started or stopped. (Do *not* change the dosage of either drug yourself; only your doctor should do this.)

---

Diazepam (**Valium**®)

Rifampin (**Rifadin**®, **Rifamate**®, **Rimactane**®)

[used in combination with at least one other drug, rifampin is used to treat tuberculosis; also used in the treatment of individuals who are carriers of meningitis]

Rifampin may lower the concentration of diazepam in the body, possibly leading to a decreased effect (i.e., inadequately control the anxiety). Diazepam is in a drug class known as benzodiazepines. The same interaction may occur when using rifampin with certain other benzodiazepines, specifically clorazepate (Tranxene®), halazepam (Paxipam®), and prazepam (Centrax®).

---

Estazolam (**ProSom**®)

Alcohol

Enhanced effect of the alcohol, such as decreased alertness, an impaired ability to concentrate, dizziness, incoordination, forgetfulness, and drowsiness.

If either one or both agents is taken in large amounts, the combination can be very dangerous, leading to impaired breathing, coma, and, in severe cases, heart failure.

Individuals on this combination should be warned not to operate heavy machinery or drive a car.

**Recommendation:** Do not drink alcoholic beverages when taking estazolam or any other benzodiazepine drug.

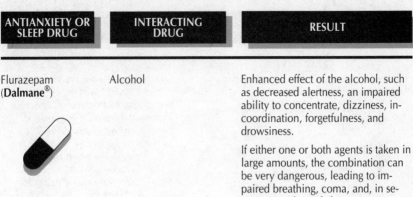

| | | |
| --- | --- | --- |
| Flurazepam (**Dalmane**®)  | Alcohol | Enhanced effect of the alcohol, such as decreased alertness, an impaired ability to concentrate, dizziness, incoordination, forgetfulness, and drowsiness. |

If either one or both agents is taken in large amounts, the combination can be very dangerous, leading to impaired breathing, coma, and, in severe cases, heart failure.
Individuals on this combination should be warned not to operate heavy machinery or drive a car.

**Recommendation:** Do not drink alcoholic beverages when taking flurazepam or any other benzodiazepine drug.

| | | |
| --- | --- | --- |
| Flurazepam (**Dalmane**®)  | Cimetidine (**Tagamet**®) [for relief of stomach and intestinal ulcers] | Cimetidine may cause an increased amount of flurazepam in the blood, possibly leading to increased sedation, decreased alertness, an impaired ability to concentrate, forgetfulness, and drowsiness. |

This interaction may be more severe in elderly persons.

**Recommendation:** If you must take cimetidine and a sleeping pill, temazepam (Restoril®) does not appear to be affected by cimetidine. Another alternative is to use the antiulcer drug ranitidine (Zantac®) or famotidine (Pepcid®) rather than cimetidine; they appear to be less likely to interact with benzodiazepines, such as flurazepam, than cimetidine.

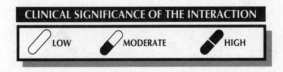

CLINICAL SIGNIFICANCE OF THE INTERACTION

LOW     MODERATE     HIGH

| ANTIANXIETY OR SLEEP DRUG | INTERACTING DRUG | RESULT |
|---|---|---|

Halazepam
(**Paxipam**®)

Rifampin (**Rifadin**®, **Rimactane**®)

[used in combination with at least one other drug, rifampin is used to treat tuberculosis; also used in the treatment of individuals who are carriers of meningitis]

Rifampin may lower the concentration of halazepam in the body, possibly leading to a decreased effect (i.e., inadequately control the anxiety). Halazepam is in a drug class known as benzodiazepines. The same interaction may occur when using rifampin with certain other benzodiazepines, specifically clorazepate (Tranxene®), diazepam (Valium®), and prazepam (Centrax®).

---

Lorazepam
(**Ativan**®)

Alcohol

Enhanced effect of the alcohol, such as decreased alertness, an impaired ability to concentrate, dizziness, incoordination, forgetfulness, and drowsiness.

If either one or both agents is taken in large amounts, the combination can be very dangerous, leading to impaired breathing, coma, and, in severe cases, heart failure.

Individuals on this combination should be warned not to operate heavy machinery or drive a car.

**Recommendation:** Do not drink alcoholic beverages when taking lorazepam or any other benzodiazepine drug.

---

Lorazepam
(**Ativan**®)

Oral contraceptives, such as **Brevicon**®, **Demulen**®, **Enovid**®, **Lo/Ovral**®, **Norinyl**®, **Ortho Novum**®, **Ovcon**®, **Ovral**®, **Tri-Norinyl**®, **Triphasil**®, and many others.

[for prevention of pregnancy]

Oral contraceptives may decrease the concentration of lorazepam in the body, possibly leading to a decreased effect (i.e., increased anxiety and agitation).

**Recommendation:** It may be necessary for your doctor to adjust the dose of lorazepam if oral contraceptives are started or stopped.

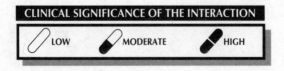

CLINICAL SIGNIFICANCE OF THE INTERACTION

LOW    MODERATE    HIGH

380

| ANTIANXIETY OR SLEEP DRUG | INTERACTING DRUG | RESULT |
|---|---|---|
| Meprobamate (**Equagesic**®, **Equanil**®, **Miltown**®) | Alcohol | Enhanced depression of the central nervous system, symptoms of which decreased alertness, an impaired ability to concentrate, dizziness, incoordination, forgetfulness, and drowsiness.<br><br>If either one or both agents is taken in large amounts, the combination can be very dangerous, leading to impaired breathing, coma, and, in severe cases, heart failure.<br><br>Individuals on this combination should be warned not to operate heavy machinery or drive a car.<br><br>**Recommendation:** Do not drink alcoholic beverages when taking meprobamate. |
| Oxazepam (**Serax**®) | Alcohol | Enhanced effect of the alcohol, such as decreased alertness, an impaired ability to concentrate, dizziness, incoordination, forgetfulness, and drowsiness.<br><br>If either one or both agents is taken in large amounts, the combination can be very dangerous, leading to impaired breathing, coma, and, in severe cases, heart failure.<br><br>Individuals on this combination should be warned not to operate heavy machinery or drive a car.<br><br>**Recommendation:** Do not drink alcoholic beverages when taking oxazepam or any other benzodiazepine drug. |
| Oxazepam (**Serax**®) | Oral contraceptives, such as **Brevicon**®, **Demulen**®, **Enovid**®, **Lo/Ovral**®, **Norinyl**®, **Ortho Novum**®, **Ovcon**®, **Ovral**®, **Tri-Norinyl**®, **Triphasil**®, and many others<br><br>[for prevention of pregnancy] | Oral contraceptives may decrease the concentration of oxazepam in the body, possibly leading to a decreased effect (i.e., increased anxiety and agitation).<br><br>**Recommendation:** It may be necessary for your doctor to adjust the dose of oxazepam if oral contraceptives are started or stopped. |

| ANTIANXIETY OR SLEEP DRUG | INTERACTING DRUG | RESULT |
|---|---|---|
| Phenobarbital (**Luminal®, Solfoton®**) | Griseofulvin (**Fulvicin® P/G, Grisactin®, and Gris-PEG®**)<br><br>[used to treat fungal infections] | Phenobarbital may reduce blood concentrations of griseofulvin, but it is not known how much this reduction inhibits the antifungal effect of griseofulvin. Not much is known about the effect of other barbiturates (e.g., amibarbital, pentobarbital, secobarbital) on griseofulvin, but they may have the same effect.<br><br>Your doctor may decide to use larger doses of griseofulvin if you are taking phenobarbital. (Do *not* change the dosage of either drug yourself; only your doctor should do this.) |
| Phenobarbital (**Luminal®, Solfoton®**) | Lidocaine (**Xylocaine®, Anestacon®**, and others)<br><br>[used to treat abnormal heart rhythms; for topical anesthesia during minor surgery; also available as an over-the-counter medication for relief of pain, itching, and inflammation, but such topical use is unlikely to interact with phenobarbital] | Phenobarbital may reduce the effectiveness of lidocaine; your doctor may need to use a slightly larger dose of lidocaine in the presence of phenobarbital. (Of course, only your doctor should alter the dosage of any medication.)<br><br>Other barbiturates may have a similar effect on lidocaine. |
| Phenobarbital (**Luminal®, Solfoton®**) | Primidone (**Mysoline®**)<br><br>[for the control of grand mal and other epileptic seizures] | This combination may result in excessive phenobarbital levels in the blood (a considerable portion of primidone is converted in the body to phenobarbital). Symptoms of high phenobarbital levels include sleepiness, lethargy, and sometimes rapid, involuntary eye movements and incoordination when walking.<br><br>**Recommendation:** It is usually best to avoid this combination. If these drugs are used together, you should be monitored for excessive phenobarbital levels. |

**CLINICAL SIGNIFICANCE OF THE INTERACTION**

LOW        MODERATE        HIGH

| | | |
|---|---|---|
| Phenobarbital (**Luminal®, Solfoton®**) | Valproic acid (**Depakene®**) [for treatment of various types of seizures] | Several studies have shown that this combination can lead to excessively high levels of phenobarbital, even to the point of phenobarbital toxicity (symptoms of which include excessive sedation, lethargy, and sometimes rapid, involuntary eye movements and incoordination when walking). |
| Prazepam (**Centrax®**) | Alcohol | Enhanced effect of the alcohol, such as decreased alertness, an impaired ability to concentrate, dizziness, incoordination, forgetfulness, and drowsiness. |

Prazepam (**Centrax®**) / Alcohol (continued):

If either one or both agents is taken in large amounts, the combination can be very dangerous, leading to impaired breathing, coma, and, in severe cases, heart failure.

Individuals on this combination should be warned not to operate heavy machinery or drive a car.

**Recommendation:** Do not drink alcoholic beverages when taking prazepam or any other benzodiazepine drug.

| | | |
|---|---|---|
| Prazepam (**Centrax®**) | Cimetidine (**Tagamet®**) [for relief of stomach and intestinal ulcers] | Cimetidine may increase the plasma concentration of prazepam, which could lead to an increased effect as evidenced by decreased alertness, an impaired ability to concentrate, dizziness, incoordination, forgetfulness, and drowsiness. |

This interaction may be more severe in elderly persons, who are more sensitive to the action of prazepam.

**Recommendation:** If you must take a benzodiazepine (i.e., a type of drug such as prazepam) for the treatment of anxiety while you are taking cimetidine, your doctor may need to monitor your response to the antianxiety medication more carefully than usual. Two antianxiety benzodiazepines that do not appear to be affected by cimetidine are lorazepam (Ativan®) and oxazepam (Serax®).

(cont.)
Prazepam | Cimetidine | Another way to reduce the risk of this interaction is to use ranitidine (Zantac®) or famotidine (Pepcid®) rather than cimetidine; they are probably less likely to interact with benzodiazepines than cimetidine.

Prazepam (**Centrax**®)

Rifampin (**Rifadin**®, **Rimactane**®)

[used in combination with at least one other drug, rifampin is used to treat tuberculosis; also used in the treatment of individuals who are carriers of meningitis]

Rifampin may decrease the effect of prazepam (i.e., inadequately control the anxiety). Prazepam is in a drug class known as benzodiazepines. The same interaction may occur when using rifampin with certain other benzodiazepines, specifically clorazepate (Tranxene®), diazepam (Valium®), and halazepam (Paxipam®).

Quazepam (**Doral**®)

Alcohol

Enhanced effect of the alcohol, such as decreased alertness, an impaired ability to concentrate, dizziness, incoordination, forgetfulness, and drowsiness.

If either one or both agents is taken in large amounts, the combination can be very dangerous, leading to impaired breathing, coma, and, in severe cases, heart failure.

Individuals on this combination should be warned not to operate heavy machinery or drive a car.

**Recommendation:** Do not drink alcoholic beverages when taking quazepam or any other benzodiazepine drug.

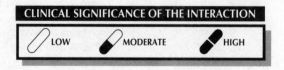

CLINICAL SIGNIFICANCE OF THE INTERACTION

LOW  MODERATE  HIGH

| ANTIANXIETY OR SLEEP DRUG | INTERACTING DRUG | RESULT |
|---|---|---|
| Temazepam (**Restoril**®) | Alcohol | Enhanced effect of the alcohol, such as decreased alertness, an impaired ability to concentrate, dizziness, incoordination, forgetfulness, and drowsiness. |
| | | If either one or both agents is taken in large amounts, the combination can be very dangerous, leading to impaired breathing, coma, and, in severe cases, heart failure. |
| | | Individuals on this combination should be warned not to operate heavy machinery or drive a car. |
| | | **Recommendation:** Do not drink alcoholic beverages when taking temazepam or any other benzodiazepine drug. |
| Temazepam (**Restoril**®) | Oral contraceptives, such as **Brevicon**®, **Demulen**®, **Enovid**®, **Lo/Ovral**®, **Norinyl**®, **Ortho Novum**®, **Ovcon**®, **Ovral**®, **Tri-Norinyl**®, **Triphasil**®, and many others<br><br>[for prevention of pregnancy] | Oral contraceptives may decrease the concentration of temazepam in the blood, possibly leading to a decreased effect of temazepam (i.e., sleeplessness). |
| Triazolam (**Halcion**®) | Alcohol | Enhanced effect of the alcohol, such as decreased alertness, an impaired ability to concentrate, dizziness, incoordination, forgetfulness, and drowsiness. |
| | | If either one or both agents is taken in large amounts, the combination can be very dangerous, leading to impaired breathing, coma, and, in severe cases, heart failure. |
| | | Individuals on this combination should be warned not to operate heavy machinery or drive a car. |
| | | **Recommendation:** Do not drink alcoholic beverages when taking triazolam or any other benzodiazepine drug. |

| ANTIANXIETY OR SLEEP DRUG | INTERACTING DRUG | RESULT |
|---|---|---|

Triazolam
(**Halcion**®)

Cimetidine (**Tagamet**®)

[for relief of stomach and intestinal ulcers]

Cimetidine may cause an increased amount of triazolam in the blood, possibly leading to increased sedation, decreased alertness, an impaired ability to concentrate, forgetfulness, and drowsiness.

This interaction may be more severe in elderly persons who are more sensitive to the action of triazolam.

**Recommendation:** If you must take cimetidine and a sleeping pill, temazepam (Restoril®) does not appear to be affected by cimetidine. Another alternative is to use the antiulcer drug ranitidine (Zantac®) or famotidine (Pepcid®) rather than cimetidine; they appear to be less likely to interact with triazolam than cimetidine.

Triazolam
(**Halcion**®)

Erythromycin (**E-Mycin**®, **Erythrocin**®, **Ilosone**®, **Wyamycin**®, and others)

[for treatment of various bacterial infections, such as pneumonia and infections of the ear and throat]

This combination can lead to a substantial increase in the concentration of triazolam in the blood, possibly increasing its sedative effect, which could lead to drowsiness, impaired ability to concentrate, and forgetfulness.

**Recommendation:** Your doctor may need to reduce your dose of triazolam when erythromycin is taken concurrently. (Of course, *never* alter the dosage of any medication without your doctor's consent and supervision.)

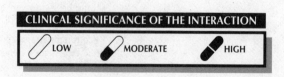

CLINICAL SIGNIFICANCE OF THE INTERACTION

LOW    MODERATE    HIGH

| ANTIANXIETY OR SLEEP DRUG | INTERACTING DRUG | RESULT |
| --- | --- | --- |
| Triazolam (**Halcion**®)  | Isoniazid (**INH**®) [used to treat tuberculosis] | Isoniazid may increase the amount of triazolam in the blood, possibly leading to drowsiness, impaired ability to concentrate, and forgetfulness. Little is known regarding the effect of isoniazid on other drugs in the same class as triazolam, known as benzodiazepines. |
| Triazolam (**Halcion**®)  | Oral contraceptives, such as **Brevicon**®, **Demulen**®, **Enovid**®, **Lo/Ovral**®, **Norinyl**®, **Ortho Novum**®, **Ovcon**®, **Ovral**®, **Tri-Norinyl**®, **Triphasil**®, and many others [for prevention of pregnancy] | Oral contraceptives may increase the concentration of triazolam in the blood, possibly leading to decreased alertness, an impaired ability to concentrate, forgetfulness, and drowsiness. |
| Triazolam (**Halcion**®) | Troleandomycin (**TAO**®) [for treatment of various bacterial infections, such as pneumonia and streptococcal infections of the throat] | Taking triazolam together with troleanadomycin can cause a substantial increase in the concentration of triazolam in the blood, leading to drowsiness, impaired ability to concentrate, and forgetfulness. |

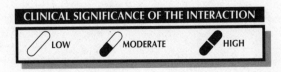

CLINICAL SIGNIFICANCE OF THE INTERACTION

LOW    MODERATE    HIGH

387

# NOTES

Chapter 2

1. Lecos, C. W. "Still a Killer: Pneumonia Targets the Ill, the Elderly." FDA Consumer 1987; 21(5):8–13.

2. National Center for Health Statistics, 1985.

3. Snider, S. "How to Take Your Medicine: Penicillin." FDA Consumer 1990; 24(6):29–31.

Chapter 3

1. Douglas, R. M., Moore, B. W., Miles, H. B., et al. "Prophylactic Efficacy of Intranasal Alpha2-Interferon Against Rhinovirus Infections in the Family Setting." New England Journal of Medicine 1986; 314(2):65–70.

2. Eggleston, P. A., Hendley, J. O., and Gwaltney, J. R., Jr. "Mediators of Immediate Hypersensitivity in Nasal Secretions During Natural Colds and Rhinovirus Infection." Acta Otolaryngology 1984; 413 (Suppl.):25–35.

3. Graham, N. M. H., Burrell, C. J., Douglas, R. M., et al. "Adverse Effects of Aspirin, Acetaminophen, and Ibuprofen on Immune Function, Viral Shedding, and Clinical Status in Rhinovirus-Infected Volunteers." Journal of Infectious Diseases 1990; 162:1277–82.

Chapter 4

1. National Asthma Education Program Expert Panel Report. Guidelines for the Diagnosis and Management of Asthma. National Heart, Lung, and Blood Institute, Bethesda, Md., Publication No. 91-3042, August 1991.

2. U.S. Public Health Service: Task Force Report: Epidemiology of Respiratory Diseases, 1980. NIH Publication No. 81-2019.

3. U.S. Department of Health and Human Services. Reducing the Health Consequences of Smoking: 25 Years of Progress. A Report of the Surgeon General. U.S. Department of Health and Human Services, Public Health Service, Centers for Disease Control, Center for Chronic Disease Prevention and Health Promotion, Office on Smoking and Health. DHHS Publication No. (CDC) 89-8411, 1989.

4. Ingram, R. H., Jr., and Davies, S. "Chronic Obstructive Diseases of the Lung." In Rubenstein, E., and Federman, D. D. (eds.). Scientific American Medicine. New York: Scientific American, Inc., Chapter 14, Subsection 3, March 1992, p. 2.

Chapter 5

1. Soll, A. H. "Pathogenesis of Peptic Ulcer and Implications for Therapy." New England Journal of Medicine 1990; 332(13):909.

2. Samloff, I. M. "Peptic Ulcer: The Many Proteinases of Aggression. Gastroenterology 1989; 96(Suppl.):586–95.

3. Soll, A. H. "Duodenal Ulcer and Drug Therapy." In Sleisenger, M. H., Fordtran, J. S. (eds.). Gastrointestinal Disease: Pathophysiology, Diagnosis, and Management, ed. 4 (Philadelphia: W. B. Saunders, 1989), pp. 814–79.

4. Kurata, J. H., Honda, G. D., Frankl, H. "The Incidence of Duodenal and Gastric Ulcers in a Large Health Maintenance Organization." American Journal of Public Health 1985; 75:625–29.

5. Graham, D. Y., Lew, G. M., Evans, D. G., Jr., Klein, P. D. "Effect of Triple Therapy (Antibiotic plus Bismuth) on Duodenal Ulcer Healing." Annals of Internal Medicine 1991; 115:266–69.

6. Gray, G. M. "Peptic Ulcer Diseases." In Rubenstein, E., Federman, D. D. (eds.). Scientific American Medicine. New York: Scientific American Inc., 1988, p. 12.

7. Pounder, R. "Silent Peptic Ulceration: Deadly Silence or Golden Silence?" Gastroenterology 1989; 96:627.

Chapter 6

1. Abramowicz, A. (ed.): "Bepridil for Angina Pectoris." The Medical Letter on Drugs and Therapeutics 1991; 33(845).

2. DeSanctis, R. W., Ruskin, J. N. "Disturbances of Cardiac Rhythm and Conduction." In Rubenstein, E., and Federman, D. D. (eds.). Scientific American Medicine. New York: Scientific American, Inc., July 1989, p. 32.

3. Ibid.

Chapter 8

1. Segal, M. "Norplant: Birth Control at Arm's Reach." FDA Consumer May 1991, p. 9.

2. Olefsky, J. M. "Diabetes Mellitus." In Wyngaarden, J. B., and Smith, L. H. (eds.). Textbook of Medicine (Philadelphia: W. B. Saunders, 1988), p. 1362.

Chapter 9

1. Potter, W. Z., Rudorfer, M. V., Manji, H. "The Pharmacologic Treatment of Depression." New England Journal of Medicine 1991; 325(9):633–42.

2. Quitkin, F. M., Rabkin, J. G., Ross, D., et al. "Duration of Antidepressant Drug Treatment: What Is an Adequate Trial?" Archives of General Psychiatry 1984; 41:238–45.

Chapter 10

1. Abromowicz, A. (ed.). "Drugs for Psychiatric Disorders." The Medical Letter of Drugs and Therapeutics 1991; 33(844):43.

2. "Drugs and Insomnia: The Use of Medications to Promote Sleep." Journal of the American Medical Association 1984; 251(18):2410–14.

3. "Benzodiazepine Dependence, Toxicity, and Abuse: A Task Force Report of the American Psychiatric Association," Washington, D.C., 1990, p. 15.

# INDEX

**Note:** Generic names of drugs begin with a lowercase letter; trade names of drugs begin with a capital letter. Page numbers shown in **bold** indicate main references to drugs. Readers are advised to check *all* page numbers.